IMMUNOBIOLOGY OF PROTEINS AND PEPTIDES · I

ADVANCES IN EXPERIMENTAL MEDICINE AND BIOLOGY

Recent Volumes in this Series

Volume 98
IMMUNOBIOLOGY OF PROTEINS AND PEPTIDES • I
Edited by M. Z. Atassi and A. B. Stavitsky

Volume 99
THE REGULATION OF RESPIRATION DURING SLEEP AND ANESTHESIA
Edited by Robert S. Fitzgerald, Henry Gautier, and Sukhamay Lahiri

Volume 100
MYELINATION AND DEMYELINATION
Edited by Jorma Palo

Volume 101
ENZYMES OF LIPID METABOLISM
Edited by Shimon Gatt, Louis Freysz, and Paul Mandel

Volume 102
THROMBOSIS: Animal and Clinical Models
Edited by H. James Day, Basil A. Molony, Edward E. Nishizawa, and Ronald H. Rynbrandt

Volume 103
HOMEOSTASIS OF PHOSPHATE AND OTHER MINERALS
Edited by Shaul G. Massry, Eberhard Ritz, and Aurelio Rapado

Volume 104
THE THROMBOTIC PROCESS IN ATHEROGENESIS
Edited by A. Bleakley Chandler, Karl Eurenius, Gardner C. McMillan, Curtis B. Nelson, Colin J. Schwartz, and Stanford Wessler

Volume 105
NUTRITIONAL IMPROVEMENT OF FOOD PROTEINS
Edited by Mendel Friedman

Volume 106
GASTROINTESTINAL HORMONES AND PATHOLOGY OF THE DIGESTIVE SYSTEM
Edited by Morton Grossman, V. Speranza, N. Basso, and E. Lezoche

Volume 107
SECRETORY IMMUNITY AND INFECTION
Edited by Jerry R. McGhee, Jiri Mestecky, and James L. Babb

IMMUNOBIOLOGY OF PROTEINS AND PEPTIDES • I

Edited by

M. Z. Atassi

Mayo Medical School
Rochester, Minnesota
and University of Minnesota
Minneapolis, Minnesota

and

A. B. Stavitsky

School of Medicine
Case Western Reserve University
Cleveland, Ohio

PLENUM PRESS • NEW YORK AND LONDON

Library of Congress Cataloging in Publication Data

International Symposium on Immunobiology of Proteins and Peptides, 1st, Minneapolis, Minn., 1977.
Immunobiology of proteins and peptides • I

(Advances in experimental medicine and biology; v. 98)
Includes index.
1. Antigens–Congresses. 2. Proteins–Congresses. 3. Peptides–Congresses. 4. Immunology–Congresses. I. Atassi, M. Z. II. Stavitsky, Abram Benjamin, 1919- III. Title. IV. Series. [DNLM: 1. Immunology–Congresses. 2. Immunochemistry–Congresses. 3. Proteins–Analysis–Congresses. 4. Peptides–Analysis–Congresses. W1 AD559 v. 98/QU55 I675 1977i]
QR186.6.P76I57 1977 599'.02'9 78-5083

DOI 10.1007/978-1-4615-8858-0

Proceedings of the First International Symposium on Immunobiology of Proteins and Peptides held in Minneapolis, Minnesota, September 25–28, 1977

Scientific Council of the symposium

M. Z. Atassi, Chairman
E. Benjamini
J. W. Goodman
A. B. Stavitsky

Support

This symposium is supported in part by:
National Cancer Institute
National Institute of Arthritis, Metabolism, and Digestive Diseases
Fogarty International Center
National Institute of Allergy and Infectious Diseases

Sponsorship

Symposium sponsors include
Kallestad Laboratories, Inc.
Beckman Instruments, Inc.
Bio-Rad Laboratories
Coulter Electronics, Inc.
Pierce Chemical Company
Minnesota Mining and Manufacturing Company

A Division of Plenum Publishing Corporation
227 West 17th Street, New York, N.Y. 10011

Preface

One of the central questions in immunology is the understanding in molecular terms of antigen-antibody interactions and of the cellular recognition of antigens. It is hoped that this understanding will extend eventually to the immunobiological basis of host defense to infectious agents and of tissue damage or deranged cell functions which stem from these reactions. A variety of natural and artificial substances have been used as models for these studies. Emphasis was placed upon substances of known and relatively uncomplicated chemical structures. These included polysaccharides, amino acid polymers, nucleic acids and haptens. On the other hand, until recently there has been very little information on protein antigens. The complexity of these molecules posed an immense chemical obstacle to precise immunochemical analysis. Indeed, it is this difficulty with proteins that spurred the synthesis and immunological studies of amino acid polymers. The control and normal regulation of the immune system at the cellular-molecular interface and the great majority of antigens associated with immune disorders are attributed to protein molecules. In the last few years great advances have been made in the analysis and synthesis of the antigenic sites of some proteins. The entire antigenic structures of myoglobin and lysozyme and the partial antigenic structures of several other proteins have been determined. Moreover, in the past seven years several biological responses resulting from the reactions of proteins and their peptides with cells of the immune system were described. Precise elucidation of the molecular features responsible for the antigenicity of certain parts of a protein molecule should pave the way to the definition of the cellular specificity and collaboration in the recognition process and the genetic control of this recognition.

The realization that proteins and peptides held great promise for molecular immunological studies and that this subject had not been reviewed in any symposium sparked the informal discussions which led to the symposium on which this book is based. The First International Symposium on the Immunobiology of Proteins and Peptides was held in Minneapolis on September 25-28, 1977. The Scientific Organizing Committee (M. Z. Atassi, E. Benjamini, J. W. Goodman, A. B.

Stavitsky) developed a program which, while emphasizing the immunology of proteins and peptides, also presented original investigations and reviewed a great deal of immunochemical and immunobiological information obtained with the traditional hapten-carrier and amino acid polymer systems. It was hoped that the presentations and discussions of diverse data obtained with such different antigens would result in appreciation of the similarities and differences among these systems and possibly in the realization of some new general principles. The invited participants included both immunochemists and cellular immunologists to encourage the exchange of information, technology, and ideas. Above all, the committee hoped that this symposium would present and integrate knowledge obtained with these diverse systems and would identify the most promising directions for future investigations.

M. Z. Atassi
A. B. Stavitsky

Contents

ANTIGENIC STRUCTURE OF PROTEINS

IMMUNOBIOLOGY OF PROTEINS AND PEPTIDES

IMMUNOBIOLOGY OF PROTEIN CONJUGATES

IMMUNE RESPONSES TO SYNTHETIC POLYMERS AND TO PROTEINS

Antigenic Structure of Proteins

INTRODUCTION

Elvin A. Kabat

Departments of Microbiology, Human Genetics
and Development and Neurology
Columbia University, New York, New York 10032
and
National Cancer Institute, Bethesda, Maryland 20014

We are entering an exciting new phase in the study of antigenic determinants of protein antigens. While much progress has been made in characterizing many or all antigenic determinants on a number of protein antigens, notably myoglobin, lysozyme, staphylococcal nuclease and cytochrome c, the heterogeneity of the antibody response has seriously complicated efforts to obtain monoclonal antiprotein antibodies directed toward single determinants although some antibodies specific for an individual determinant have been obtained by suitable adsorption and we shall hear about these tonight. While myeloma proteins have yielded a considerable number of monoclonal antibodies, these have been largely to carbohydrate determinants, phosphocholine, DNP, etc. To date only one monoclonal myeloma with antiprotein specificity has been identified - namely, MOPC 467 with antiflagellin activity. This myeloma protein has not yet been sequenced beyond the first 23 residues.

A very important class of antiprotein antibodies are the idiotypic antibodies directed against determinants on the variable regions of immunoglobulins. At the moment we know nothing of how many different anti-idiotypic determinants can be formed to a single monoclonal immunoglobulin nor can we specify even a single amino acid in the V-region as involved in idiotypic specificity.

Recent developments have opened the way to a ready solution of such problems. Köhler and Milstein found that hydribds of a B cell myeloma and a spleen cell from an immunized animal will continue to secrete the antibody formed by the splenic B cell. Such hybrid cell lines can be propagated indefinitely and if injected into mice will produce plasmacytomas. Ascites from one such animal can yield quantities of the order of 5 mg antibody per ml. The antibody from each hybridoma is monoclonal. One thus has the possibility of preparing monoclonal antibodies of any desired specificity. One may also determine how many different clones can be formed to a given antigen and how many different idiotypic specificities a given monoclonal antibody can induce. We shall have a set of reagents capable of recognizing almost any type of structure. When such antiprotein and anti-idiotypic antibodies are characterized as to their site sizes and shapes, crystallized and studied by high resolution X-ray crystallographic methods, we shall really begin to understand the structural basis of antibody complementarity and be able to define more readily the spectrum of antigenic determinants.

IDENTIFYING ANTIGENIC DETERMINANTS ON CYTOCHROME *C* FOR B AND T CELLS

Morris Reichlin and Jerald Eng

SUNY at Buffalo School of Medicine
Veterans Administration Hospital
3495 Bailey Avenue, Buffalo, New York 14215

INTRODUCTION

Localization of the antigenic determinants on the cytochrome *c* molecule reactive with rabbit antibodies has depended on the antigenic comparison of cytochromes *c* of known structure by quantitative cross reactions. In addition, antibodies to these regions can be isolated by affinity chromatography methods and the specificity of these "site specific" antibodies determined by their pattern of reactivity with cytochromes *c* of known structure. Such studies lead to the conclusion that a limited number of antigenic regions elicit antibodies when various cytochromes *c* are injected into rabbits. While the precise number of amino acids contributing to the structure of the antigenic determinant is not known, certain amino acids can be identified which make a decisive contribution to the specificity. In trying to obtain similar information about the location on cytochrome *c* of the antigenic determinants reactive with receptors on thymus derived cells one encounters limitations. Assays do not exist which can yield the type of molecular information about antigenicity that immunochemists have been able to obtain from a study of the antigen-antibody reaction.

A model system is described involving the immunization of guinea pigs with horse cytochrome *c* and the elicitation of a pure delayed hypersensitivity reaction. Lymphocytes from such guinea pigs respond to antigen in culture with a molecular specificity at least as exquisite as the specificity manifest in the reaction of rabbit antibodies to the same antigen.

Brief Summary of Published Results

It was inferred from early cross reaction data with rabbit antisera to the horse and human proteins that antigenic determinants were located in sequence positions where the horse and human proteins differed in sequence. The reciprocal cross reactions were weak and the sequence differences between the two proteins are concentrated in four regions of the linear sequence. These regions are listed in Table 1 which also contains the sequences of several

TABLE 1

			I						II			
	11	12	13	14	15	44	45	46	47	48	49	50
Human	I	M	K	C	S	P	G	Y	S	Y	T	A
Monkey												
Horse	V	Q	K	C	A	P	G	F	T	Y	T	D
Donkey									S			
Rabbit	V	Q	K	C	A	V	G	F	S	Y	T	D
Mouse	V	Q	K	C	A	A	G	F	S	Y	T	D
Guanaco	V	Q	K	C	A	V	G	F	S	Y	T	D
Beef	V	Q	K	C	A	P	G	F	S	Y	T	D

			III				IV			
	58	59	60	61	62	83	89	90	91	92
Human	I	W	G	E	D	V	E	E	R	A
Monkey	T									
Horse	T	W	K	E	E	A	T	E	R	E
Donkey										
Rabbit	T	W	G	E	D	A	D	E	R	A
Mouse	T	W	G	E	D	A	G	E	R	A
Guanaco	T	W	G	E	E	A	G	E	R	A
Beef	T	W	G	E	E	A	G	E	R	E

Horse and donkey proteins are identical at all positions except 47.

Human and monkey proteins are identical at all positions except 58.

The single letter code employed is isoleucine, I; methionine, M; Lysine, K; cysteine, C; serine, S; proline, P; glycine, G; tyrosine, Y; phenylalanine, F; threonine, T; valine, V; glutamine, Q; glutamic acid, E; aspartic acid, D; alanine, D; tryptophan, W; arginine, R.

cytochromes c. Eleven of the twelve sequence differences that distinguish the human and horse proteins are clustered in these four regions which account for about 20% of the 104 residues of cytochrome c. The differences among all these cytochromes c are in the same regions. Evidence linking such regions with antigenic determinants was derived from comparing two cytochromes c which differed by a single amino acid residue in reaction with antiserum in quantitative complement fixation or radioimmunoassay tests. Thus with anti-human cytochrome c, the donkey protein was antigenically superior to the horse protein and the human protein reacted more strongly than the monkey protein implicating residue 47 and 58 respectively in antigenic determinants in human cytochrome c. By studying the cross reactions of the closely related rabbit, whale, and mouse cytochromes c with anti-human cytochrome c, position 89 could be implicated in an antigenic determinant. Similar experiments with rabbit anti-horse cytochrome c provided evidence for antigenic determinants influenced by residue positions 58 and 92 respectively. A detailed discussion of these findings can be found in a recent review[1].

An approach has been recently reported by Urbanski and Margoliash which simplifies the problem of antigenicity by the immunization of animals (rabbits and mice) by cytochromes c (rabbit, mouse, and gaunaco) which differ from the cytochrome c of the immunized animal by only 2 amino acid residues[2]. By separating purified antibodies prepared by affinity chromatography methods with the appropriate cytochrome c sepharose columns, fractions could be separated which in each case corresponded to a single antibody population related to a limited region of amino acid sequence. The analytical methods used for the determination of stoichiometry and specificity were fluorescence quenching and radioimmunoassay respectively. Description of the data obtained with guanaco cytochrome c serum prepared in rabbits suffice to illustrate the approach. Purified rabbit anti-guanaco antibodies bind to guanaco cytochrome c with stoichiometry of 2.0. One of these two populations binds rabbit cytochrome c and can be separated on a rabbit cytochrome c sepharose column. The fraction binding the rabbit protein with a stoichiometry of one also binds the mouse, beef, and guanaco proteins. It failed to bind the horse protein presumably because of the interference of lysine 60 with the binding. Inspection of the appropriate sequences leads one to the conclusion that the crucial residue determining specificity is glutamic acid 62. The fraction failing to bind to the rabbit cytochrome c sepharose column bound only the mouse and the guanaco proteins and failed to bind the horse, beef, and rabbit proteins. The sequence region shared by the guanaco and mouse proteins which was different in the unreactive proteins was the region from 88-92. Thus a specificity study of the two separated antibody populations permitted molecular assignment of the corresponding antigenic

TABLE 2

Sequence Position Implicated in Antigenicity

Species to Which Rabbit Antiserum Produced	Region of Sequence I	II	III	IV
Human[1]		47	58	89,92
Horse[1]			58	89,92
Guanaco[2]			62	89,92
Mouse[2]		44	62	89,92

Data from References 1 and 2

determinants. Table 2 then summarizes the literature data on the localization of antigenic determinants in various cytochromes *c* reactive with homologous rabbit antisera. It is seen that residue positions in regions III and IV are implicated in antigenicity in all these antisera. Data to be presented will also show that some but not all rabbits produce antibodies reactive with region II of horse cytochrome *c* influenced by proline 44.

No direct evidence supports the existence of antibodies reactive with region 1. However, an antibody fraction can be isolated from rabbit antisera to human cytochrome *c* which when bound to the human protein in a 1:1 complex, blocks the oxidation of ferrocytochrome *c* by cytochrome *c* oxidase. Since chemical modification of lysine 14 of region 1 diminishes the interaction between ferrocytochrome *c* and cytochrome *c* oxidase[3] it has been postulated that this "antioxidase" antibody fraction is directed toward region 1[4].

Resolution of the Heterogeneity of Rabbit Anti-Horse Cytochrome *c*

Affinity chromatography utilizing cytochrome *c*-sepharose columns has been used to resolve the antibodies into fractions specific for different determinant regions on horse cytochrome *c*. Two patterns of specificity were noted with the total antibodies isolated from a horse cytochrome *c*-sepharose column. Preparation of Fab fragments and the fluorescence quenching technique were performed as previously described[5]. Tables 3 and 4 lists the maximum quenching levels (Q) achieved with various cytochromes *c*. Table 3 lists the data from a study of antibodies isolated from rabbit 614 which shows that horse, bovine, human, and rabbit

TABLE 3

Cross Reactions of Cytochromes c with Rabbit Anti-Horse c (614) by Fluorescence Quenching

Species Cytochrome c	% Q Maximum
Horse	42.8
Beef	29.9
Human	25.7
Rabbit	7.8

TABLE 4

Cross Reactions of Cytochromes c with Rabbit Anti-Horse c (645) by Fluorescence Quenching

Species Cytochrome c	% Q Maximum
Horse	46.0
Beef	34.0
Rabbit	18.8
Human	18.8
Dogfish	18.6
Tuna	12.5

cytochromes c quench these antibodies in the order of effectiveness listed. Notable here is the poor reaction of the rabbit protein. Table 4 contains data from a second rabbit (645) in which the horse and bovine proteins bear the same quantitative antigenic relationship as in Table 3. However, the antibodies from rabbit 645 react in equivalent fashion with rabbit and human cytochromes c.

These two types of antibodies were resolved on a series of affinity chromatography columns and the individual fractions characterized by their reactivity with various cytochromes c in both fluorescence quenching and radioimmunoassay experiments. For the resolution of the antibodies prepared from rabbit 614 the following series of columns were used: human, rabbit, beef, and horse cytochromes c sepharose. The effluent from each column was passed sequentially onto the next column. Fractions from each column were eluted with a stepwise gradient utilizing pH 4.0, pH 3.0, and pH 2.2 acid buffers solutions which were .1 M acetate buffer, .1 M and 1.0 M acetic acid solutions respectively. In the case of rabbit 614, fractions were obtained from the human, bovine, and horse cytochrome c columns which could be characterized. Little material was isolated from the rabbit cytochrome c sepharose column.

TABLE 5

Binding of 1.0 M Acetic Acid Fraction From Human Cyt. c Sepharose Column (Rabbit 614) with Various Cytochromes c

Cytochrome c	% Q Max 1.0 M Acetic Acid Fx
Horse	46.8
Beef	45.9
Kangaroo	47.4
Human	45.3
Samia Cynthia	31.0
Rabbit	22.0
Whale	18.0
Turkey	0.0

Table 5 lists the maximum quenching levels achieved with various cytochromes c and the fraction eluted with 1.0 M acetic acid from the human cytochrome c sepharose column. The horse, beef, kangaroo, and human proteins were equivalent in their binding yielding a linear titration curve and a stoichiometry of unity. The samia cynthia protein quenched the fluorescence of this fraction linearly and with unitary stoichiometry but only quenched 75% as well as the other four proteins. The rabbit and whale proteins bound the fractions weakly as evidenced by a hyperbolic titration curve and the turkey protein was unreactive. The

TABLE 6

Correlation of Amino Acid at Position 44 and Reactivity with 1.0 M Acetic Acid Fraction From Human Cytochrome c Sepharose (Rabbit 614)

Species Cytochrome c	No. Amino Acid Differences From Horse c	Reaction with Fx-Human Cyt. c Sepharose	Residue at Position 44
Horse	0	Strong	Proline
Beef	3	Strong	Proline
Kangaroo	7	Strong	Proline
Human	12	Strong	Proline
Samia Cynthia	29	Strong	Proline
Whale	5	Weak	Valine
Rabbit	6	Weak	Valine
Turkey	11	None	Glutamic Acid

only residue position common to the horse, beef, kangaroo, human, and samia cynthia protein which is different in the whale, rabbit, and turkey proteins is position 44 where the shared residue is proline. These data are summarized in Table 6. It is concluded that proline 44 plays a key role in determining the structure of one antigenic determinant in horse cytochrome c.

Study of the fractions eluted from the beef cytochrome c column revealed the following properties. They bound to horse cytochrome c with a stoichiometry of 1.0 and yielded a linear titration curve. Beef cytochrome c bound these fractions with a lower affinity than the horse protein. From 10^3 to 6.25×10^4 as much beef protein as horse protein was required to achieve equal binding to the various fractions isolated from the beef cytochrome c sepharose column. These are listed in Table 7. Human, rabbit, whale, kangaroo, and turkey cytochromes c did not bind any of these fractions. The only residue position in which beef and horse are identical and the other cytochromes c are different is position 92 where the horse and beef proteins carry glutamic acid. It is likely that position 89 also contributes to the binding specificity to account for the weaker binding of the beef protein to these antibody

TABLE 7

Concentrations of Cold Horse and Beef Cytochromes *c* Required to Displace 50% of ^{131}I Horse Cytochrome *c* from Fractions Isolated From Beef Cytochrome *c* Sepharose

Fraction	Horse	Beef	Horse/Beef
pH 4.0	.004	250	6.25×10^4
pH 3.0	.01	12.6	1.26×10^3
1.0 M Acetic Acid	.01	10.0	1.0×10^3

Concentrations are in μg/ml

fractions. At this position the beef protein carries glycine while the horse protein carries threonine. It is not likely that the other two positions where horse and beef differ (position 47 and 60) contribute to the horse-beef difference since there are other cytochromes *c* with structures identical to the beef protein at those positions which do not bind these antibody fractions. These data suggest that both glutamic acid 92 and threonine 89 contribute to the structures forming an antigenic determinant in horse cytochrome *c*.

Antibodies eluted from the horse cytochrome *c* sepharose column reacted equally well with horse and donkey cytochromes *c* and reacted with no other cytochromes *c*. Beef cytochrome *c* in molar excesses of 10^6 failed to displace ^{131}I labelled horse cytochrome *c* from these "horse specific" antibodies. Since the beef and horse proteins differ at only positions 47, 60, and 89 it is worth considering those differences. Position 47 cannot be involved in the binding since donkey and beef cytochromes *c* carry the same residue at position 47. It is not likely that position 89 is involved in the difference between the horse and beef proteins since the fractions from the beef cytochrome *c* column also depend on position 89 for their antigenicity. If position 89 were required for the structure of the "horse specific" determinant it would mean that two antibodies could bind to the same amino acid residue simultaneously. This seems highly unlikely. This leaves only lysine 60 of the three residue positions that distinguish the horse and beef proteins as being the residue which influences the structure of the "horse specific" fraction.

These three antibody fractions account for all the specificity in serum 614. Two of these three fractions were also found in two other rabbits studied in this way. The fractions occurring in the other rabbits were those designated glutamic acid 92, threonine 89, (eluted from beef cytochrome c sepharose) and lysine 60 (eluted from horse cytochrome c sepharose). The proline 44 fraction was not found in the other two rabbits. Instead, a fraction was eluted from a rabbit cytochrome c column which accounted for slightly more than 50% of the total antibody and had the property of binding to all tested cytochromes c. For sera of this type the sequence of sepharose columns utilized was rabbit-beef-horse through which the sera were passed sequentially. As would be expected, horse cytochrome c bound the fractions eluted from the rabbit cytochrome c sepharose column most effectively and the heterologous proteins required from 1 to 500 times more protein than the horse protein for equivalent inhibition. The ability of various cytochromes c to bind this fraction is listed in Table 8. It is postulated that such antibodies bind to regions of the cytochromes c sequence which are very similar and are outside the foci of sequence differences listed in Table 1.

It is also likely that these antibodies bind to several regions since the fluorescence quenching titrations suggest a stoichiometry between 3 and 4. Thus no sequence positions have been assigned to these antibodies with apparent specificity for common regions of

TABLE 8

Specificity of Fractions Isolated From Rabbit Cytochrome c Sepharose

Cytochrome c	Rabbit 662	Rabbit 645
Horse	.12	.84
Beef	1.0	1.0
Rabbit	3.4	8.0
Dogfish	n.d.	10.0
Duck	9.0	13.0
Human	64.0	25.0

Numbers listed are concentration in µg/ml required to displace 50% of ^{131}I labelled horse cytochrome c from fractions eluted from rabbit cytochrome c sepharose with 1.0 M acetic acid.

TABLE 9

Column	Stoichiometry	Residue Assignment	Rabbit Sera
Human c Sepharose	Unity	Proline 44	614
Beef c Sepharose	Unity	Glutamic 92 Threonine 89	614, 662, 645
Horse c Sepharose	Unity	Lysine 60	614, 662, 645
Rabbit c Sepharose	3 to 4	---	662, 645

Stoichiometries, residue assignments, and rabbit sera of fractions isolated from immunoabsorbent columns as listed.

the cytochrome c sequence. Some data on the four types of antibody fractions isolated from rabbit antisera to horse cytochrome c are listed in Table 9.

Specificity of the Blastogenic Response to Horse Cytochrome c in Guinea Pigs

Studies have been undertaken to obtain molecular information about the specificity of structures in cytochrome c reactive with receptors on thymus derived cells. Guinea pigs immunized with horse cytochrome c in complete Freund's adjuvant develop classical delayed hypersensitivity skin reactions when challenged with antigen but produce no measurable antibody[6]. Lymphocytes isolated from sensitized animals undergo brisk antigen dependent DNA synthesis in short term culture. Preliminary studies with nylon wool columns indicate that removal of more than 90% of the B cells from isolated peripheral blood lymphocytes does not diminish the proliferative responses of these lymphocytes to antigen. Such blastogenic responses are apparently due to T cells. Table 10 lists data from 2 animals which illustrates the ability of various cytochromes c to activate peripheral blood lymphocytes from guinea pigs sensitized to the horse protein. It is seen that only the horse, donkey, and beef proteins activate the cells and do so in a graded fashion. There is a large difference between the horse and donkey proteins and a correspondingly large difference between the donkey and beef

TABLE 10

Animal	T2		NM	
Ag	23.1 μg/ml	579 μg/ml	23.1 μg/ml	579 μg/ml
Horse	43.7 ± 9.9	108 ± 5.3	23.8 ± 1.1	56.0 ± 6.3
Donkey+	8/84 ± 2.28	34.9 ± 0.70	2.26 ± 0.46	16.4 ± 2.9
Beef	9.24 ± 0.78	18.9 ± 4.13	1.16 ± 0.50	8.47 ± 3.53
Rabbit	1.36 ± 0.19	2.81 ± 1.09	1.13 ± 0.56	1.57 ± 0.29
Turkey	2.13 ± 0.16	3.17 ± 0.39	0/99 ± 0.29	0.83 ± 0.34
Tuna	1.36 ± 0.12	0.52 ± 0.31	0.90 ± 0.22	0.30 ± 0.06
Saline	33.3 ± 2.75 C.P.M.		40.4 ± 9.2 C.P.M.	
Cell No./well	3 x 10^5		1.5 x 10^5	
PHA	596 ± 95 S.I.		813 ± 127 S.I.	

+The donkey concentration in the second column is 281 μg/ml rather than 579 μg/ml.

Saline values are counts per minute per well. All other numbers are the stimulation indices ± one standard derivation. The stimulation index is the ratio of the CPM incorporated with antigen divided by the CPM incorporated with saline.

proteins. Rabbit cytochrome c fails to activate the cells at the highest concentrations tested. In addition, experiments were conducted in which a 10-fold excess of the rabbit protein was mixed with the horse protein to see if the blastogenic response to the horse protein could be inhibited. These experiments failed to show any effect of the rabbit cytochrome c. The entire specificity of the blastogenic response to horse cytochrome c is related to the six amino acid differences existing between rabbit and horse cytochromes c. These are the same differences which determine the specificity of the antigenic determinants in horse cytochrome c related to binding with antibody. Since there is a large difference between the horse and donkey proteins, residue 47 is implicated in one determinant. Because there is a large difference between the donkey and beef proteins either or both positions 60 and 89 also contribute to structures controlling determinants reactive with receptors activating these cells. The antigenic distinction between the horse and donkey proteins which is apparent in these lymphocyte transformation experiments cannot be demonstrated with rabbit antibodies to the horse protein. Indeed, if one compares the ability of various cytochromes _c_ to activate guinea pig lymphocytes sensitized to horse cytochrome _c_ with their ability to bind rabbit anti-horse cytochrome _c_ antibody a sharper discrimination is made by the cellular assay. These data are illustrated in Figure 1 in which the lymphocyte transformation response to antigen is compared to the binding of antibody by antigen in quantitative complement fixation tests as a function of the amino acid difference existing between the heterologous protein and the horse protein.

DISCUSSION

Studies of rabbit antibodies to the cytochrome _c_ molecule suggest that there are a small number of antigenic determinants, the majority of which are closely related to the regions of cytochrome _c_ which are the loci of variation among cytochromes _c_. Thus it is apparent that the sequence from 89-92 is antigenic in the human, horse, guanaco, and mouse proteins. Antibodies of unique specificities arise in rabbits who respond to the human and the horse proteins while antibody of a similar specificity arises in response to both the mouse and guanaco proteins which are identical in that region of the sequence. It is convenient to picture the specificity of these determinants and their corresponding antibodies as being related to the sequence differences between the structure of the immunogen and the rabbit protein in that portion of sequence. Similarly, sequence positions 44-50 and 58-62 are frequently antigenic in the system studied thus far. In addition to determinants related to sequence differences among cytochromes _c_, there also arise in some rabbits antibodies which bind all the cytochromes _c_ tested and whose specificity must therefore relate to sequences shared by these cytochromes _c_. Cross reaction studies are not very useful in localizing such determinants in cytochrome _c_ to any specific molecular region. Other techniques such as a search for reactive peptides or chemical modification studies will be necessary to analyze the specificities of these regions.

Initial studies of antigen receptors on guinea pig T cells for cytochrome _c_ indicate that the specificity of these reactions are related to the same sequence differences that determine the specificity of rabbit antibodies to horse cytochrome _c_. Only further study will reveal if the proliferative response to

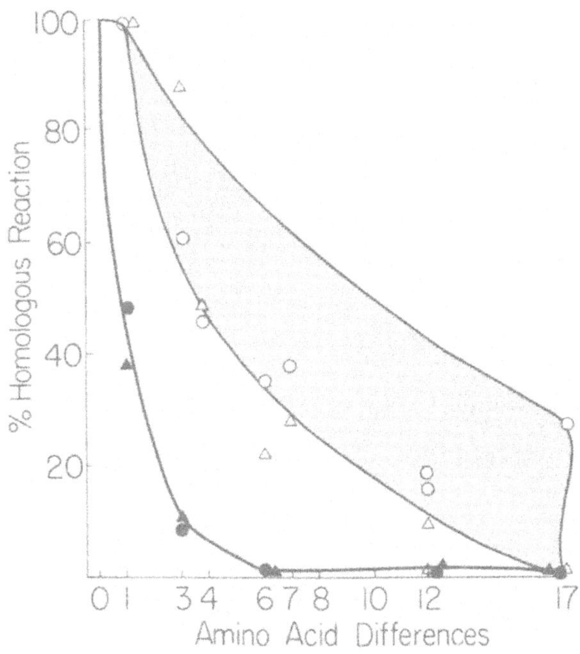

FIGURE 1

The stimulation index for a given cytochrome c is divided by the stimulation index for the horse cytochrome c at the same antigen dose for 2 animals for various heterologous cytochromes c (•,▲). Data from Reference 7. Two rabbit antisera (o,Δ) have been studied by quantitative complement fixation with various cytochromes c. The percentage reactivity at the maximum of the complement fixation curve of the heterologous to the homologous antigen is plotted for various heterologous cytochromes c. Data from Reference 8.

cytochrome c in various species is equally sensitive to variations in cytochrome c structure as is the guinea pig. The first published abstract of such studies suggests that the proliferative response of nylon wool purified mouse lymphocytes is indeed sensitive to the small numbers of amino acid changes existing among closely related cytochromes c[9]. These initial studies suggest that the antigen receptors on T cells for cytochrome c have a specificity which is very similar to the specificities exhibited by antibodies to cytochrome c.

BIBLIOGRAPHY

1. Reichlin, M. Advances in Immunology 20:71, 1975.

2. Urbanski, G.J. and Margoliash, E. J. Immunol. 118,1170, 1977.

3. Smith, L., Davies, H.C., Reichlin, M. and Margoliash, E. J. Biol. Chem. 248:237, 1973.

4. Wada, K. and Okunuki, K. J. Biochem. (Tokyo) 66:249, 1969.

5. Noble, R.W., Reichlin, M., Gibson, Q.H. J. Biol. Chem. 244: 2403, 1969.

6. Reichlin, M. and Turk, J.L. 251:335, 1974.

7. Wolff, M. and Reichlin, M. Immunochemistry, in press.

8. Margoliash, E., Nisonoff, A. and Reichlin, M. J. Biol. Chem. 245:931, 1970.

9. Corradin, G., Chiller, J. Fed. Proc. 36:1187, 1977 abstract.

The work of the authors of this paper is supported by USPHS AM10428 and funds from the Veterans Administration.

FIRST CONSEQUENCES OF THE DETERMINATION OF THE ENTIRE ANTIGENIC STRUCTURE OF SPERM-WHALE MYOGLOBIN

M. Zouhair Atassi and A. Latif Kazim

Department of Immunology, Mayo Medical School
Rochester, Minnesota 55901
and
Department of Biochemistry, University of Minnesota
Minneapolis, Minnesota 55455

SUMMARY

By using the antigenic structure of sperm-whale Mb as a model we have established that the antigenicity of its sites is independent of any sequence identities between the injected myoglobin and the Mb of the immunized animal. Furthermore, the ability to produce in rabbits autoantibodies to rabbit Mb and the successful extrapolation of the antigenic structure of sperm-whale Mb to human hemoglobin strongly demonstrated that the antigenicity of certain parts of a protein molecule is primarily dependent on the uniqueness of their conformational locations.

INTRODUCTION

Knowledge of the molecular features responsible for the antigenicity of certain parts of native protein molecules lies at the basis of understanding, in molecular terms, the cellular events of the immune response. The majority of antigens associated with immunological disorders are proteins and therefore defining the antigenic sites of these protein antigens will be critical for the molecular elucidation of the mechanisms of these disorders. From a purely chemical perspective, the interaction between protein antigens and their antibodies and the elegant specificity of this recognition phenomenon remains one of the most fascinating and challenging frontiers in biochemistry.

Abbreviations: Mb, myoglobin; Hb, hemoglobin.

In 1975, I reported (Atassi, 1975), the first precise determination of the entire antigenic structure of a protein - that of sperm-whale myoglobin. This represented the culmination of intensive research over an 11-year period.

I had considered at the outset that the antigenic structure of a protein cannot be deduced by the exclusive application of a single chemical approach. Our strategy, therefore, relied on five approaches (Atassi, 1972) which first enabled us to achieve the precise determination of the entire antigenic structure of Mb (Atassi, 1975), and which we subsequently found to be equally effective in scoring a similar achievement with lysozyme (Atassi, 1978). These approaches were: (1) to study the effect of conformational changes on the immunochemistry of the protein; (2) to study the immunochemistry and conformation of chemical derivatives of the protein, specifically modified at appropriate amino acid locations; (3) to isolate and characterize immunochemically-reactive fragments that can quantitatively account for the total reaction of the native protein; (4) to study the effect of chemical modification at selected amino acid locations on the immunochemistry and conformation of immunochemically-reactive peptides; (5) after hopefully narrowing down each of the antigenic sites by approaches (1-4) to a conveniently small size, the final delineation would rely on studying the immunochemistry of synthetic peptides corresponding to many overlaps around this region. It is critical to note that each of these chemical approaches has advantages as well as shortcomings. The application, usefulness and shortcomings of these approaches to protein immunochemistry have recently been discussed in considerable detail (Atassi, 1975, 1977a, 1977b). It is also necessary to stress here that none of these approaches by itself is capable of yielding the full antigenic structure. We invariably used the results from one approach to confirm and correct those from the others. The complete structure is a composite, logical coordination of all the information.

A highly pertinent aspect of this strategy is that the precise definition of the antigenic sites of this protein, and the unequivocal demonstration of the absolute non-involvement of the remaining portions of the Mb molecule with respect to the specificity of the humoral response has been an important asset in our *in vitro* cellular studies. These have been aimed at comparing the specificities of different lymphocyte populations in immune recognition and response to protein antigens. These studies are presented in part in an accompanying report (Stavitsky *et al.*, this volume).

SPECIAL FEATURES OF THE ANTIGENIC STRUCTURE

Our precise determination of the entire antigenic structure of sperm-whale Mb has been reviewed elsewhere (Atassi, 1975; or in

Region	Structure and Location	No. of Residues
Region 1	15 16 21 22 (Ala)-Lys-Val-Glu-Ala-Asp-Val-(Ala)	6 (or 7)
Region 2	56 62 Lys-Ala-Ser-Glu-Asp-Leu-Lys	7
Region 3	94 99 Ala-Thr-Lys-His-Lys-Ile	6
Region 4	113 119 His-Val-Leu-His-Ser-Arg-His	7
Region 5	145 146 151 (Lys)-Tyr-Lys-Glu-Leu-Gly-Tyr	6 (or 7)

Fig. 1. Primary structures of the five antigenic reactive regions of sperm-whale Mb. Residues in parentheses are part of the reactive region only with some antisera. Thus for region 1, the reactive region invariably occupies sequence 16-21 and with some antisera alanine 15 is part of the region (which will then correspond to sequence 15-21) while with other antisera alanine 22 is an essential part of the region (which will then correspond to sequence 16-22). This region occupies either 6 or 7 residues depending on antiserum. For regions 2,3 and 4 no such 'displacement' or 'shift' to one side or the other has been observed (at least with the antisera so far studied). In the case of region 5, lysine 145 can be part of the reactive region only with some antisera and this region will therefore comprise 6 or 7 residues, depending on the antiserum (from Atassi, 1975).

more detail, Atassi, 1977b). This section summarizes the main features of the antigenic structure of Mb:

Five antigenic reactive regions are present in the native protein (Figs. 1 and 2) and are situated on: (Site 1) Sequence 16-21, +1 or 0 residue one side only of this segment depending on the antiserum. This antigenic region exhibits a certain degree of 'shift' or 'displacement' and minor variability in size (limited to $\pm$ 1 residue only) from one antiserum to the next. Its location in the three-dimensional structure is on the bend between helices A and B. (Site 2) Sequence 56-62, on the bend between helices D and E. This reactive region has exhibited no variability in size with the antisera so far studied. (Site 3) Sequence 94-99 on the bend between helices F and G. (Site 4) Sequence 113-119, on the end of helix G and only part of the bend GH. (Site 5) Sequence 146-151 (+ lysine 145 with some antisera). This reactive region is situated on the end of helix H and part of the randomly-

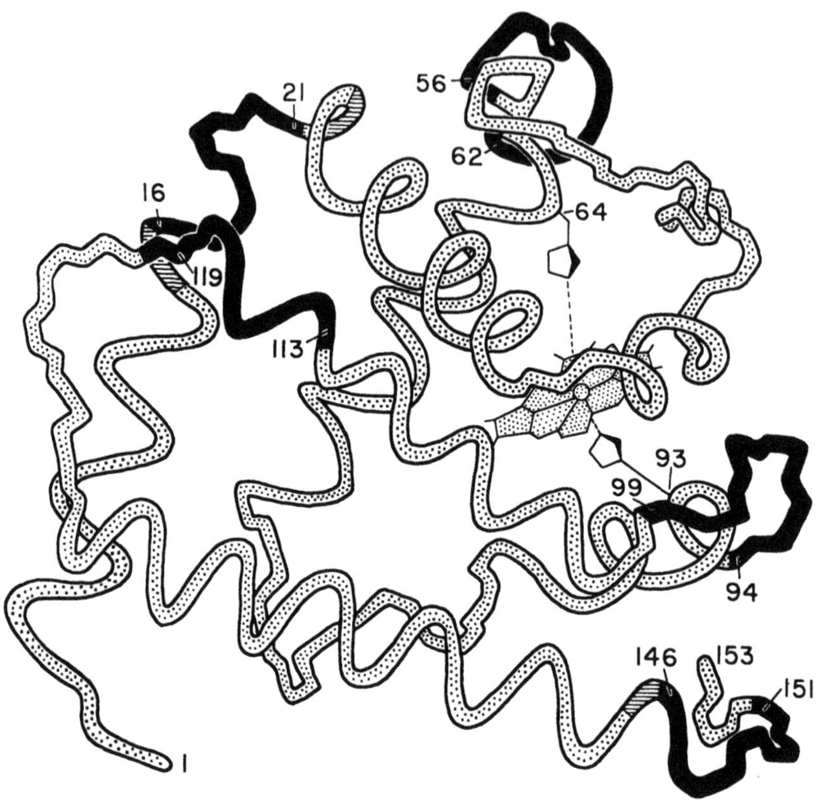

Fig. 2. A schematic diagram showing the mode of folding of Mb and its antigenic structure. The solid black portions represent segments which have been shown to comprise accurately entire antigenic reactive regions. The striped parts, each corresponding to one amino acid residue only, can be part of the antigenic reactive region with some antisera. The dotted portions represent parts of the molecule which have been shown exhaustively to reside outside reactive regions (from Atassi, 1975).

coiled C-terminal pentapeptide. The primary structures of the five antigenic reactive regions are shown in Fig. 1. The locations of the reactive regions in the three-dimensional structure of native Mb are shown in a schematic diagram in Fig. 2.

We have previously cautioned (Atassi, 1975; Atassi and Pai, 1975) against the likely formulation of an erroneous conclusion that every bend constitutes a reactive region. No such statement is made or implied here and indeed examination of Fig. 2 immediately reveals that the bends B-C, C-D and E-F do not carry reactive regions. Also, region 4 (i.e. 113-119) is located mostly on a helical portion.

The antigenic reactive regions are surprisingly small (6-7 residues) and possess sharp boundaries. They may exhibit limited variability in boundaries with various antisera which, when it exists, will be ± 1 residue. The size, surface locations and shape of these reactive regions make them quite accessible for binding with antibody combining sites.

The types of amino acids present in the reactive regions is to be expected for their surface locations (Atassi, 1972). Lysine is present in four regions (Fig. 1) and in the fifth arginine is present. Three out of five reactive regions contain aspartic acid or glutamic acid or both. Two regions contain histidine. From this and the demonstrated detrimental effect of appropriate modifications of these polar residues on the antigenic reactivity, it may be concluded (Atassi, 1972, 1975) that interactions of the Mb reactive regions with antibody must be predominantly polar in nature. Stabilizing effects are contributed by hydroxy and non-polar amino acids through hydrogen bonding and hydrophobic interactions (Atassi, 1972). The sequence and three-dimensional structural features that confer immunogenicity on these regions are not too clear.

Any immunochemical interaction between <u>antigenic reactive regions</u> that are distant in sequence but close in three-dimensional structure to form <u>antigenic reactive sites</u> (previously suggested by (Atassi and Saplin, 1968) has been difficult to investigate (Atassi, 1975). Very recently, however, it has been shown (Atassi and Koketsu, 1975) that this type of interaction, if it occurs, must be quite minimal for this antigen in its early course antisera. However, the situation may be different on prolonged immunization and variation of the immunization schedule. In this case, antigenic <u>regions</u> and antigenic <u>sites</u> are synonymous. At equivalence no more than an average of four antibody molecules can sterically fit on the protein, even though five antigenic sites are present in Mb (Atassi, 1967a).

The affinity of a reactive region or its share of the total reactivity of Mb may vary with the antiserum. However with all the antisera studied so far (at least eight), a reactive region is invariably a reactive region, but its potency or efficiency varies with the individual animal immunized (Atassi, 1972). Significantly, antibodies produced in both rabbits and goats to native Mb recognized the same antigenic sites on Mb.

The findings that purely conformational changes in Mb will influence its reaction with antisera to the native protein (Atassi,

1967b; Andres and Atassi, 1970) and the immunochemical results on numerous peptide fragments have enabled us to conclude (Atassi and Thomas, 1969) that the primary antibody response, at least in early-course antisera, is directed against the native three-dimensional structures of proteins.

An intact antigenic reactive region free of extraneous non-reactive residues would usually react less in solution than when it is isolated as part of a longer peptide (Atassi, 1972; Koketsu and Atassi, 1973, 1974a, 1974b). The non-reactive parts may assist the achievement of the correct folding for binding of the reactive region with antibody combining site (Atassi and Saplin, 1968). On the other hand, recent evidence (Koketsu and Atassi, 1974a, 1974b; Atassi and Pai, 1975) has revealed that non-reactive parts composed of bulky residues linked to a reactive region may exert a detrimental effect on the reactivity due to unfavorable steric or conformational effects.

ANTIGENICITY OF THE SITES IS INHERENT IN THEIR THREE-DIMENSIONAL LOCATION

Having precisely located the antigenic sites of Mb, we have been able to direct our attention to examining the factors which confer antigenicity on these particular regions of the Mb molecule. As illustrated in Fig. 2, in spite of the complexity of its structure, the Mb antigenic sites are restricted to discrete and conformationally distinct surface regions of the polypeptide chain.

Our observations that both rabbit and goat antibodies recognize the same five antigenic sites on sperm-whale Mb (Atassi, 1975, 1977b) suggested that the antigenicity of these sites is inherent in their three-dimensional location and is independent of any sequence identities between the injected myoglobin antigen and the myoglobin of the immunized host. Our recent studies have strongly confirmed this conclusion and are described below.

Antigenic Sites that are Structurally Identical to the Corresponding Locations in Rabbit Myoglobin: Autoreactivity of Rabbit Antibodies to Sperm-Whale Myoglobin.

In view of the conservation of the overall three-dimensional structure among globin chains and occasionally extensive homologies in their primary structures, we investigated (Kazim and Atassi, 1977a) whether, in responding to sperm-whale Mb, the host animal will make antibodies to regions of the sperm-whale Mb molecule which are similar or identical to the corresponding regions in the animal's own Mb. The recent availability of the primary structure of rabbit Mb (Romero-Herrera *et al.*, 1976) afforded us the opportunity for such studies.

SITE 1 of	15							22
Sperm-Whale Mb	[Ala]	Lys	Val	Glu	Ala	Asp	[Val]	Ala
Rabbit Mb	[Gly]	Lys	Val	Glu	Ala	Asp	[Leu]	Ala

SITE 2 of	56						62
Sperm-Whale Mb	Lys	Ala	Ser	Glu	Asp	Leu	Lys
Rabbit Mb	Lys	Ala	Ser	Glu	Asp	Leu	Lys

SITE 3 of	94					99
Sperm-Whale Mb	Ala	Thr	Lys	His	Lys	Ile
Rabbit Mb	Ala	Thr	Lys	His	Lys	Ile

SITE 4 of	113						119
Sperm-Whale Mb	His	Val	Leu	His	Ser	[Arg]	His
Rabbit Mb	His	Val	Leu	His	Ser	[Lys]	His

SITE 5 of	145						151
Sperm-Whale Mb	[Lys]	Tyr	Lys	Glu	Leu	Gly	[Tyr]
Rabbit Mb	[Gln]	Tyr	Lys	Glu	Leu	Gly	[Phe]

Fig. 3. A diagram showing the primary sequences of the five antigenic sites of sperm-whale Mb and the corresponding regions of rabbit Mb. The sequences shown occupy identical positions in the respective protein chains. Identical positions having different amino acids in the two chains are indicated by blocks (from Kazim and Atassi, 1977a).

A comparison of the primary structure of sperm-whale Mb with that of rabbit Mb shows that both have identical chain lengths (153 amino acids), and differ in sequence at 22 amino acid locations. Of the 22 residues by which sperm-whale and rabbit Mb differ, only 5 of these fall within the boundaries of the antigenic sites recognized by rabbit antibodies to sperm-whale Mb. In Fig. 3 the primary sequences of the five antigenic sites of sperm-whale Mb are shown together with the corresponding regions from rabbit Mb. The amino acid replacement which occur in the corresponding rabbit Mb sequences are: $Ala^{15} \longrightarrow Gly$ and $Val^{21} \longrightarrow Leu$ in region 15-22, $Arg^{118} \longrightarrow Lys$ in region 113-119, and $Lys^{145} \longrightarrow Gln$ and $Tyr^{151} \longrightarrow Phe$ in region 145-151. Two regions, 56-62 and 94-99, are identical in both myoglobins.

The close similarity of the two myoglobins in these regions was surprising to us in view of the belief that the antigenic sites of proteins would not be in regions of a protein antigen which were identical to equivalent regions in the animal's own homologous protein (Reichlin, 1972). These similarities also

TABLE I: INHIBITORY ACTIVITIES OF RABBIT Mb IN THE SPERM-WHALE Mb-ANTI SW Mb PRECIPITIN REACTION+

Antisera were raised against sperm-whale Mb in rabbits (77) and goats (G3, G4). Inhibition values are expressed as maximum per cent inhibition by rabbit Mb of the precipitin reaction of sperm-whale Mb with the antisera shown. Each value is an average of at least three determinations which varied ± 1.5% or less.

Antiserum	Maximum inhibition (%)	Molar ratio (R Mb/SW Mb) at ½ max. inhibn.*
77	72	19
G3	76	12
G4	90	3

* These values represent the rabbit Mb/sperm-whale Mb molar ratios at 50% maximum inhibition. R Mb, rabbit Mb; SW Mb, sperm-whale Mb.

+ Table is from Kazim and Atassi (1977a).

suggested that barring any drastic conformational differences rabbit antibodies to sperm-whale Mb could also react with rabbit Mb. Since both rabbit and goat antibodies to sperm-whale Mb recognize identical antigenic sites (shown in Figs. 1 and 2) on the sperm-whale Mb molecule, goat antibodies to sperm-whale Mb may also be expected to react with rabbit Mb.

It was most significant that rabbit Mb cross-reacted extensively with rabbit antisera to sperm-whale Mb (Kazim and Atassi, 1977a). Although rabbit Mb did not give immune precipitates with either rabbit or goat antisera to sperm-whale Mb, it was quite effective in inhibiting the quantitative precipitin reaction of sperm-whale Mb with rabbit or goat antibodies to sperm-whale Mb (Table I). The large inhibitions obtained with these antisera indicate that rabbit Mb interacts effectively with both rabbit and goat antisera to sperm-whale Mb, but the affinity for rabbit Mb varied with the antiserum (Table I). The reactivity of rabbit Mb with antisera to sperm-whale Mb was also measured by examining the ability of an immunoadsorbent of rabbit Mb to bind antibodies from antisera to sperm-whale Mb (Kazim and Atassi, 1977a). Table II summarizes the results with antisera from two rabbits (77 and 80) and one goat (G4) and shows that a substantial portion of the antibodies to sperm-whale Mb could be adsorbed by the rabbit Mb adsorbent.

The extensive ability of rabbit Mb to interact with antibodies to sperm-whale Mb leads to a consideration of the sites

TABLE II: SUMMARY OF IMMUNOADSORBENT STUDIES+

Antisera are the same as those referred to in Table I except No. 80 which is a rabbit antiserum to sperm-whale Mb (SW Mb). Values are expressed as per cent of the total antibodies adsorbed by a rabbit Mb (R Mb) adsorbent relative to those bound by a sperm-whale Mb adsorbent as 100%.

Antiserum	Anti SW Mb adsorbed by SW Mb - Sepharose (%)*	Anti SW Mb adsorbed by R Mb - Sepharose (%)*
77	100%	42.9%
80	100%	65.8%
G4	100%	49.6%

* These values have been corrected for non-specifically adsorbed protein retained on a Lysozyme-Sepharose adsorbent.

+ Table is from Kazim and Atassi (1977a).

through which the rabbit Mb may interact with these antisera (Kazim and Atassi, 1977a). Regions 56-62 and 94-99 are identical in both myoglobins (Fig. 3), and unless their conformations have been altered through amino acid replacements not located in these regions, these two sites would be expected to react completely. However, ORD and CD studies (Kazim and Atassi, unpublished results) have revealed no conformational differences between sperm-whale Mb and rabbit Mb. With respect to regions 15-22 and 113-119, our previous studies have shown that the binding of the Mb antigenic sites with antibodies is primarily effected through polar interactions, with non-polar amino acids providing more of a stabilizing role through hydrophobic interactions (Atassi, 1972). Based on these considerations and on the conservative character of the amino acid substitutions in region 15-22 and 113-119, these two regions in rabbit Mb would not be expected to be completely unreactive. However, it cannot be excluded that subtle and undetectable conformational changes in these regions directed by these replacements as well as by replacements elsewhere in the rabbit molecule, could diminish the affinity of these sites for their respective antibodies. Although Lys-145 is included in the reactive region 145-151, it plays only a marginal role with some antisera and, of those studied, is required only for the reaction of the free peptide 145-151 with antiserum G4, but is not part of the reactive region in intact, native sperm-whale Mb (Koketsu and Atassi, 1973; Atassi _et al._, 1973). Therefore, the replacement of Lys-145 by glutamine in rabbit Mb should be without consequence to the reactivity of this region in native rabbit Mb. However, Tyr-151 has been shown to be absolutely essential for the reactivity of this region, and its replacement by phenylalanine completely obliterates its reactivity (Atassi and Saplin, 1971). Rabbit Mb is, therefore, not expected to react with antibodies to sperm-whale Mb through region 145-151. The expected diminished reactivities for region 15-22 and 113-119 together with the complete unreactivity of region 145-151 would account for the lack of total cross-reactivity of these two myoglobins mentioned above.

The foregoing studies clearly indicate that rabbits respond to immunization with sperm-whale Mb by producing antibodies that are directed against regions of the sperm-whale Mb molecule which are both identical (regions 56-62 and 94-99) and closely similar (regions 15-22 and 113-119) to the corresponding sequences in the rabbit's own Mb. Furthermore, these antibodies will extensively cross-react with rabbit Mb through these equivalent regions. As mentioned above both rabbits and goats make antibodies directed against regions of the sperm-whale Mb molecule which are identical in their structures and locations (Koketsu and Atassi, 1973, 1974a, 1974b; Pai and Atassi, 1975; Atassi and Pai, 1975). Pertinent, in this regard, is that hen egg-white lysozyme, the second protein whose antigenic structure has been completely determined (Lee and Atassi, 1977a, 1977b; Atassi and Lee, 1978a, 1978b), is also recognized through identical antigenic sites by both rabbit and goat antisera. In a pilot experiment we have also observed that goat Mb is extremely effective in inhibiting the precipitin reaction of sperm-whale Mb with goat antisera to sperm-whale Mb (unpublished results). Although the sequence of goat Mb is not available for comparison at the present time, we predict that similar identities exist between the reactive regions of sperm-whale Mb and the corresponding regions of goat Mb.

The fact that both rabbits and goats recognize identical antigenic sites on sperm-whale Mb, together with the results of our studies with rabbit Mb, indicate that the antigenicity of at least some regions of Mb is inherent in their three-dimensional location and is independent of sequence differences between the immunizing Mb and that of the host (Kazim and Atassi, 1977b).

As previously mentioned, these observations are in contrast to conclusions from studies on hemoglobin (Reichlin, 1972), that the antigenic sites of proteins are not located at sequence positions that are identical in the immunizing and the homologous host protein; and from chemically polymerized cytochrome c (Urbanski and Margoliash, 1977) that the antigenic sites of proteins are not peculiar to the protein but are defined by the animal species in which the immune response is elicited. In this regard, rabbits immunized with heterologous cytochrome c from various species consistently gave antibodies that reacted with the homologous, rabbit cytochrome c to a large extent (Margoliash _et al_., 1970). Although the antigenic structures of these cytochromes _c_ are not known, the authors overlooked the implication that the rabbits were responding to regions on the heterologous cytochrome c which are identical to the rabbit's own cytochrome c. More recently, these authors found that in both of the two species immunized with chemically polymerized, heterologous cytochrome c, antibodies were directed to regions which differed in sequence, as well as to a region identical in both host and immunogen cytochrome c (Urbanski and Margoliash, 1977). The persistent expression of this invariable region supports our concept of structurally-inherent antigenic sites, and is inconsistent with the conclusion that the locations of antigenic sites are not inherent to the protein but are defined by the species in which the immune response is elicited. It is relevant to stress here that, as observed for sperm-whale Mb, both rabbits and goats also recognize the same antigenic sites on hen egg-white lysozyme (Atassi and Habeeb, 1977). However, it should be cautioned that these studies on cytochrome c may not be applicable to those of myoglobin. Cytochrome c is frequently observed to be weakly or entirely non-immunogenic in its native monomeric state. The high degree of chemical cross-linking in the polymers of cytochrome c used to enhance the antibody response to this protein might have not only altered its antigenic potency, but also the sites recognized as being antigenic in the immunized host.

It is worthwhile to note here that while Mb is an intramuscular protein thought to be sheltered from exposure to the immune system its presence in normal serum has been demonstrated (Stone *et al.*, 1975). In fact, there is increasing evidence to indicate that antigens previously thought to be sequestered from the immune system are indeed present in the circulation (Allison and Denman, 1976), although in low amounts.

The induction of autoreactive antibodies to "sequestered" antigens by immunization with a cross-reacting antigen is not unprecedented. In fact, it has been suggested that suppressive and tolerizing influences on the immune response to autologous proteins may be circumvented by stimulating helper effects specifically with cross-reacting antigens (Allison and Denman, 1976). However, the lack of knowledge concerning the molecular structures and locations of protein antigenic sites has lead to uncertainty regarding the precise regions of the proteins through which these cross-reactions are effected. This is the first system to be described in which the structures of the antigenic sites of the cross-reacting protein are completely known, and provides an excellent model for studying some of the molecular aspects of immunologic tolerance to auto-antigens and its termination.

Autoantibodies Produced by Immunization with Rabbit Mb

As an extension of our findings that the antigenic sites of

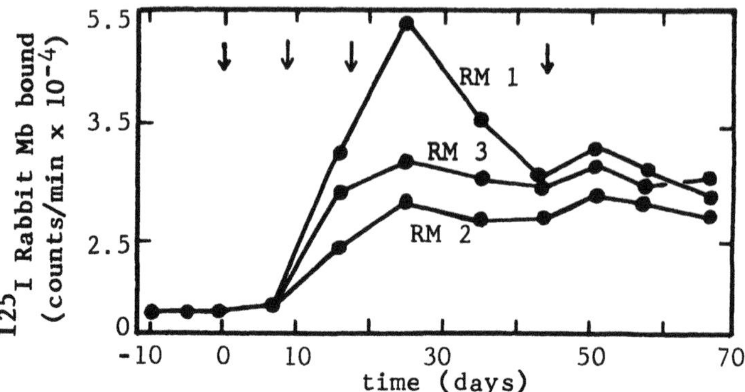

Fig. 4. Screening of ^{125}I-rabbit Mb binding by antisera obtained from serial bleedings of three rabbits (RM 1, RM 2 and RM 3) immunized with rabbit Mb. Arrows indicate times of immunization (from Kazim and Atassi, 1978).

myoglobin are not dependent on sequence differences between the immunizing Mb and that of the host, we reasoned (Kazim and Atassi, 1978) that rabbits immunized with rabbit Mb should produce antibodies against this protein.

Our recent studies (Kazim and Atassi, 1978) clearly demonstrate that rabbits, when immunized with rabbit Mb, do make antibodies against this autologous protein. The results are outlined in Figs. 4 and 5. A summary of these observations follow: 1) No significant binding of ^{125}I-rabbit Mb occurred with the preimmune sera (Fig. 4). 2) Sera from immunized rabbits show a dramatic increase in the binding of ^{125}I-rabbit Mb, the appearance of binding being consistent with the "lag" observed in humoral responses (Fig 4). 3) The binding is associated entirely with the immunoglobulins of these antisera as demonstrated by the quantitative ability of a goat anti-rabbit antibody (with specificity only for heavy and light chains of rabbit immunoglobulins) to precipitate labeled antigen bound by these antisera. 4) The binding of ^{125}I-rabbit Mb could be completely inhibited by unlabeled rabbit Mb and partially by unlabeled sperm-whale Mb - a related cross-reacting protein (Fig. 5). No inhibition was obtained by human hemoglobin at comparable concentrations, indicating that the inhibitions by rabbit Mb and sperm-whale Mb were specific and not due to non-specific protein effects (Fig. 5). 5) Two of the three rabbits immunized gave characteristic precipitin curves upon reaction of antisera taken 25 days after the initial immunization with rabbit Mb. 6) The fact that all three rabbits responded to rabbit Mb either with precipitating or non-precipitating antibodies and the similarities in the overall profiles of the response curves

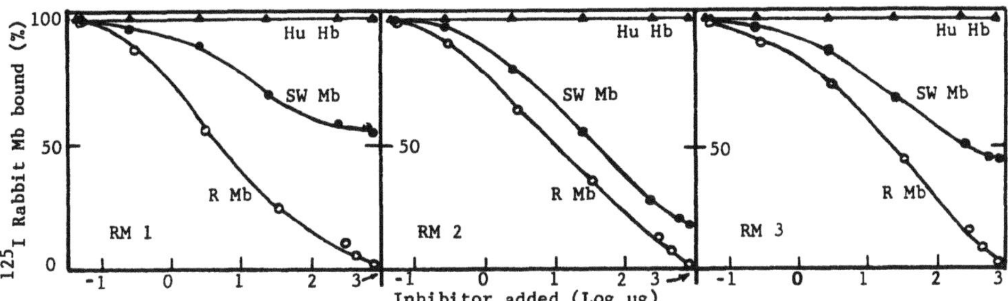

Fig. 5. Inhibition of ^{125}I-rabbit Mb binding by unlabelled rabbit Mb, sperm-whale Mb and human hemoglobin. The antisera used in these assays were obtained from the 25-day bleedings. In each case, the amount of antisera present bound 20-30% of the total ^{125}I-rabbit Mb added in the absence of competing, unlabeled protein (from Kazim and Atassi, 1978).

(Fig. 4) indicate that these rabbits do not represent isolated cases of response to this autologous antigen. The Mb used in these studies was the major chromatographic component of the combined muscle extracts of two unrelated rabbits and had an amino acid composition identical to that of rabbit Mb isolated in England (Romero-Herrera et al., 1976). Therefore, it is unlikely that this Mb preparation differs from the major Mb component of these immunized rabbits. Accordingly, we believe these antibodies to be true autoantibodies.

Somewhat low antibody titres were observed with these antisera (ca. 0.25 mg/ml) and may be accounted for (Kazim and Atassi, 1978) by the formation of complexes of these antibodies with circulating Mb. As mentioned, myoglobin has been found to exist in serum of normal humans to the extent of 6-85 ng/ml (Stone et al., 1975). The fast renal clearance of Mb (Kagen, 1973), facilitated by its small size, suggests a somewhat higher rate of entrance into the circulation than is reflected by the net concentration in the serum. By analogy with the human system, the binding of these rabbit antibodies to this small, yet constant supply of circulating Mb would enable the antibodies bound to escape detection. The possibility of more direct attenuating influences on the antibody response should not, however, be overlooked.

Our studies on the antigenic structure of sperm-whale Mb showed that antibodies to this protein elicited by immunization with sperm-whale Mb emulsified in Freund's complete adjuvant were directed against its native three-dimensional structure (Atassi and Thomas, 1969). Furthermore, the reactivity of these antibodies with sperm-whale Mb were shown to be extremely sensitive to slight conformational distortions intentionally imposed on the native structure of sperm-whale Mb by modifications which were clearly outside antigenic sites (Atassi, 1967b; Andres and Atassi, 1970). Similar observations have been made for lysozyme (Atassi and Habeeb, 1977). Obviously, emulsification in Freund's adjuvant did not alter the native conformation of these proteins. We therefore expect that the autoantibodies to rabbit Mb (obtained by immunization with emulsions of rabbit Mb in Freund's complete adjuvant) are similarly directed against the native conformation of rabbit Mb.

The efficiency with which sperm-whale Mb cross-reacts with these antisera to rabbit Mb, as judged by the comparable concentrations of sperm-whale and rabbit Mb required for maximal inhibition of the binding of ^{125}I-rabbit Mb (Fig. 5), indicate that the cross-reacting antigenic sites on rabbit Mb to which these antibodies are directed exist in an identical or near-identical form in sperm-whale Mb (Kazim and Atassi, 1978). These cross-reacting sites are, of course, expected to be located away from regions which carry amino acid replacements between the two myoglobins. This would be especially true of regions carrying non-conservative amino acid replacements which have alterations in their electrostatic characteristics, since we have previously shown that polar interactions predominate over non-polar interactions in the binding of antigenic sites to their antibodies (Atassi, 1972, 1975). Sperm-whale Mb, however, did not completely inhibit the binding of ^{125}I-rabbit Mb to these anti-rabbit Mb antibodies, although for one antiserum (RM2) the inhibition was greater than 80% (Fig. 5). The individual variations in the extent of inhibition by sperm-whale Mb with these antisera probably reflect differences in the relative amounts of antibodies directed against sites on rabbit Mb which have cross-reacting counterparts on sperm-whale Mb (Kazim and Atassi, 1978).

It was pointed out (Kazim and Atassi, 1978) that the inability of sperm-whale Mb to completely cross-react with the antisera to rabbit Mb indicates that antigenic sites, peculiar to rabbit Mb, are undoubtedly recognized. However, these sites are not necessarily excluded from being located at similar structural positions to those of sperm-whale Mb. Similarities in the amino acid sequences between the two myoglobins in the regions of the antigenic sites of sperm-whale Mb (Kazim and Atassi, 1977a), and the ability of rabbit Mb to react extensively with rabbit antibodies to sperm-whale Mb have been mentioned above. However, there is no guarantee that antibodies directed against the same structural locations in rabbit Mb, but bearing the new amino acid substitutions will react with sperm-whale Mb.

Autoantibody responses to immunization with autologous proteins have been previously described. For example, auto-reactive antibodies to thyroglobulin have been observed upon immunization with autologous thyroglobulin in Freund's complete adjuvant or heterologous thyroglobulin in the absence of adjuvant (Allison and Denman, 1976). Immunization with structurally altered autologous proteins have also been shown to result in autoantibody formation (Williams and Kunkel, 1963). For example, rabbits immunized with papain-digested autologous γ-globulins formed auto-reactive precipitating antibodies to these proteins. Similarly, rabbits did not respond to native rabbit cytochrome c, but made antibodies to highly chemically polymerized rabbit cytochrome c preparations (Reichlin et al., 1970). However, such findings were not substantiated by these authors in subsequent trials (Urbanski and Margoliash, 1977).

Clearly the results show that the potential for auto-recognition of rabbit Mb is present, and that this potential is expressed when rabbits are immunized with rabbit Mb (Kazim and Atassi, 1978). Furthermore, no "structural alterations" of rabbit Mb were necessary in order to induce these autoantibodies. Regardless of whether or not the autoantigenic sites of rabbit Mb lie in the same structural locations as the antigenic sites of sperm-whale Mb, these autoantigenic sites are clearly not dependent on sequence differences between the immunogen and the corresponding host protein. The relative ease with which autoantibodies to Mb were induced suggests that autoimmunity to Mb may play a role in the pathogenesis of muscle diseases.

Prediction and Synthesis of Two Antigenic Sites in Hemoglobin by Extrapolation from the Mb Antigenic Structure

Compelling evidence to support our concept that the antigenicity of protein antigenic sites is inherent in their three-dimensional locations has been our recent prediction and synthesis of two antigenic sites of hemoglobin by extrapolation from the Mb antigenic structure (Kazim and Atassi, 1977b). Previously we had shown that the structure of antigenic sites of proteins are directed by their amino acid sequences as well as by the three-dimensional arrangement of the participating amino acid residues (Habeeb and Atassi, 1971; Atassi, 1975; Atassi et al., 1976a, 1976b; Lee and Atassi, 1976). The results obtained during our delineation of the entire antigenic structure of sperm-whale Mb also suggested that the antigenic sites of other myoglobins are located at similar structural positions in their respective chains (Atassi and Saplin, 1971). Since the primary antibody response to a native protein is directed against its native three-dimensional structure (Atassi

Residue Location:	A_{13}	A_{14}	A_{15}	A_{16}	AB_1	B_1	B_2	B_3	B_4	B_5
Site 1 of Mb:	Ala[15]	Lys	Val	Glu	Ala	Asp	Val	Ala[22]		
Hb α (15-23):	Gly[15]	Lys	Val	Gly	Ala	His	Ala	Gly	Glu[23]	
Hb β (16-23):	Gly[16]	Lys	Val	Asn	...	...	Val	Asp	Glu	Val[23]

Fig. 6. Diagram showing the sequence and structural location of antigenic site 1 of sperm-whale Mb and the corresponding regions of the adult human Hb α and β chains. For the letter/number notation used to designate the structural locations of the amino acid residues, and for the alignment of the Hb α and β chains with sperm-whale Mb see Dickerson and Geis (1969) (from Kazim and Atassi, 1977b).

and Thomas, 1969), we were prompted to examine whether conformationally homologous, yet more complex globins would possess antigenic sites at similar locations in their three-dimensional structure (Kazim and Atassi, 1977b). The many structural features which the α and β chains of Hb share with Mb (Perutz _et al._, 1968) made the Hb molecule particularly suitable for examining whether it is possible to extrapolate, and thereby predict, the antigenic sites of a large, multisubunit protein from those of a smaller member of the same protein family.

In a very recent study (Kazim and Atassi, 1977b) we have focused on the Mb antigenic site 1 (region 15-22). The sequences and structural locations of the corresponding regions in the α and β chains of human Hb are shown in Fig. 6. To examine whether these extrapolated regions of the α and β chains (α 15-23, β 16-23) were immunochemically active, they were synthesized and their immunochemical reactions with antisera to human Hb studied (Kazim and Atassi, 1977b). Antigenic site 1 of sperm-whale Mb invariably included the sequence 16-21 with all antisera tested (Koketsu and Atassi, 1974a). However, some antisera also required either Ala-15 or Ala-22 for full reactivity. Accordingly, site 1 was taken here to comprise the sequence 15-22 in order to accommodate the individual variabilities of different antisera. Sequence 15-22 of sperm-whale Mb occupies the helix positions A13 through B3, and is located at the highly exposed bend between helices A and B (Watson, 1969; also see Fig. 5 for explanation of structural notations). The three-dimensional counterpart of the Mb antigenic site 1 in the Hb α chain also spans residues α 15-22 (Perutz _et al._, 1968). In our studies we chose to extend this region to include Glu-23 in order to increase the solubility of the synthetic peptide α 15-23 in aqueous solvents. The Hb β chain varies in its alignment with the α chain in this region by not having the corresponding AB1 and B1 positions (Perutz _et al._, 1968). Therefore, we extended the synthetic region of the β chain to Val-23 in order to compensate for the deficiency in length which would occur from a precise structural extrapolation of this region. By examination of the three-dimensional structures of human deoxyhemoglobin (Fermi, 1975) and of horse oxyhemoglobin (Perutz _et al._, 1968) these regions (α 15-23 and β 16-23) are not involved in either chain-heme or chain-chain interactions in the native Hb molecule, and they occupy highly accessible positions in their respective α and β chains in the native Hb tetramer. Thus these regions were considered (Kazim and Atassi, 1977b) ideally suited for examining whether the structural extrapolation of antigenic sites are possible.

We found (Kazim and Atassi, 1977b) that the synthetic peptides were unable to inhibit the precipitin reaction of Hb with its antisera, even at molar excess of 1000-fold, either individually or in combination. This was not entirely unexpected. Although the synthetic antigenic sites of Mb inhibit its immune reaction quantitatively, other workers have reported that Hb fragments will not inhibit the Hb immune reaction (Reichlin, 1972). Also, antibodies to a region around Val-6 in Hb S, obtained from anti-Hb S by an immunoadsorbent of the synthetic peptide β 1-13 of Hb S, accounted for only about 5% of the total antibodies to Hb S. Furthermore, the peptide, which was initially used to obtain this antibody population by immunoadsorption was not fully effective in displacing Hb S bound to these antibodies (Young _et al._, 1975). These results may in part be accounted for by the large size of Hb, and conceivably an increased number of antigenic sites, and the decreased affinity which immunochemically active peptides in a non-native conformation exhibit for their antibodies (Atassi and Saplin, 1968). These observations suggested to us that, not withstanding the structural alterations which would occur upon being covalently coupled to Sepharose, quantitative immunoadsorption would be the most suitable approach for studying the immunochemical activities of these extrapolated peptides (Kazim and Atassi, 1977b).

The results of the immunoadsorption studies (Table III) showed (Kazim and Atassi, 1977b) that these peptides are immunochemically active with antisera to native Hb, accounting for a significant portion of the reactivities of Hb and of the respective α and β chains. The immunochemical activities of these peptides are further illustrated by comparing them to the activity of a reference peptide, α 1-15, which does not fall within the boundaries of an antigenic site that could be predicted from Mb. This peptide showed no significant immunochemical activity (Kazim and Atassi, 1977b). The calculated sum of the reactivities of the α

TABLE III: QUANTITATIVE IMMUNOADSORPTION OF ^{125}I-ANTI HEMOGLOBIN+

Results represent the average of three determinations which varied ± 1.5% each. They have also been corrected for protein non-specifically bound to lysozyme-Sepharose. This correction amounted to no more than 1-2% of the total counts bound to Hb-Sepharose. Amount of labelled antibody applied to each immunoadsorbent was 102,000 c.p.m. (1.099 x 10^{-12} moles).*

Immunoadsorbent	Amount antibody bound (CPM)	% Rel. to HbA	% Rel. to Chain
HbA	98006	100	
α chain	82138	83.8	
β chain	57801	59.0	
α (15-23)	10842	11.1	13.2
β (16-23)	7132	7.28	12.3
α (1-15)	133	0.14	0.16

* Peptides on the immunoadsorbents were present in a vast molar excess (approx. 600,000) relative to the labelled antibody applied.

\+ Table is from Kazim and Atassi (1977b).

and β chains was greater than that of Hb. Similar observations have recently been made by others (Tan-Wilson et al., 1976) and were attributed to cross-reactivities between the chains.

The aforementioned results clearly indicate that by extrapolation of the structural location of antigenic site 1 of sperm-whale Mb, we were able to predict and confirm antigenic sites for a larger, more complex member of the same protein family (Kazim and Atassi, 1977b). Based on these results we stated (Kazim and Atassi, 1977b) that when similar extrapolations of antigenic sites of Mb are made to other homologous proteins, the predicted regions will also be shown to be immunochemically active. However, we cautioned that not all structural counterparts of the antigenic sites of one protein are expected to be immunochemically active in a homologous protein. Thus, in the tetrameric hemoglobin molecule, for example, obstructions due to subunit interactions, and conformational adjustments effected by amino acid substitutions (both within and outside the predicted regions) as well as by the influence of neighboring subunits may alter the antigenic expression of these regions. For similar reasons, new antigenic sites on individual subunits or combinations thereof, without antigenic counterparts in the myoglobin molecule, should not be unexpected in the hemoglobin molecule.

CONCLUSION

In summary, by comparing the precisely delineated structure of sperm-whale Mb with the primary structure of rabbit Mb we have shown that the locations of antigenic sites of this protein are not dependent on sequence differences between the immunizing and host myoglobins. Also, the ability of rabbit antisera against sperm-whale Mb to cross-react with rabbit Mb, and the immunogenicity of rabbit Mb in rabbits may implicate the participation of auto-reactive clones in the antibody response to heterologous proteins. This may in fact be a general phenomenon with protein antigens, and serves to emphasize the need for caution and critical evaluation of approaches relying on the notion that antigenic sites on a protein are located in parts of the molecule that are different in sequence from the corresponding protein in the immunized host.

Furthermore, these observations, together with our successful extrapolation of the antigenic structure of sperm-whale Mb to human hemoglobin demonstrate that the antigenicity of certain regions of a native protein molecule is primarily dependent on the uniqueness of their conformational locations. This property will be independent of whether or not such sites are recognized as being autologous or present on immunochemically unrelated proteins. We would like to refer to these antigenic sites as "structurally inherent antigenic sites".

The utility of "structurally inherent" antigenic sites to the immune system is that the overall complementarity between the shape of the antibody combining site and the antigenic site can be maintained with minimal amino acid replacements in the combining site and without a drastic overhaul. This affords a biological advantage in that it may reduce the information load and time lag necessary for recognition and antibody response to protein antigens.

ACKNOWLEDGEMENTS

The work was supported by a grant (AM 18920) from the Institute of Arthritis and Metabolic Diseases, National Institutes of Health, U.S. Public Health Service and by a grant (AI 13181) from the National Institute of Allergy and Infectious Diseases.

REFERENCES

Allison, A.C. and Denman, A.M. (1976) Br. Med. Bull. 32, 124.

Andres, S.F. and Atassi, M.Z. (1970) Biochemistry 9, 2268.

Atassi, M.Z. (1967a) Biochem. J. 102, 478.

Atassi, M.Z. (1967b) Biochem. J. 103, 29.

Atassi, M.Z. (1972) in "Specific Receptors of Antibodies, Antigens and Cells", 3rd International Convocation of Immunology, June 12-15, (Edited by Pressman, D., Tomasi, T.B., Grossberg, A.L. and Rose, N.R.) p. 118-136, Karger, Basel.

Atassi, M.Z. (1975) Immunochemistry 12, 423.

Atassi, M.Z. (1977a) in Immunochemistry of Proteins (Atassi, M.Z., Ed.) Vol. 1, pp. 1-161, Plenum, New York.

Atassi, M.Z. (1977b) in Immunochemistry of Proteins (Atassi, M.Z., Ed.) Vol. 2, pp. 77-176, Plenum, New York.

Atassi, M.Z. (1978) Immunochemistry, in press.

Atassi, M.Z. and Habeeb, A.F.S.A. (1977) in Immunochemistry of Proteins (Atassi, M.Z., Ed.) Vol. 2, pp. 177-264, Plenum, New York.

Atassi, M.Z. and Koketsu, J. (1975) Immunochemistry 12, 741.

Atassi, M.Z. and Lee, C.-L. (1978a) Biochem. J., in press.

Atassi, M.Z. and Lee, C.-L. (1978b) Biochem. J., in press.

Atassi, M.Z. and Pai, R.-C. (1975) Immunochemistry 12, 735.

Atassi, M.Z. and Saplin, B.J. (1968) Biochemistry 7, 688.

Atassi, M.Z. and Saplin, B.J. (1971) Biochemistry 10, 4740.

Atassi, M.Z. and Thomas, A.V. (1969) Biochemistry 8, 3385.

Atassi, M.Z., Perlstein, M.T. and Staub, D.J. (1973) Biochim. Biophys. Acta 328, 278.

Atassi, M.Z., Koketsu, J. and Habeeb, A.F.S.A. (1976a) Biochim. Biophys. Acta 420, 358.

Atassi, M.Z., Lee, C.-L. and Pai, R.-C. (1976b) Biochim. Biophys. Acta 427, 745.

Dickerson, R.E. and Geis, I. (1969) in The Structure and Action of Proteins, p. 52, Harper & Row, New York.

Fermi, G. (1975) J. Mol. Biol. 97, 237.

Habeeb, A.F.S.A. and Atassi, M.Z. (1971) Biochim. Biophys. Acta 236, 131.

Kagen, L.J. (1973) in Myoglobin: Biochemical, Physiological and Clinical Aspects, p. 91, Columbia University Press, New York.

Kazim, A.L. and Atassi, M.Z. (1977a) Biochim. Biophys. Acta 494, 277.

Kazim, A.L. and Atassi, M.Z. (1977b) Biochem. J. 167, 275.

Kazim, A.L. and Atassi, M.Z. (1978) Immunochemistry, in press.

Koketsu, J. and Atassi, M.Z. (1973) Biochim. Biophys. Acta 328, 289.

Koketsu, J. and Atassi, M.Z. (1974a) Immunochemistry 11, 1.

Koketsu, J. and Atassi, M.Z. (1974b) Biochim. Biophys. Acta 342, 21.

Lee, C.-L. and Atassi, M.Z. (1976) Biochem. J. 159, 89.

Lee, C.-L. and Atassi, M.Z. (1977a) Biochem. J. 167, 571.

Lee, C.-L. and Atassi, M.Z. (1977b) Biochim. Biophys. Acta 495, 354.

Margoliash, E., Nisonoff, A. and Reichlin, M. (1970) J. Biol. Chem. 245, 931.

Pai, R.-C. and Atassi, M.Z. (1975) Immunochemistry 12, 285.

Perutz, M.F., Muirhead, H., Cox, J.M. and Goaman, L.C.G. (1968) Nature 219, 131.

Reichlin, M. (1972) J. Mol. Biol. 64, 485.

Reichlin, M., Nisonoff, A. and Margoliash, E. (1970) J. Biol. Chem. 245, 947.

Romero-Herrera, A.E., Lehmann, H. and Castillo, O. (1976) Biochim. Biophys. Acta 439, 51.

Stone, M.J., Willerson, J.T., Gomez-Sanchez, C.E. and Waterman, M.R. (1975) J. Clin. Invest. 56, 1334.

Tan-Wilson, A.L., Reichlin, M. and Noble, R.W. (1976) Immunochemistry 13, 491.

Urbanski, G.J. and Margoliash, E. (1977) J. Immunol. 118, 1170.

Watson, H.C. (1969) in Progress in Stereochemistry (Aylett, B.J. and Harris, M., Eds.) p. 299-333, Butterworth, London.

Williams, R.C., Jr. and Kunkel, H.G. (1963) Proc. Soc. Exp. Biol. Med. 112, 554.

Young, N.S., Curd, J.G., Eastlake, A., Furie, B. and Schechter, A.N. (1975) Proc. Natl. Acad. Sci. 72, 4759.

THE PRECISE AND ENTIRE ANTIGENIC STRUCTURE OF LYSOZYME: IMPLICATIONS OF SURFACE-SIMULATION SYNTHESIS AND THE MOLECULAR FEATURES OF PROTEIN ANTIGENIC SITES

M. Zouhair Atassi

Department of Immunology, Mayo Medical School
Rochester, Minnesota 55901
and
Department of Biochemistry, University of Minnesota
Minneapolis, Minnesota 55455

SUMMARY

Intensive research in the author's laboratory over a 10-year period has now culminated in the precise determination of the entire antigenic structure of native hen egg-white lysozyme. The protein carries three antigenic sites. Each site is made up of spatially adjacent surface residues that are not in direct peptide linkage. The residues of each site describe an imaginary line which circumscribes part of the surface topography of the protein and act functionally towards the antibody as if they are in direct peptide bond linkage. The reactivity of each site is fully satisfied by an appropriate surface-simulation synthetic peptide, and the three synthetic sites account for the full immunochemical reactivity of the native protein. Each site is subject to conformational restrictions and exhibits directionality which is a function of side chain orientations. The antigenic sites of myoglobin and lysozyme are compared. It is proposed that antigenic sites of the type found in myoglobin are called "continuous sites", while antigenic sites of the type seen in lysozyme are defined as "discontinuous sites".

The unorthodox and novel concept of "surface-simulation" synthesis, which we developed for the precise definition of the antigenic sites of lysozyme, links the spatially adjacent residues constituting a site directly via peptide bonds with appropriate spacers where necessary. Application of this concept has enabled us to mimick synthetically, at least in terms of binding function, the antibody combining sites to lysozyme antigenic sites. The implications and potential applications of surface-simulation synthesis are discussed.

I. INTRODUCTION

The antigenic structures of disulfide-containing proteins (e.g. lysozyme, ribonuclease, albumin, etc.) have been extremely difficult to study. The covalent cross-linking of the protein by the disulfide bonds imparts on the molecule a high structural stability and a 'tight' mode of folding which renders it almost completely inaccessible to cleavage procedures. It has already been shown (Atassi, 1972, 1975) that one of the useful approaches which was instrumental in our elucidation of the entire antigenic structure of sperm-whale myoglobin (Atassi, 1975) depends on the isolation of a large variety of overlapping peptide fragments representing various parts of the protein molecule. However, because of the inaccessibility of these tight proteins it has not been possible to apply the cleavage approach in a systematic and effective manner. Although some limited information was derived from peptic and similar fragments, these accounted only for a very small portion of the reactivity of the intact protein (see Section IV-A). Accordingly, for lack of a better alternative, many investigators resorted to studying the immunochemistry of protein derivatives with broken disulfide bonds since such derivatives are completely accessible to cleavage procedures. Unfortunately, these unfolded preparations do not show any immunochemical cross-reaction with the native parent protein (Brown *et al.*, 1959; Brown, 1962; Gerwing and Thompson, 1968; Young and Leung, 1970; Lee and Atassi, 1973; Atassi *et al.*, 1973). In order to understand the complex primary and three-dimensional structural features of protein antigenic sites, only the native protein is the appropriate model for investigation, even though it posed a major chemical challenge.

Lysozyme represents a typical member of this class of disulfide-containing tight proteins. When this work started early in 1967, the covalent structure of hen egg-white lysozyme had been previously determined (Canfield, 1963a, 1963b; Jollès *et al.*, 1963, 1964; Canfield and Liu, 1965). Also, its three-dimensional structure had been elucidated (Blake *et al.*, 1965, 1967). Lysozyme is a single polypeptide chain of 129 amino acid residues and is internally cross-linked by four disulfide bonds.

I wish to report here the precise determination of the entire antigenic structure of native hen egg-white. This is the second antigenic structure of a native protein antigen to be thus fully determined, with the first being that of sperm-whale myoglobin

(Atassi, 1975). The work commenced in June 1967 (Atassi and Habeeb, 1969) and was fully completed in July 1977 (Atassi and Lee, 1978b). These long and extensive investigations and the logical processes of the delineation as well as its impact on protein immunochemistry in particular and protein chemistry in general will be narrated here in a summary fashion. Readers desiring more detail may consult the original articles cited here. The delineation was carried out with early-course antisera which were raised against native lysozmye in rabbits and goats as previously described for myoglobin (Atassi, 1967a).

Our strategy of attack at the antigenic structure relied on the five approaches which previously had been extremely effective in the determination of the entire antigenic structure of myoglobin (Atassi, 1972, 1975). These approaches were: (1) to study the effect of conformational changes on the immunochemistry of the protein; (2) to isolate and characterize immunochemically-reactive fragments that can quantitatively account for the total reaction of the native protein; (3) to study the immunochemistry and conformation of chemical derivatives of lysozyme specifically modified at appropriate amino acid locations; (4) to study the effect of chemical modification of selected amino acid locations on the immunochemistry and conformation of immunochemically-reactive peptides; (5) after hopefully narrowing down each of the antigenic sites by approaches (1-4) to a conveniently small region, the final delineation would rely on studying the immunochemistry of synthetic peptides corresponding to many overlaps around this region. The application, usefulness and shortcomings of these approaches to protein immunochemistry have recently been discussed in considerable detail (Atassi, 1977b). It is also necessary to mention here that none of these approaches by itself is capable of yielding the full antigenic structure. We invariably used the results from one approach to confirm and correct those from the others. The complete structure is a composite logical synthesis of all the information. In the following sections, the findings derived from each of these approaches will first be presented very briefly, following which the information will be coordinated to derive the precise and entire antigenic structure of native lysozyme.

II. IMMUNOCHEMISTRY AND CONFORMATION OF LYSOZYME DERIVATIVES WITH BROKEN DISULFIDE BONDS

Very recent studies from our laboratories (Atassi *et al.*, 1973, 1976b, 1976c, 1976d) have shown that the disulfides are extremely important in bringing into conformational proximity various parts of each antigenic site from otherwise distant (in sequence) parts of the molecule.

The complete cleavage of the disulfide bonds in lysozyme gives rise (antigenically speaking) to a new protein antigen that is entirely unrelated to the parent native protein (Gerwing and Thompson, 1968; Young and Leung, 1970; Lee and Atassi, 1973). Antisera to lysozyme will not react with the reduced S-carboxymethylated derivative (SCM-lysozyme). Similarly, antisera to SCM-lysozyme will not react with lysozyme.

The foregoing studies show that cleavage of the disulfides effects a complete disruption of the conformation and immunochemical properties of the protein in spite of the directive force of long-range interactions. Clearly, a satisfactory approach of the previously disulfide-linked regions is prevented by like-charge repulsion or by steric obstruction of the substituent or by both. We investigated (Lee and Atassi, 1973) the possibility of improving the reapproach of regions previously linked by disulfide bonds by eliminating the like-charge repulsion and minimizing the effect of steric hindrance by the substituents. Two lysozyme derivatives were prepared (Lee and Atassi, 1973) one in which the disulfides were reduced and then the resultant thiol groups carboxymethylated (SCM-lysozyme), and in the other reduction was followed by methylation (SM-lysozyme). ORD and CD measurements in water showed that both derivatives were greatly unfolded relative to native lysozyme, although the CD results indicated that SM-lysozyme was somewhat more folded than SCM-lysozyme. Conformational studies in increasing concentrations of methanol suggested that SM-lysozyme assumed, around 35% methanol, some stabilized structure whose ORD parameters approximated those of native lysozyme. In contrast, SCM-lysozyme showed no discretely stabilized structure in the range 0-60% methanol. This was further confirmed by immunochemical studies. SCM-lysozyme showed no reaction (0%) with antisera to lysozyme, while SM-lysozyme had appreciable (35-38%) cross-reaction with these antisera. However, neither derivative had any enzymatic activity, suggesting that more rigid structural requirements are needed for this property than for immunochemical cross-reaction. These findings indicated that it was indeed feasible, at least to a limited extent, to effect a stabilized structure in SM-lysozyme due to the ability of the S-methyl groups to participate in non-polar interactions. In SCM-lysozyme, the directive effect of long-range interactions is ineffective because a refolded, stabilized structure is prevented by the like-charge repulsion and steric hindrance of the carboxymethyl anions as they approach one another (Lee and Atassi, 1973).

III. IMMUNOCHEMISTRY AND CONFORMATION OF SPECIFIC CHEMICAL DERIVATIVES OF LYSOZYME

Determination of the structural features responsible for the antigenicity of the native protein and correlation of these with the three-dimensional structure was our prime goal, and it was apparent from the foregoing that only the intact protein can be studied. Critical information for the delineation of the antigenic structure of lysozyme has been obtained from the immunochemical results of pure and well-characterized chemical derivatives of lysozyme, and which suffered no conformational changes from the modification. Table 1 summarizes the results and a comprehensive account of these derivatives was given in a recent review (Atassi and Habeeb, 1977). The advantages and shortcomings of this approach have been critically analyzed and discussed and the chemistry of chemical modification and cleavage reactions has been reviewed in detail (Atassi, 1977a). In this section, the findings from the chemical derivatives of lysozyme (see Table I) will be briefly discussed.

Lysozyme was modified at the amino groups by guanidination, acetylation, succinylation or maleylation (Habeeb and Atassi, 1971b). Guanidination of five amino groups did not alter the conformation, enzymatic activity or the antigenic reactivity with antisera to lysozyme. The acetylated, succinylated, or maleylated derivatives showed small, but measurable, conformational changes. The enzymatic activity was abolished upon modification of four or more amino groups and this loss was attributed to changes in electrostatic interactions between the modified enzyme and the negatively charged bacterial cell wall. Significantly, the two acetyl derivatives showed identical immunochemical reactivity (78% relative to lysozyme) despite the esterification of seven and fifteen aliphatic hydroxyl groups (Habeeb and Atassi, 1971b). From the foregoing results, it was concluded that at least eight aliphatic hydroxyl groups and about three amino groups are not parts of antigenic sites in native lysozyme (Habeeb and Atassi, 1971b).

From a heterogeneous succinylated product of lysozyme six homogeneous derivatives were isolated by column chromatography (Lee, Atassi and Habeeb, 1975). The locations of the modifications in each derivative are shown in Table 1. Only derivatives IV, V and VI showed no conformational changes by ORD and CD measurements and by accessibility of their disulfide bonds to reduction. Of the six succinyl derivatives, only derivative VI possessed some (10%) enzymatic activity. The reactivity of each of the derivatives with antisera to lysozyme was lower than the homologous reaction. Since conformational changes in succinyl derivatives IV, V and VI were virtually absent, it was concluded (Lee _et al._, 1975) that lysines 33, 96 and 116 are parts of antigenic reactive sites in lysozyme.

In another study, the reaction of lysozyme with diketene and tetrafluorosuccinic, maleic and citraconic anhydrides was

TABLE 1: Summary of Results from Some Chemical Derivatives of Lysozyme

Derivative	Residues modified	Conformational change	Immunochemical change	Conclusion
A. Derivatives with broken disulfides				
1) SCM-lysozyme[a]	The 4 disulfides, reduced and carboxy-methylated	large	total	none made because of the large conformational change
2) SM-lysozyme[a]	The 4 disulfides, reduced and methylated	large	total	
B. Tyrosyl derivatives				
1) NT_2-lysozyme[b,c]	Tyr-20 & -23, nitrated	present	present	Tyr -20 and/or -23 at or near an antigenic site
2) AT_2-lysozyme[b,c]	Tyr-20 & -23, to aminotyrosine	present	none	
C. Tryptophan derivatives				
1) NPS_6-lysozyme[d,c]	6 tryptophans, with 2-nitrophenylsulfenyl chloride	large	very large	none made because of large conform. change
2) DISA-lysozyme[e]	Trp-123, with 2,3-dioxo-5-indolinesulfonic acid	none	none	Trp-123 not in antigenic site
D. Methionine derivatives				
1) CNBr-lysozyme[f]	Cleavage at Met-12 & -105, with CNBr	large	present	none made due to large conform. change
2) CE-lysozyme[g]	Met-12 & -105, carboxyethylated	none	none	Met-12 & -105 not in antigenic site
E. Arginine derivatives				
1) CHD-lysozyme I[h]	10 arginines, with cyclohexanedione in 0.1N NaOH	large	very large	none made because of large conform. change
2) CHD-lysozyme II[h]	10 arginines, with cyclohexanedione in 0.1M triethylamine	large	very large	
3) PG-lysozyme[h]	Arg-61, with phenylglyoxal	minor	none	Arg-61 not in antigenic site

F. Amino group derivatives				
1) Gu_5-lysozyme[i]	5 amino groups, guanidinated	none	none	none, modification does not alter charge
2) AC_7-lysozyme[i]	7 amino groups, acetylated	large	large	none made
3) ML_7-lysozyme[i,j]	7 amino groups, maleylated	large	large	because of
4) Su_7-lysozyme[i]	7 amino groups, succinylated	large	large	the large
5) Su-lysozyme I[k]	Lys-1(α-&ε-), 13, 97 & 116; -OH at 43 (or 36 or 40), succinylated	large	large	conformational
6) Su-lysozyme II[k]	Lys-1(α-&ε-), 13, 96 & 116, succinylated	considerable	large	change
7) Su-lysozyme III[k]	Lys-1(α-&ε-), 13, 97 & 116, succinylated	considerable	large	
8) Su-lysozyme IV[k]	Lys-1(α-NH_2), 33, 96 & 116, succinylated	minor or none	present	one or more of Lys-33, -96 & -116 in antigenic sites
9) Su-lysozyme V[k]	Lys-1(α-NH_2), 33, 96, succinylated	minor or none	present	Lys-33 & -96 in antigenic sites
10) Su-lysozyme VI[k]	Lys-33 and 116, succinylated	minor or none	present	Lys-33 & -116 in antigenic sites
G. Carboxyl group derivatives				
1) BH_3-lysozyme[l]	Asp-119 & Leu-129, reduced by BH_3	minor	none	Asp-119 & Leu-129 not in antigenic sites
2) GME_2-lysozyme[m]	Asp-119 & Leu-129, coupled to Gly-methyl ester	minor	none	
3) HME_2-lysozyme[m]	Asp-119 & Leu-129, coupled to His-methyl ester	large	large	none made because of large conform. change

For the immunochemical results with antisera to lysozyme and antisera to the derivatives, see references cited below.

References: (a) Lee and Atassi, 1973; (b) Atassi and Habeeb, 1969; (c) Atassi *et al.*, 1971; (d) Habeeb and Atassi, 1969; (e) Atassi and Zablocki, 1976; (f) Johnson *et al.*, 1978; (g) Atassi *et al.*, 1976b; (h) Atassi *et al.*, 1972; (i) Habeeb and Atassi, 1971b; (j) Habeeb and Atassi, 1971b; (k) Lee *et al.*, 1975; (l) Atassi *et al.*, 1975a; (m) Atassi *et al.*, 1974; Atassi and Rosemblatt, 1974.

Table from Atassi (1977c).

investigated (Habeeb and Atassi, 1970). The results have been reviewed elsewhere (Atassi and Habeeb, 1972) and will be mentioned here only briefly. Studies on unmasking of the amino groups showed that only citraconyl derivatives gave homogeneous preparations with full (100%) recovery of amino groups, enzymatic activity, immunochemical properties and native conformation. Citraconylated lysozyme exhibited conformational changes (Habeeb and Atassi, 1970) which formed the basis for a novel approach (Atassi _et al._, 1973) to obtain all the tryptic peptides from lysozyme with intact disulfide bonds (see Section IV-B).

Lysozyme derivatives in which 10 arginine residues were modified (by 1,2-cyclohexanedione) showed large conformational changes, no enzymatic activity and very little immunochemical resemblance to lysozyme (Atassi _et al._, 1972). The extensive nature of the modifications and the accompanying large conformational changes precluded a definite assignment of residues to antigenic (and enzymatic) sites (Atassi _et al._, 1972). A homogeneous lysozyme derivative, that was modified at one arginine (residue 61) (Atassi _et al._, 1972), was prepared from reaction with phenylglyoxal. The derivative showed no conformational changes and had equal antigenic reactivity to that of lysozyme, both with antisera to lysozyme or to the derivative. It was concluded that arginine 61 is not located in an antigenic site of lysozyme (Atassi _et al._, 1972). Also, the findings demonstrated that not all conformational changes will influence antigenic reactivity. This phenomenon was subsequently observed with other derivatives of lysozyme.

Carboxyl groups were modified (Atassi _et al._, 1974) by activation with carbodiimide and coupling with glycine methyl ester (GME) or with histidine methyl ester (HME) followed by column chromatography. The two homogeneous derivatives were modified at the carboxyl groups of Asp-119 and the _C_-terminal leucine. Little or no conformational differences were observed between lysozyme and GME_2-lysozyme while HME_2-lysozyme suffered large conformational changes (Atassi and Rosemblatt, 1974). The enzymatic activities of both derivatives were drastically decreased. Lysozyme and GME_2-lysozyme had equal antigenic reactivities, both with antisera to the native protein or with antisera to the derivative, while HME_2-lysozyme reacted much lower with these antisera. It was concluded that the carboxyl groups of Asp-119 and leucine 129 are not essential parts of an antigenic site in lysozyme (Atassi _et al._, 1974). This conclusion was confirmed by reduction of the same two carboxyl groups.

Diborane reduction followed by reoxidation of the reduced disulfides and chromatography on CM-cellulose yielded a homogeneous lysozyme derivative in which the carboxyl groups of Asp-119 and the end-chain leucine residue were reduced to their corresponding alcohols (Atassi *et al.*, 1975a). Conformational differences between the derivative and lysozyme were almost undetectable by ORD and CD measurements, but were readily detected by chemical monitoring of the conformation and appeared to be small. The lytic activity of the derivative decreased (to 52%) but retained the same pH optimum. Lysozyme and the derivative possessed identical antigenic reactivities, with antisera to either protein. These findings further confirmed that Asp-119 and the *C*-terminal leucine are not part of an antigenic site in lysozyme (Atassi *et al.*, 1975a). Again it may be noted here that the slight conformational change had no effect on the immunochemical properties.

The two methionine residues in lysozyme were specifically carboxyethylated by reaction with β-propiolactone (Atassi *et al.*, 1976b), a reagent of high specificity for methionine (Taubman and Atassi, 1968; Atassi, 1969). The electrophoretically homogeneous derivative showed no conformational changes by ORD and CD measurements, but exhibited a slight increase in disulfide reducibility relative to native lysozyme. Its lytic activity was about half that of native lysozyme, probably as a result of the slight conformational change. The derivative and native lysozyme had identical antigenic reactivities with eight different rabbit and goat (both early-course and late-course) lysozyme antisera and unequivocally demonstrated that methionines 12 and 105 are not involved in interaction of lysozyme with its antibodies (Atassi *et al.*, 1976b). Our conclusion derived from the carboxyethyl lysozyme derivative was further confirmed by evidence obtained from immunochemical study of synthetic peptides (see Section IX-A).

Lysozyme was modified at the six tryptophan residues by reaction with 2-nitrophenylsulfenyl chloride in 98% formic acid (Habeeb and Atassi, 1969). This solvent effected the esterification of 12 (out of 17) hydroxy amino acids. The derivative suffered large conformational changes (Atassi *et al.*, 1971) and its reactivity with lysozyme antisera was minor (9-12%). The presence of large conformational changes precluded an unequivocal conclusion regarding the role of the tryptophans in antigenic sites.

Lysozyme was reacted (Atassi and Zablocki, 1976) with 2,3-dioxo-5-indolinesulfonic acid, a reagent highly specific for tryptophan (Atassi and Zablocki, 1975). The homogeneous derivative which was modified at Trp-123 showed no conformational changes by ORD and CD measurements, and some slight changes by increases in accessibility to tryptic hydrolysis and in disulfide reducibility. Its lytic activity was greatly decreased (50%), probably as a result of the conformational change. However, with several antisera to lysozyme the derivative and the native protein possessed equal reactivities, indicating that the small conformational change had no detrimental effect on the antigenic reactivity. From this derivative it was concluded that Trp-123 is not part of an antigenic site in native lysozyme (Atassi and Zablocki, 1976).

Two derivatives of lysozyme modified at tyrosines 20 and 23 in more than one way were prepared (Atassi and Habeeb, 1969). In one derivative, tyrosines 20 and 23 were nitrated (NT_2-lysozyme) and in the other the nitrotyrosine residues were reduced to aminotyrosine (AT_2-lysozyme). Conformational changes were revealed by ORD and CD measurements in the pH range 7 to 3, by increase in disulfide reducibility and in accessibility to tryptic attack, and by the effect of sodium dodecyl sulfate on the availability of the disulfide bonds to reduction (Atassi _et al._, 1971). The results indicated that the tyrosyl derivatives had closely similar, if not identical, conformations which differed from that of lysozyme (Atassi _et al._, 1971). Comparable enzymic activities were observed in NT_2-lysozyme (50%) and AT_2-lysozyme (56%), which may be explained by the similar conformational changes. The antigenic reactivity decreased slightly in nitrated lysozyme (77-90% relative to homologous reaction) but was entirely recovered upon reduction of the nitrotyrosine residues to aminotyrosine despite the fact that conformational changes still existed (Atassi and Habeeb, 1969; Atassi _et al._, 1971). Conversely, lysozyme and AT_2-lysozyme reacted equally but less efficiently with antisera to NT_2-lysozyme than the homologous antigen (Atassi and Habeeb, 1969). From the foregoing results it was concluded (Atassi and Habeeb, 1969) that one or both of tyrosines 20 and 23 is located in or very close to an antigenic site.

IV. IMMUNOCHEMISTRY OF PEPTIDE FRAGMENTS

The immunochemistry of a large number of peptide fragments with a variety of overlaps and representing various parts of the protein molecule affords a very effective approach for narrowing down of the antigenic reactive sites of the protein (Atassi, 1972, 1975). The shortcomings of this approach and precautions to be observed in its application have been discussed in detail, together with a review and critical analysis of chemical cleavage reactions for proteins at given amino acid locations (Atassi, 1977a).

A. Peptides Obtained by Peptic and Other Cleavage Procedures

Lysozyme can be digested by pepsin (Canfield and Liu, 1965) and many investigators have exploited this susceptibility to isolate fragments from peptic digests and study their immunochemistry (Shinka _et al._, 1967; Fujio _et al._, 1968a,b; Komatsu _et al._, 1975; Ha _et al._, 1975; Arnon and Sela, 1969; Maron _et al._, 1971). Some synthetic parts of such peptides have been studied (Arnon *et al.*, 1971; Geiger and Arnon, 1974). Also, peptides prepared from digestion of lysozyme with thermolysin have been studied (Sakato *et al.*, 1972). The results of these investigations (reviewed in detail by Atassi and Habeeb, 1977), show that they have been troubled by work with impure peptides, often yielding confusing and contradictory results. Also, the broad selectivity of the peptic digestion produced many intermediates which varied considerably with the conditions and made reproducibility difficult. Furthermore, these peptides accounted additively for only a small part (38%) of the lysozyme immune reaction (Fujio *et al.*, 1968b). This situation has been frustrating in the search for immunochemically-reactive peptides from lysozyme.

B. A Novel Cleavage Approach that Yielded Fragments Accounting for the Full Antigenic Reactivity

To break the aforementioned deadlock, a reproducible cleavage procedure of high specificity was needed that can yield a variety of peptides directly from the native protein without rupturing the disulfide bonds. Based on the observation (Habeeb and Atassi, 1970) that reversible masking of the amino groups by citraconylation induced in the protein conformational changes which rendered it accessible to tryptic attack at the arginyl peptide bonds we introduced a novel cleavage approach for obtaining fragments with intact disulfide bonds from "tight" (i.e. disulfide-containing, proteolytically inaccessible) proteins (Atassi *et al.*, 1973). The tryptic cleavage may be terminated, after scission of the arginyl bonds, by adding trypsin inhibitor before removal of the citraconyl masking groups at pH 4. If no trypsin inhibitor is added then, following the removal of the protecting groups, cleavage of the lysyl bonds may be continued, if desired. By this approach, it was possible to effect the complete tryptic hydrolysis of lysozyme without rupturing the disulfide bonds (Atassi *et al.*, 1973). The total tryptic hydrolysate showed substantial inhibitory activity (85-89%) of the reaction of lysozyme with its antibodies. The fragments responsible for this inhibition were identified mainly as the three disulfide-containing tryptic peptides: 22-23-(Cys 30-Cys 115)-115-116; 62-68-(Cys 64-Cys 80)-74-97-(Cys 76-Cys 94); and 6-13-(Cys 6-Cys 127)-126-128 (see Fig. 1). This remarkably high inhibitory activity of the three peptides enabled us to account for the first time for almost all the immune reaction of native lysozyme.

The approach is not limited to lysozyme and has proved to be of general applicability. We have employed it to obtain disulfide-containing fragments from bovine serum albumin (Habeeb *et al.*, 1974; Atassi *et al.*, 1976a) and bovine ribonuclease A (Habeeb and Atassi, unpublished results). Also, the cleavage reaction can be

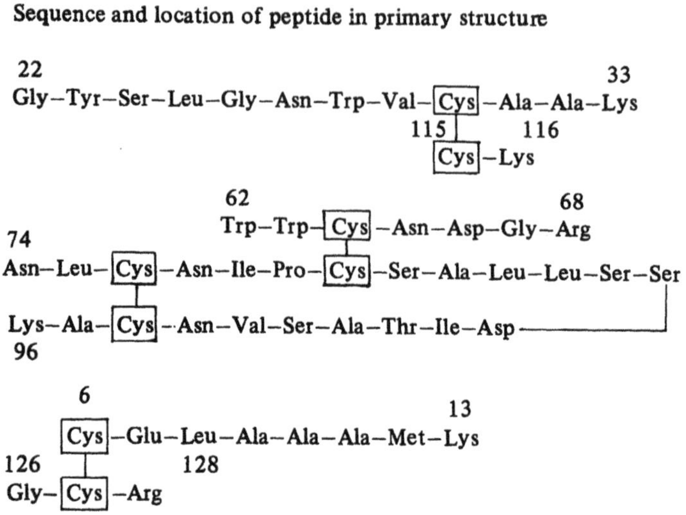

Sequence and location of peptide in primary structure

```
22                                              33
Gly–Tyr–Ser–Leu–Gly–Asn–Trp–Val–[Cys]–Ala–Ala–Lys
                                 115|       116
                                  [Cys]–Lys

                 62                          68
74               Trp–Trp–[Cys]–Asn–Asp–Gly–Arg
Asn–Leu–[Cys]–Asn–Ile–Pro–[Cys]–Ser–Ala–Leu–Leu–Ser–Ser
          |                                          |
Lys–Ala–[Cys]–Asn–Val–Ser–Ala–Thr–Ile–Asp ------------
96

      6                               13
    [Cys]–Glu–Leu–Ala–Ala–Ala–Met–Lys
126   |         128
Gly–[Cys]–Arg
```

Fig. 1. Covalent structure of the three peptides that are responsible for inhibition (85-89%) of the reaction of native lysozyme with its antisera. (From Atassi et al., 1973).

used to determine the correct disulfide pairing in proteins (Atassi et al., 1973, 1975a).

V. SPECIFIC CHEMICAL DERIVATIVES OF IMMUNOCHEMICALLY-REACTIVE PEPTIDES

Identification of the residues involved in binding with antibody and further narrowing down of antigenic reactive sites in an immunochemically-reactive peptide is best achieved (Atassi, 1968) by immunochemical studies of chemical derivatives of the peptide modified at specific amino acid locations. The advantages and shortcomings of the approach have previously been outlined (Atassi, 1972, 1975). The chemistry of chemical modification reactions for proteins has recently been reviewed in detail (Atassi, 1977a).

A. Derivatives of the Two-Disulfide Peptide

The peptide corresponding to sequence 62-68-(Cys 64-Cys 80)-74-96-(Cys 76-Cys 94), isolated by the approach described in Section IV-B, had a strong immunochemical reactivity which accounted for about one-third (see Table 2) of the total reactivity of native lysozyme with its early-course antisera (Atassi et al., 1973, 1975a). The peptide was also isolated with lysine 97 attached to it (Lee and Atassi, 1975) and ORD measurements showed that it was greatly unfolded in solution relative to its expected mode of

TABLE 2: Inhibitory Activitives of the Two Disulfide Peptide and Its Derivatives

Results are expressed in maximum percent inhibition of the precipitin reaction of native lysozyme with its antisera. Each value represents the average of six or more replicate determinations which varied ± 0.8% or less. Antisera G9 and G10 are goat antisera against native lysozyme.

Peptide or derivative*	Antiserum G9		Antiserum G10	
	Max. inhibitory activity	Molar ratio at ½ max. inhibn**	Max. inhibitory activity	Molar ratio at ½ max. inhibn**
$(SS)_2$-peptide[a,b]	26.4	14.2	32.7	4.5
DISA-peptide[a]	12.0	14.5	14.5	7.0
Succinyl-peptide[a]	12.2	14.3	14.7	4.5
Succinyl-DISA-peptide[a]	2	52	2.5	40
HME_4-peptide[b]	11.6	13.7	16.1	6.5
CHD-peptide[b]	3.2	43	4.6	40
PG-peptide[b]	13.2	19	15.2	4.8
Pre-protected PG-peptide[b]	26.5	14.2	32.6	4.5
Chymotryp.-cleaved peptide[a+]	3	40	3.5	35
S-Carboxymethyl-peptide[a]	0	310‡	0	300‡

*Abbreviations: $(SS)_2$-peptide, the two-disulfide peptide corresponding to the sequence 62-68-(Cys 64-Cys 80)-74-97-(Cys 76-Cys 94); DISA-peptide, derivative of the $(SS)_2$-peptide modified at tryptophans 62 and 63 by reaction with 2,3-dioxo-5-indolinesulfonic acid; Succinyl-peptide, derivatives succinylated at the amino groups and succinyl-DISA-peptide, a succinylated DISA-peptide; HME_4-peptide, derivative coupled to histidine methyl ester at the four carboxyl groups; CHD-peptide, derivative modified with cyclohexanedione at arginine 68, the two tryptophans, the two lysine and the N-terminal asparagine 74; PG-lysozyme, derivative modified by phenylglyoxal at Arg-68, Trp-62, Asn-74 and one ε-amino group; Pre-protected PG-peptide, derivative in which the NH_2-groups were first protected by citraconylation and after reaction with phenylglyoxal the protecting groups were removed giving a derivative modified only at Arg-68.

**These values represent peptide/antigen molar ratio at 50% of the maximum inhibition.

+Similar results were obtained either with the total chymotryptic hydrolysate or with peptide 64-68-(Cys 64-Cys 80)-76-83-(Cys 76-Cys 94)-94-97.

‡These values represent the maximum molar excess of peptide relative to lysozyme in the inhibition reaction.

References: (a) Lee and Atassi, 1975; (b) Atassi et al., 1976c.

Table is from Atassi (1977c).

folding within the intact lysozyme molecule. Despite its unfolding the peptide exhibited a surprising binding efficiency which can be seen from the relatively low molar excess required to achieve half the maximum inhibition (Table 2). This was attributed to the covalent linkage of the relevant parts of the antigenic site by the two disulfide bonds (Atassi et al., 1973; Lee and Atassi, 1975).

For identification of the residues involved in binding with antibody, several chemical derivatives of the peptide were prepared, purified, and characterized and their conformations studied. The antigenic reactivities of the derivatives are shown in Table 2. The derivatives suffered no conformational change relative to the unmodified peptide. However, modification of the two tryptophans by reaction with 2,3-dioxo-5-indolinesulfonic acid resulted in the loss of about half the immune reaction of the peptide (Lee and Atassi, 1975). Also succinylation of the amino groups caused the loss of about half of immunochemical reactivity (Lee and Atassi, 1975). Modification of the two tryptophans followed by succinylation of the amino groups abolished the antigenic reactivity almost completely (Lee and Atassi, 1975). From these results it was concluded that the antigenic site in this part of lysozyme incorporates one or both of tryptophans 62 and 63 as well as one or both of lysines 96 and 97. This agreed with previous results (Lee et al., 1975) derived from modification of these lysines in intact lysozyme (see Section III). Since reduction and carboxymethylation of the disulfides abolished the antigenic reactivity of the peptide (Atassi et al., 1973; Lee and Atassi, 1975), it was concluded that the two disulfides 64-80 and 76-94 bring these two parts of the lysozyme molecule into a single antigenic site. The intactness of the disulfides is essential for maintenance and reactivity of the site. On modification of all the carboxyl groups in the peptide by activation with carbodiimide followed by coupling with histidine methyl ester the homogeneous derivative retained only less than half of the immunochemical reactivity of the peptide (Table 2) (Atassi et al., 1976c). Reaction of the peptide with phenylglyoxal after protection of the free amino groups by citraconylation followed by removal of the protecting groups resulted in the modification of arginine 68 only. The derivative retained the full immunochemical reactivity of the unmodified peptide (Atassi et al., 1976c). From these studies it was concluded that one (or both) of aspartic acids 66 and 87 is part of the antigenic site, whereas arginine 68 is not located in this site on the peptide (Atassi et al., 1976c).

Studies on the chemical derivatives of the peptide, which are summarized diagramatically in Fig. 2, enabled us in fact to define the complex boundaries of the antigenic site in this part of the molecule with considerable accuracy (Atassi et al., 1976c). This definition directed us to the formulation of a novel synthetic

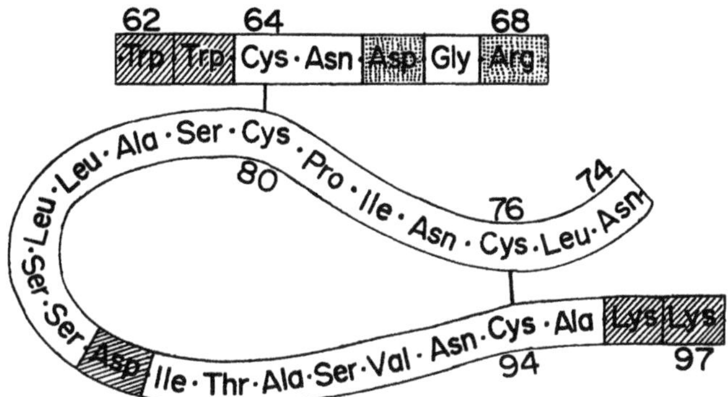

Fig. 2. Schematic diagram showing the primary structure of the $(SS)_2$-peptide. The marked residues are those whose involvement or otherwise in antigenic reactivity has been derived from their chemical modification. Striped residues (Asp 87; one or both of Trp 62 and Trp 63; Lys 96 and Lys 97) are part of the antigenic site while the dotted residues (Arg 68 and Asp 66) are outside the antigenic site. (From Atassi et al., 1976c).

strategy for the final delineation of the site. These results are described and coordinated in Section VIII.

VI. PEPTIDE SYNTHESIS FOR FINAL DELINEATION OF ANTIGENIC SITES

Following the accurate narrowing down of antigenic sites in our laboratories by the foregoing chemical approaches, the final delineation of the sites was accomplished by the organic synthesis and immunochemistry of peptides representing different parts of each site. The precautionary measures that must be employed in the application of this approach to problems of protein antigenic structures have been outlined elsewhere (Atassi, 1977b).

The foregoing chemical approaches demonstrated that the antigenic sites were located around disulfide bonds. The strategy, therefore, required the synthesis of disulfide-containing peptides. Such a synthetic scheme was employed in the delineation of the reactive site around the disulfide 6-127 (i.e. site 1) and for which nine disulfide peptides (Fig. 7) were synthesized by Atassi et al. (1976b). This approach proved to be extremely time-consuming and laborious and was not subsequently employed in the delineation of the other two antigenic sites of lysozyme. For these, and subsequently for antigenic site 1, an entirely novel and unorthodox concept was introduced (Atassi *et al.*, 1976d) and an extremely powerful and unique synthetic approach was devised. The various peptides synthesized in our laboratory for the delineation of the three antigenic sites are shown in Figs. 3, 5, 6, 7 and 9. The rationale behind the choice of these peptides is best handled in the following section which deals with the accurate assignment of the antigenic sites.

VII. ACCURATE DELINEATION OF THE ANTIGENIC SITE AROUND THE DISULFIDES 64-80 AND 76-94 (SITE 2)

In this and Sections VIII and IX, the information obtained from our chemical and synthetic approaches will be coordinated to derive the accurate location of the antigenic sites of native lysozyme. It has recently been shown (Atassi *et al.*, 1976c) that lysozyme has only three antigenic sites.

The delineation of antigenic site 2 will be described first because it was the first such site that we defined precisely. Also, historically, it was in the process of the delineation of this site that we introduced major novel and basic concepts into protein chemistry, most profound of which has been the ability to study protein interactions by "surface-simulation" synthesis.

A. Assignment of the Antigenic Site

Of our immunochemical studies on specific chemical derivatives of native lysozyme that are of direct relevance here are the findings that arginine 61 is not part of an antigenic site (Atassi *et al.*, 1972), whereas lysine 96 is located within an antigenic site in native lysozyme (Lee *et al.*, 1975). Subsequently, we showed that the two-disulfide peptide 62-68-(Cys 64-Cys 80)-74-97-(Cys 76-Cys 94)[i.e. $(SS)_2$-peptide] accounted for about a third of the total antigenic reactivity of native lysozyme (Atassi *et al.*, 1973, 1975a). Immunochemical studies of derivatives of the $(SS)_2$-peptide (see Section V-A) showed that Arg-68 and Asp-66 are not part of the antigenic site (Atassi *et al.*, 1976c) but that either one (or both) of tryptophans 62 and 63 and one (or both) of lysines 96 and 97 are located in the antigenic site (Lee and Atassi, 1975), in agreement with the results we obtained (Section III) from derivatives of the intact protein (Lee *et al.*, 1975). It was demonstrated that the tryptophan(s) and the lysine(s) are parts of the same antigenic site (Lee and Atassi, 1975), which requires intactness of the disulfide bonds to effect its three-dimensional construction (Lee and Atassi, 1975). Furthermore, it was shown that the region around Asp-87 was essential for the full reactivity of the site (Atassi *et al.*, 1976c). After modification of Asp-87, the antigenic site, however retained about half of its reactivity (Atassi *et al.*,

1976c). It became clear, therefore that this site begins (or ends) at tryptophan 62 or 63, requires lysine 96 or 97 (or both) and some or all of the region 84-93 (Lee and Atassi, 1975; Atassi *et al.*, 1976c). Since the $(SS)_2$-peptide carries a single antigenic site and the total of its reactivity together with the two smaller single-disulfide peptides (Atassi *et al.*, 1973) accounts for 90% of the entire antigenic reaction of native lysozyme, it became clear at this stage that lysozyme has only three major antigenic sites (Atassi *et al.*, 1976c).

B. Novel Synthetic Peptides with Diglycyl Bridges Instead of Disulfides

Chemical modification and cleavage studies will not yield any further delineation of this antigenic site. Accordingly, we then focused our effort on the organic synthesis and immunochemical studies of peptides related to the $(SS)_2$-peptide. From studies of novel synthetic peptides designed to simulate the sequences 62-64, 76-80 and 94-97, which were linked in that order by diglycyl bridges instead of disulfides (Fig. 3) we were able to differentiate the individual roles of Trp-62, Trp-63, Lys-96 and Lys-97 (Lee *et al.*, 1976). The peptides in Fig. 3 showed differences in their immunochemical activities which were not due to effects of peptide size. Peptide III exhibited the highest inhibitory activity which approximated the expected value (Lee *et al.*, 1976). From comparison of the inhibitory activities of the peptides, we succeeded in demonstrating unambiguously that both Lys-96 and Lys-97, but only Trp-62 (and not Trp-63) were essential parts of the antigenic site (Lee *et al.*, 1976). Furthermore, phenylalanine substituted for tryptophan with equal immunochemical efficiency. Therefore, the residues Asp-87, Lys-96, Lys-97 and Trp-62 are essential parts of the antigenic site in this part of the molecule (Atassi *et al.*, 1976c).

The remarkable effectiveness of the substitution by diglycyl segments for the disulfide bonds may be applicable to the solution of other similar problems in proteins and should merits consideration in certain studies.

C. "Surface-Simulation" Synthesis: A Novel Concept Directly Linking the Conformationally Adjacent Residues Forming the Site

Examination of the three-dimensional structure of lysozyme enabled us to explain the manner in which the aforementioned four residues construct the antigenic site, and we proposed (Atassi *et al.*, 1976c) that it comprised the residues: Asp-87, Thr-89, Asn-93, Lys-96, Lys-97 and Trp-62 (Fig. 4). From the foregoing description it can be seen that residues 87, 96, 97 and 62 were

A

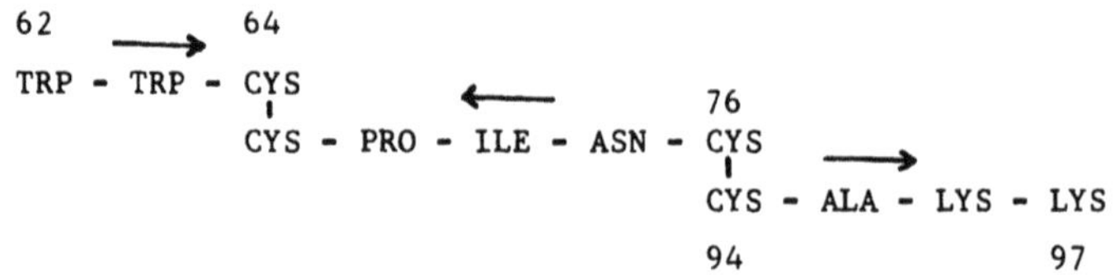

```
            62          64
            TRP - TRP - CYS
                         |       <---       76
                        CYS - PRO - ILE - ASN - CYS
                                                 |       --->
                                                CYS - ALA - LYS - LYS
                                                94               97
```

B

I	TRP - TRP -	GLY - GLY	- PRO - ILE - ASN -	GLY - GLY	- ALA - LYS - LYS
II	TRP -	GLY - GLY	- PRO - ILE - ASN -	GLY - GLY	- ALA - LYS - LYS
III	PHE - PHE -	GLY - GLY	- PRO - ILE - ASN -	GLY - GLY	- ALA - LYS - LYS
IV	PHE -	GLY - GLY	- PRO - ILE - ASN -	GLY - GLY	- ALA - LYS - LYS
V		GLY - GLY	- PRO - ILE - ASN -	GLY - GLY	- ALA - LYS - LYS
VI	PHE - PHE -	GLY - GLY	- PRO - ILE - ASN -	GLY - ALY	- ALA - LYS
VII	PHE - PHE -	GLY - GLY	- PRO - ILE - ASN -	GLY - GLY	- ALA

Fig. 3. Amino acid sequence of: (A) The disulfide-linked sequences (62-64) (76-80) (94-97) of native lysozyme. (B) The peptides synthesized in our laboratory. The arrows indicate the direction (N to C) of the peptide chains. The vertical dashed lines used to outline the diglycyl segments which were used to substitute for the disulfides in peptide A. (From Lee et al., 1976).

directly implicated in the active interaction with the antibody. The possible involvement of the residues Thr-89 and Asn-93 in the site was only concluded from examination of the three-dimensional structure. In the three-dimensional structure of lysozyme, Thr-89 and Asn-93 lie reasonably well in an imaginary plane (or line) bearing the other residues. However, since the two end and two middle residues were unambiguously assigned, the boundaries of the site were therefore clearly defined.

Although we had anticipated the existence of protein antigenic sites (i.e. spanning residues that are close in three-dimensional structure but distant in sequence) relatively early (Atassi and Saplin, 1968), this was in fact the first such site ever to be described (Atassi et al., 1976c) at the time these studies were completed. The antigenic structure of only one protein (i.e. sperm-whale myoglobin) had been precisely elucidated (for review, see Atassi, 1975; a more extensive review is in Atassi, 1977b) and did not reveal the existence of such sites. The structural features conferring immunogenicity on certain parts of a protein molecule were (and continue to be) unclear (Atassi, 1975). Accordingly, a very conclusive proof for the structure of the site was needed which had to be independent of the above findings. For this, we

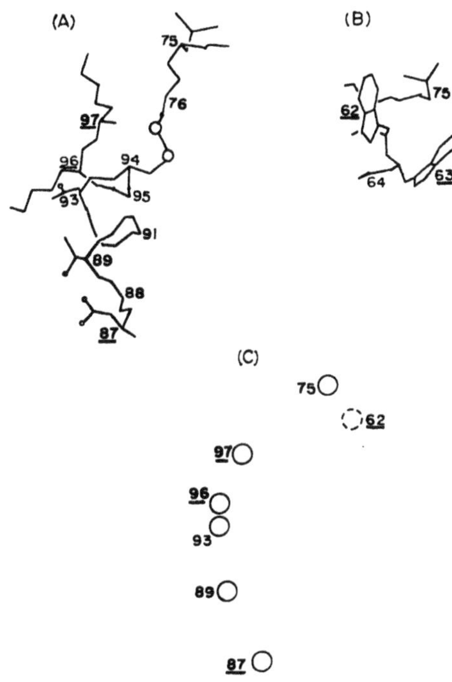

Fig. 4. A schematic diagram showing the relative conformational arrangement of the residues in antigenic site 2. Residues that we have shown by chemical modification to be part of the antigenic site are underlined. (A) shows the mode of folding and the relative arrangement of the residues in the antigenic site. To avoid overcrowding the diagram, only the side chains of the residues that are part of the antigenic site are shown. Aspartic 87 is closest to the observer and the residues 89, 93, 96, 97 and 75 steadily recede away from the observer so much that Trp-62 is well behind the plane of the paper and is not shown in (A) and is continued in (B). The view in (A) is from the opposite face to that in which the enzyme's cleft is located. In going from 87 to 62, the antigenic reactive site moves from one side of the cleft (from behind it though) to the other. (B) shows only the relative positions and proximity of Leu-75, Trp-62 and Trp-63 and is obtained by looking at the molecule from the surface of the enzyme's cleft (i.e. the opposite surface to that in (A). Residues 62, 63 and 75, in that order, gradually recede away from the observer. (C) is a simplified diagram showing the relative positions of the α-carbons, only of the residues constituting the antigenic reactive site. This is quite useful since the positions of the side-chains can fluctuate to adjust themselves to the antibody combining site. From 87 to 62, the residues are receding steadily from the observer so that in fact Trp-62 is behind the plane of the paper and is therefore shown as a broken circle. Residues 87, 96, 97 and 62 have been shown by specific chemical derivatives of the $(SS)_2$-peptide (see text) to be part of the antigenic site. Residues 89 and 93 are intervening residues that must, because of their three-dimensional location, constitute part of the site. However, the boundaries of the site are well defined since the residues at the two ends of the site have been well characterized The dimensions of the antigenic site are given in Figures 5 and 10. (From Atassi et al., 1976c).

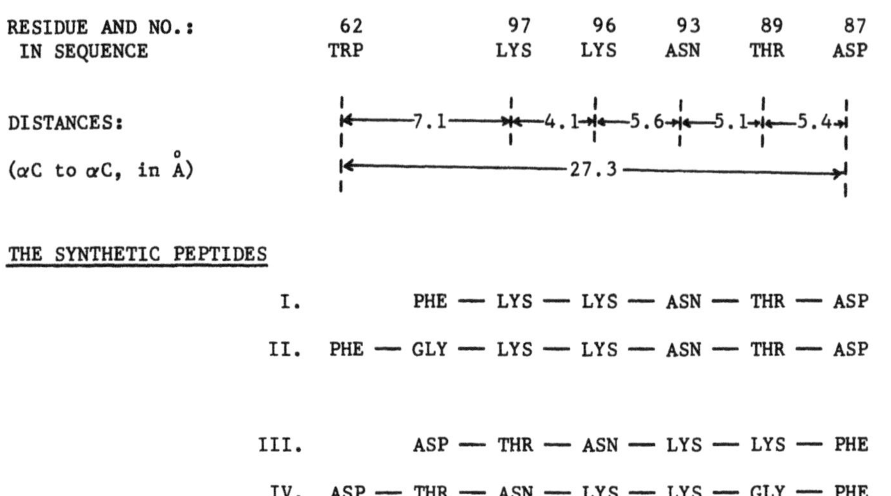

Fig. 5. A diagram showing the spatially contiguous surface residues constituting antigenic site 2 and their numerical position in the primary structure of lysozyme. The distances (in Å) separating the consecutive residues of the site are given as C^{α}-to-C^{α} distances together with the overall extended dimension of the site. Below, the primary structures of the synthetic peptides studied here are given. Previously we had shown (Lee *et al.*, 1975) that tryptophan can be replaced by phenylalanine with equal efficiency. (From Lee and Atassi, 1977b).

devised (Atassi *et al.*, 1976d) a novel and entirely unorthodox approach which linked the relevant conformationally-adjacent residues constructing the site into a single peptide. From examination of the three-dimensional structure of lysozyme, the distances between the contiguous residues of the site were measured (see Fig. 5). The residues Trp-62, Lys-97, Lys-96, Asn-93, Thr-89 and Asp-87 described an imaginary line circumscribing part of the surface topography of the native protein molecule. Accordingly, a peptide was initially synthesized (Atassi *et al.*, 1976d), carrying phenylalanine instead of tryptophan and having a glycine spacer between phenylalanine and lysine (peptide II in Fig. 5) in order to obtain the correct separation between their side chains. These studies established (Atassi *et al.*, 1976d) for the first time and most conclusively and accurately an antigenic site which clearly comprised spatially adjacent residues that are distant in the sequence reacting as if in direct peptide linkage. Since this approach attempts to mimic part of the surface of a protein molecule, we subsequently defined it (Lee and Atassi, 1976) by the appropriately-descriptive term, "surface-simulation" synthesis.

Very recently, in our precise delineation of another antigenic site in native lysozyme around the disulfide bonds 30-115 (site 3), also by "surface-simulation" synthetic peptides, we have found (Lee and Atassi, 1977a) that antigenic site 3 was subject to conformational constraints. Also, it exhibited a preferred 'direction' by surface-simulation synthesis. The surface-simulation synthetic peptides in Fig. 5 were therefore designed (Lee and Atassi, 1977b) to study the conformational restrictions of site 2 and to investigate if the site has a preferred 'direction' in order to achieve a more precise description of this site and consequently of the antigenic structure of lysozyme.

Accurate definition and conformational restrictions of the site

The results of immunochemical studies (Lee and Atassi, 1977b) with the surface-simulation synthetic peptides are summarized in Table 3. Peptide II showed the highest immunochemical reactivity with each of the antisera studied. The immunochemical reactivity of the peptides improved both in terms of maximum inhibitory activity and of the peptide excess required to achieve that maximum (Table 4). The higher immunochemical efficiency of the peptides obtained with the IgG fractions was attributed to avoiding any proteolytic and/or binding effect excerted by serum proteins when the whole antisera were employed. Omission of the glycine spacer between phenylalanine and lysine (peptide I) resulted in a large detrimental effect on the immunochemical reactivity. This demonstrates the limitations on the conformational alterations that can be tolerated by such antigenic sites composed of conformationally adjacent residues that are distant in sequence (Lee and Atassi, 1977b). These restrictions on the conformational degrees of freedom are more stringent than we had expected. The results explain the sensitivity of the antigenic structure of lysozyme to conformational changes in several chemically-modified analogues that we have previously reported and in evolutionarily-substituted homologous proteins (for review, see Atassi and Habeeb, 1977). The electrostatic inductive effect that we recently observed (Lee and Atassi, 1977a) exerted by modifications or substitutions on a neighboring antigenic site (see Section VIII-B) is also further rationalized.

When the sequence of the surface-simulation synthetic site was reversed (i.e. peptide IV), the immunochemical reactivity decreased drastically with goat antisera to native lysozyme but was unaltered with rabbit antisera (Lee and Atassi, 1977b). This indicated that the antigenic site has a preferred direction towards goat antisera, at least by surface-simulation synthesis.

Table 3: Inhibitory Activity of the Pure Surface-Simulation Peptides

Results are expressed in maximum per cent inhibition by the peptide of the precipitin reaction of native lysozyme with various antisera. Each value is the average of at least three determinations which varied ± 0.7% or less. Values in parentheses represent peptide/lysozyme molar ratio at 50% of the maximum inhibition. G9 and G10 are goat antisera, L7 and L21 are rabbit antisera against native lysozyme.

Surface-Simulation Peptides	Percent inhibitory activity with whole antisera			
	G9	G10	L7	L21
A. Peptides of Site 1[a] (Fig. 9)				
I	25.1 (160)	12.8 (300)	6.67 (400)	8.50 (380)
II	30.0 (100)	23.3 (260)	9.00 (320)	10.7 (310)
III	26.8 (100)	18.6 (270)	7.7 (320)	9.12 (800)
IV	32.5 (90)	33.3 (150)	22.2 (260)	21.3 (280)
B. Peptides of Site 2[b] (Fig. 5)				
I	15.4 (330)	6.5 (360)	n.d.*	5.0 (660)
II	35.7 (170)	32.3 (1290)	12.7 (460)	18.2 (1538)
III	25.0 (200)	11.1 (450)	n.d.*	13.3 (360)
IV	14.3 (310)	7.7 (900)	12.8 (540)	17.9 (1700)
C. Peptides of Site 3[c] (Fig. 6)				
I	14.5 (240)	16.7 (1360)	8.3 (210)	4.2 (380)
II	20.8 (160)	23.3 (640)	n.d.*	13.7 (380)
III	27.8 (90)	26.3 (560)	18.2 (730)	16.7 (360)
IV	25.0 (50)	25.0 (890)	17.2 (180)	15.9 (120)
V	18.9 (150)	14.7 (340)	12.8 (80)	12.5 (100)
VI	33.3 (40)	28.8 (940)	19.2 (260)	22.2 (380)

References: (a) Atassi and Lee, 1978a; (b) Lee and Atassi, 1977b; (c) Lee and Atassi, 1977a.

*n.d. not determined.

TABLE 4: Inhibitory Activities of Peptide II (Fig. 5) with Whole Antisera and with Their IgG Fractions: Comparison with the Expected Reaction of the Site

Results are given in maximum per cent inhibition by the peptide of the precipitin reaction of native lysozyme with the respective antiserum. Each value is the average of six replicate analyses which varied ± 0.8% or less. Values in parentheses represent peptide/lysozyme molar ratio at half the maximum inhibition. G9 and G10 are goat antisera, L7 and L21 are rabbit antisera each against native lysozyme.

Antiserum	Inhibitory activity (%)		Expected reaction of the site
	Whole antiserum	IgG fraction of antiserum	
G9	35.7 (170)	n.d.	26.4
G10	32.3 (1290)	34.5 (170)	32.7
L7	12.7 (460)	28.6 (190)	n.d.
L21	18.2 (1538)	28.9 (210)	n.d.

Table from Lee and Atassi (1977b).

The other two antigenic sites of lysozyme behaved similarly in that they exhibited a preferred directionality (see Sections VIII-B and IX-B). From the findings with antigenic site 3 (Lee and Atassi, 1977a), where longer surface-simulation peptides were synthesized (see Section VIII-B) in the two opposite directions, it was quite evident (Lee and Atassi, 1977b) that the preferred direction of the site was not due to an adverse effect of a free α-NH_2 group or a terminal-COOH group on binding of the first or last amino acid residues. Obviously, antigenic site 2 has a preferred direction on the surface of the globular protein. However, rabbit antisera were indifferent to the inversion of direction of site 2. The existence of a preferred direction even with goat antisera is significant in view of the fact that on the surface of an ideal spherical molecule, all directions are presumably equivalent, and that in solution the protein has an unrestricted rotational freedom. Nevertheless, the antigenic site may be accepted by the antibody combining site, only if it is presented in one way. This is indeed striking in view of the fact that only the side chains should be involved in antigen-antibody interaction (Lee *et al.*, 1976). However, the orientations of the side chains will differ in the two peptides and may alter the free energy of binding. Directionality is therefore a function of side-chain orientations (Lee and Atassi, 1977b). The indifference of rabbit antisera to the change in the direction of this site may reflect a lower conformational specificity by these antisera relative to goat antisera. Since only two rabbits and two goats were studied, we have cautioned (Lee and Atassi, 1977b) against generalizing at the present time about the species dependency of the directionality of this site. It can now be stated, in a more conservative manner, that with the antisera so far studied, the extent of sensitivity to the direction of the surface-simulation synthetic site appears to depend on the antigenic site and for a given site may be dependent on the immunized species. Attention should be paid to this in application of the surface-simulation synthesis of antigenic sites (and perhaps other binding sites) in proteins. The synthetic site made in both directions should be examined (Lee and Atassi, 1977b).

Finally, it is sometimes felt that the inhibitory activity of a peptide may not be a true representative of its immunochemical reactivity. Accordingly, we determined (Lee and Atassi, 1977b) the ability of the synthetic site (peptide II) on an immunoadsorbent to bind with lysozyme antibodies. The amount of antibody from a given antiserum that was directly bound by the peptide affinity column relative to the amount bound by lysozyme was in excellent agreement with the maximum inhibition value exhibited by the free peptide and with the maximum expected reactivity of the site (compare Tables 9 and 10). It is thus obvious that the maximum inhibition value affords a faithful measure of the immunochemical reactivity of the peptide. This agreement is not an isolated finding and has been observed with the surface-simulation synthetic peptides representing antigenic sites of myoglobin (Atassi and Koketsu, 1975) and for the two large inhibitory fragments of bovine serum albumin (Atassi _et al._, 1976a; Habeeb and Atassi, 1976).

In conclusion, our findings clearly show that antigenic site 2 of lysozyme (Fig. 10) is constructed from the alignment of the six surface residues: Trp-62, Lys-97, Lys-96, Asn-93, Thr-89 and Asp-87. These spatially adjacent surface residues describe an imaginary line which circumscribes part (27.3 Å) of the surface topography of the globular protein (Atassi _et al._, 1976d) (see plate 1). Upon binding with antibody these residues behave functionally as if in direct peptide bond linkage (Atassi _et al._, 1976d). In fact the immunochemical reactivity is fully expressed by a surface-simulation synthetic peptide (Fig. 10) in which these residues are directly linked via peptide bonds. The site exhibits considerable conformational restrictions since the inclusion of a spacer between phenylalanine and lysine is critical for the achievement of full reactivity. The site has a preferred direction with goat antisera but, surprisingly, not with rabbit antisera. Tryptophan 62 is present at the hexasaccharide binding site of the enzyme (Imoto _et al._, 1972) and therefore antigenic site 2 overlaps with the enzymic binding site (Atassi _et al._, 1976c).

VIII. ACCURATE DELINEATION OF THE ANTIGENIC SITE AROUND THE DISULFIDE 30-115 (SITE 3)

A. Assignment of the reactive site

From the immunochemical and conformational studies of specific chemical derivatives of lysozyme (see Section III) it was shown that one or both of tyrosines 20 and 23 is located in, or very close to, an antigenic site in lysozyme (Atassi and Habeeb, 1969; Atassi _et al._, 1971). Also, from the three homogeneous succinylated derivatives of lysozyme which showed no conformational changes but had a decreased antigenic reactivity with antisera to native lysozyme, we concluded (Lee _et al._, 1975) that both lysines 33 and 116 are parts of an antigenic site. The loss in antigenic reactivity that could be attributed to succinylation of Lys-33 alone (19.9 and 10.9% with antisera G9 and G10 respectively) was lower than observed upon modification of both lysines 33 and 116 (33.6 and 31.1% with antisera G9 and G10). This behaviour pointed to Lys-33 being at the 'end' of the antigenic site and is reminiscent of results obtained with some myoglobin derivatives modified at end residues of an antigenic reactive site (Atassi _et al._, 1975b). Finally, a disulfide peptide corresponding to the sequence 22-33-(Cys 30-Cys 115)-115-116 possessed a substantial inhibitory activity toward the immune reaction of lysozyme and was specifically bound by immunoadsorbents carrying lysozyme antibodies (Atassi _et al._, 1973). These findings provided strong evidence that an antigenic site in native lysozyme, incorporating both Lys-33 and Lys-116 and possibly one or both of Tyr-20 and Tyr-23, was situated around the disulfide bond 30-115. It was therefore suggested (Lee and Atassi, 1976) that Lys-33 is at one end and the tyrosine residues are at the other end of the antigenic site.

B. Surface-Simulation Synthesis of the Antigenic Site

The assignment of the site and description of its location were achieved (Lee and Atassi, 1976) by application of the 'surface-simulation' synthetic concept which was first devised in our laboratory for the delineation of antigenic Site 2 in native lysozyme (Atassi _et al._, 1976d). This approach linked the relevant spatially adjacent residues constructing the site into a single peptide. Examination of the three-dimensional structure of lysozyme revealed that the residues Tyr-20, Tyr-23, Lys-116 and Lys-33 can be accommodated, with other intervening residues, in an imaginary line (or plane) circumscribing part of the surface topography of the protein (Lee and Atassi, 1976). The surface-encircling line passes through the following residues: Tyr-20, Arg-21, Tyr-23, Lys-116, Asn-113, Arg-114, Phe-34 and Lys-33. The distances between these contiguous residues are shown in Fig. 6. Two peptides were initially synthesized (Lee and Atassi, 1976) with glycine spacers where necessary

RESIDUES COMPRISING THE ANTIGENIC REACTIVE SITE

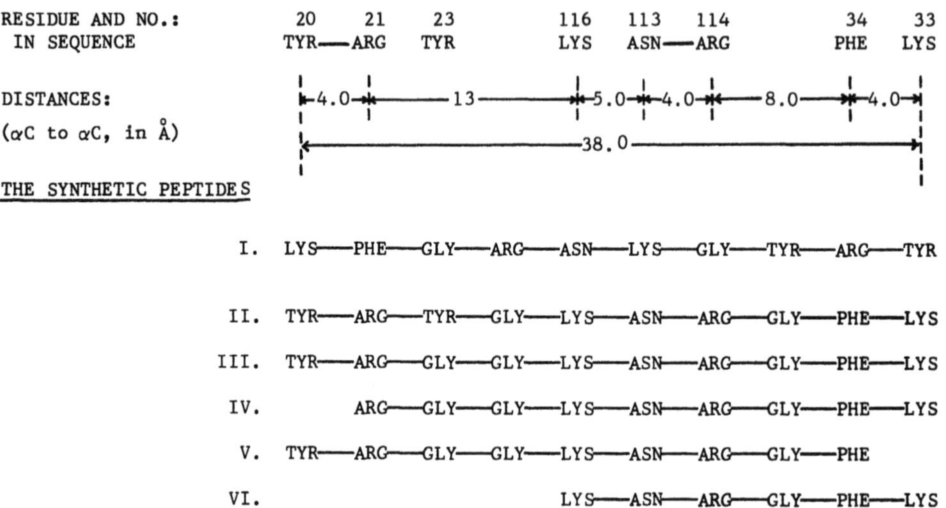

Fig. 6. Diagram showing the spatially adjacent residues within which antigenic site 3 is located and their numerical position in the primary structure of lysozyme. The distances (in Å) separating the consecutive residues of the reactive site are given as C^{α}-to-C^{α} distances, together with the overall extended dimension of the site. Below, the primary structures of the 'surface-simulation' synthetic peptides designed to mimic the antigenic site are given. (From Lee and Atassi, 1977a).

(peptides II and III in Fig. 6) in order to achieve the correct separations between their side chains. These studies established for the first time that the site was indeed formed by conformationally adjacent residues on the surface that are not necessarily in direct peptide linkage with one another (Lee and Atassi, 1976). The studies also showed that the contribution of Tyr-23 can be fully satisfied by a glycine spacer, which is in agreement with the fact that Tyr-23 is much less exposed than Tyr-20.

Subsequent studies were designed (Lee and Atassi, 1977a) to narrow down with accuracy the exact boundaries of the antigenic site and to investigate if this spatially constructed site has a preferred "direction". Several surface-simulation peptides representing various parts of the established surface region were synthesized (Fig. 6) and their immunochemistry studied in detail

(Table 3). With each of the antisera studied, peptide I had a substantially lower inhibitory activity than either of peptides II or III. In fact with some antisera (L21, Table 3), peptide I had only a negligible inhibitory activity. Clearly, therefore, the antigenic site had a preferred direction on the surface of the globular protein molecule. The antigenic site may be accepted by the antibody-combining site, only if it is presented in one way. This is of course not entirely unexpected in specific protein-protein interactions, where certain complementary side chains must attain favourable proximity. Even though only the amino acid side chains should participate in the antigen-antibody binding (Lee et al., 1976), the side chain orientations will be different in the two synthetic directions. Therefore, directionality of site 3 (like that of site 2) is a function of side-chain orientation.

The immunochemical results (Lee and Atassi, 1977a) showed that deletion of the residue equivalent to Tyr-20 (peptide IV) had no adverse effect on the immunochemical reactivity with any of the antisera (Table 3). Deletion of Lys-33 while adding back Tyr-20 (peptide V), so that the sizes of peptides IV and V are equal, caused a substantial loss in immunochemical reactivity of the peptide. Clearly Tyr-20 is not part of the antigenic site, whereas Lys-33 makes an important contribution to the reactivity of the site. With this conclusion, it became questionable whether Arg-21 is in fact part of the site. Arg-21 was implicated because it is an intervening residue in the imaginary line between Lys-116, Tyr-23 and Tyr-20. But since Tyr-23 and Tyr-20 were shown to make no contribution to the reactivity of the site, there remained no reason why Arg-21 should be implicated. Investigation of peptide VI was therefore undertaken and its immunochemical behavior demonstrated unequivocally that Arg-21 is not part of the antigenic site. It is significant that the immunochemical reactivity of peptide VI, which improved greatly with the IgG fraction of the antisera (Table 5), accounted quantitatively for the full contribution of that site (see Table 5), as can be derived from the effect of modifying both Lys-33 and Lys-116 in lysozyme (Lee et al., 1975).

To ascertain that the maximum inhibitory activity of peptide was a true representation of its immunochemical reactivity, its direct binding of anti-lysozyme antibody was examined (Lee and Atassi, 1977a) using an immunoadsorbent of the peptide. The amount of antibody from a given antiserum that was bound by the peptide-Sepharose relative to the amount bound by lysozyme was in excellent agreement with the value of 30.3% found for the inhibitory activity of the peptide (compare Tables 9 and 10). Clearly therefore, the inhibition values (as we have seen with surface-simulation synthetic site 2) provide a faithful measure of the immunochemical reactivity of the peptide.

TABLE 5: Inhibitory Activities of Surface-Simulation Site 3 (Peptide VI, Fig. 6) with Whole Antisera and with IgG Fraction of the Antisera: Comparison with Expected Reaction of the Site

Results are expressed in maximum percentage inhibition by peptide VI of the precipitin reaction of native lysozyme with various antisera or their IgG fractions. Values in parentheses represent peptide/lysozyme molar ratio at 50% of the maximum inhibition. Results are the average of six replicate analyses which varied ± 0.9% or less. G9 and G10 are goat antisera and L7 and L21 are rabbit antisera, each against native lysozyme.

	Maximum inhibitory activity (%)		Expected reaction* of the site
	Whole antiserum	IgG fraction of antiserum	
G9	33.3 (40)[a]	n.d.**	33.6
G10	28.8 (940)[a]	30.3 (200)[a]	31.1
L7	19.2 (260)[a]	33.3 (180)[a]	n.d.
L21	22.2 (380)[a]	35.2 (190)[b]	n.d.

* Calculated from the decrease in antigenic reactivity of lysozyme derivatives that can be attributed to the succinylation of both Lys-33 and Lys-116 (Lee *et al.*, 1975).

** n.d., not determined.

References: (a) Lee and Atassi, 1977a; (b) Atassi and Lee, 1978b .

Comments concerning tyrosine 20

As outlined in the preceding section we had originally concluded (Atassi and Habeeb, 1969; Atassi *et al.*, 1971) that one or both of Tyr-20 and Tyr-23 is located in, or very close to, an antigenic site in lysozyme. In fact in the first 'surface-simulation' synthesis of this site (Lee and Atassi, 1976), they were incorporated into the synthetic scheme. Even then, when Tyr-23 was found to make no contribution to the reaction of the site, Tyr-20 was believed to be at one extreme end of the site. However, since the subsequent findings (Lee and Atassi, 1977a) unequivocally showed that Tyr-20 is not part of the site, it is pertinent to present briefly here the rationalization (Lee and Atassi, 1977a) for the findings.

In the three-dimensional structure of native lysozyme, the phenolic ring of Tyr-20 is extremely close (3-4 Å) to the hydrocarbon chain of Lys-96 which is a critical residue in site 2 (Lee and Atassi, 1975, 1977b; Atassi et al., 1976c, d). The immunochemical effect of nitrating Tyr-20 may, therefore, be due to a secondary effect exerted on the ability of a neighbouring residue (Lys-96), itself in an antigenic site, to participate in binding. On nitration of a tyrosine residue at the ortho position, the inductive effect of the nitro group on the aromatic nucleus will increase the acidity of the phenolic OH, thus promoting its ionization and the resultant anion will be stabilized by the electron-withdrawing mesomeric effect (Atassi, 1968). The increased acidity is shown by a decrease of the pKa value from 10.1 for tyrosine to 7.2 for 3-nitrotyrosine (Sokolovsky et al., 1967). The pKa value for 3-aminotyrosine is 10.0 (Sokolovsky et al., 1967). Obviously the presence of a newly created negatively charged group within interaction distance of Lys-96 should be expected to disturb drastically its ionic environment and consequently its immunochemical interaction properties. This effect is completely removed, as indeed was shown to be the case (Atassi and Habeeb, 1969), when the nitrotyrosine residues are reduced to aminotyrosine.

That Tyr-20 is not part of an antigenic site makes for a more acceptable antigenic structure. If Tyr-20 were indeed part of antigenic site 3, this would mean that sites 2 and 3 will be untenably close. It will then be sterically impossible for two antibody molecules to occupy those two sites simultaneously on a given lysozyme molecule.

It was pointed out (Lee and Atassi, 1977a) that the immunochemical effect of nitrating Tyr-20 brings forth another facet, hitherto unsuspected in protein immunochemistry. Thus immunochemical changes, observed as a result of selective chemical modification of a residue in a derivative that suffers no conformational change do not necessarily imply the participation of the modified residue in an antigenic site. This face-value interpretation is no longer valid unless independent data lend it additional weight. Furthermore, it is not hard to see similar situations being generated by single amino acid evolutionary substitutions outside an antigenic site but sufficiently close to influence its ionic and binding characteristics. The immunochemical relationships of related proteins from various species are not necessarily linearly related to sequence similarities and we had previously consistently attributed this to considerable or even local and subtle conformational differences (Atassi, 1970; Atassi et al., 1970a, 1970b; Habeeb and Atassi, 1971a). Now a new factor, that is the ionic or inductive effect of a substitution on another very close residue which is a critical part of an antigenic site, has to be taken into consideration in the interpretation of the immunochemistry of protein mutants (Lee and Atassi, 1977a).

To sum up, antigenic site 3 is made up (Fig. 10) of the alignment of the side chains of the five residues Lys-116, Asn-113, Arg-

114, Phe-34 and Lys-33. The line described by these residues, which encircles part of the surface of the native protein (plate 2) has an overall extended dimension of 21 Å [taking $C_{(\alpha)}$-to-$C_{(\alpha)}$ distances]. In interaction with antibody, these residues of the site function as if in direct peptide-bond linkage (Lee and Atassi, 1976). Site 3 is analogous in spatial construction to antigenic site 2. The carbonyl group of Phe-34 and the side chain of Arg-114 make contact with the hexasaccharide substrate on binding of the latter with the enzyme (Imoto et al., 1972). Therefore antigenic site 3 overlaps with the enzymic binding site (Lee and Atassi, 1976).

IX. THE PRECISE DEFINITION OF THE ANTIGENIC SITE AROUND THE DISULFIDE BOND 6-127 (SITE 1)

A. Assignment of the Antigenic Site Chemically and by Classical Synthesis

From the immunochemical and conformational studies on derivatives of the intact protein, it was shown (see Section III) that Asp-119 and Leu-129 were not parts of an antigenic site in native lysozyme (Atassi et al., 1974; Atassi and Rosemblatt, 1974; Atassi et al., 1975a). Also modification of Trp-123 (Atassi and Zablocki, 1976) or Met-12 (as well as Met-105) (Atassi et al., 1976b) demonstrated that these residues were not located in an antigenic site. The peptide 6-13-(Cys 6-Cys 127)-126-128 carried substantial antigenic reactivity which, with two other disulfide-containing peptides (see Fig. 1), jointly accounted for almost all (90%) of the antigenic reactivity of native lysozyme (Atassi et al., 1973). These results indicated the presence of an antigenic site around the disulfide bond 6-127. On one side of the disulfide, the antigenic site clearly begins after Trp-123 and ends at or before Arg-128. On the other side of the disulfide, the second part of the site must end at or close to Met-12.

Having accomplished this degree of delineation chemically, the final narrowing down was achieved by immunochemical studies of synthetic peptides corresponding to various parts of the site. The aforementioned results were critical in that they pointed to the appropriate regions to be synthesized for the final delineation of the site. We therefore synthesized and studied the immunochemistry of nine disulfide peptides comprising various overlaps of the sequences 3-14 and 125-129 around the disulfide bond 6-127 (see Fig. 7) (Atassi et al., 1976b). None of the peptides 3-14, 5-14, or 125-129 (representing either one side or the other of the disulfide-linked antigenic site) had an inhibitory effect on the lysozyme immune reaction (Table 6). However, each of the disulfide peptides inhibited to varying degrees the reaction of lysozyme with its antisera (Atassi et al., 1976b). These results confirmed our previous findings that the integrity of the disulfide bond is essential for bringing the two distant (in sequence) parts of the site together. The behaviors of each of the peptides with three

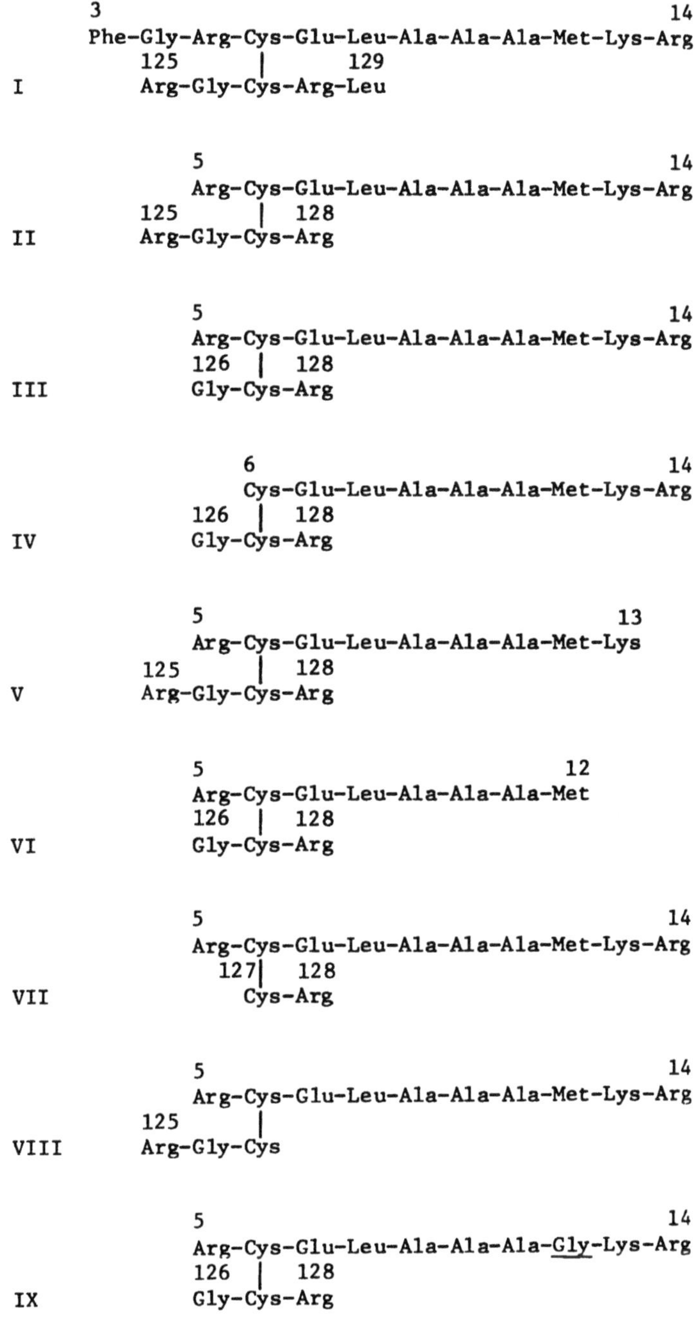

Fig. 7. Structure of the disulfide peptides that we synthesized to correspond to various regions around the disulfide bond 6-127. Peptide IX is an analogue containing glycine at position 12 instead of methionine. (From Atassi et al., 1976b).

TABLE 6: Inhibitory Activities of the Pure Synthetic Peptides Around the Disulfide 6-127 (Fig. 7)

Results are expressed in maximum percent inhibition of the precipitin reaction of native lysozyme with various antisera. Each value represents the average of four or more replicate determinations which varied ± 0.8% or less. Peptides denoted by Roman numerals refer to the disulfide peptides in Fig. 7. Linear peptides denoted by their locations in the primary structure are in the S-sulfonated form. L1 is a rabbit antiserum and G9 and G10 are goat antisera, each against native lysozyme.

Peptide	Antiserum L1		Antiserum G9		Antiserum G10	
	Max. inhib. act. (%)	Molar ratio, peptide/antigen	Max. inhib. act. (%)	Molar ratio, peptide/antigen	Max. inhib. act. (%)	Molar ratio, peptide/antigen
I	28.0	19*	26.8	17*	32.1	10*
II	27.4	18*	27.2	18*	31.9	11*
III	28.3	20*	26.5	16*	31.6	10*
IV	27.5	18*	27.0	17*	31.5	11*
V	14.6	28*	9.9	26*	21.7	23*
VI	6.3	39*	7.7	43*	8.9	38*
VII	7.5	45*	7.3	40*	8.5	38*
VIII	17.6	23*	15.8	25*	31.7	21*
IX	27.9	18*	27.1	18*	31.8	11*
3-14	0	730**	0	650**	0	610**
5-14	0	740**	0	655**	0	620**
125-129	0	735**	0	645**	0	625**

* These values represent peptide/lysozyme molar ratio at 50% of the maximum inhibition.

** These values represent the maximum molar excess of peptide, relative to lysozyme, which was employed in the inhibition experiment.

(From Atassi *et al.*, 1976b).

different antisera are given in Table 6. The antigenic site was found to be made up of residues on the two regions (6-14) and (126-128). These studies enabled us to describe the covalent structure of the antigenic site (Fig. 8) and from examination of the three-dimensional structure, we proposed (Atassi et al., 1976b) that the residues: Arg-14, Lys-13, Glu-7, Ala-10, Gly-126 and Arg-128 have the spatial possibility to form the antigenic site. Also, the sulfur of Cys-6 may come in contact with the antibody combining site. Furthermore, Met-12 (as well as Met-105), which in the three-dimensional structure is completely buried within the interior of the molecule, does not participate in interaction of lysozyme with its antibodies (Atassi et al., 1976b) and could be replaced in a synthetic peptide by a glycine without an immunochemical effect.

The above delineation of antigenic site 1 by chemical and finally by a classical synthetic approach, presented the ultimate level that could be achieved by the 'state of the art' of protein chemistry. Although it afforded an excellent and, until then, unequalled level of delineation of an antigenic site composed of conformationally contiguous residues, it came a little short of an unequivocal proof. Thus the residues presumed to be involved in direct binding of the synthetic disulfide-containing site (Fig. 8) with antibody, were deduced from examination of the three-dimensional structure of native lysozyme. No matter how compelling this evidence may have been, the fact remained that the identity of the exact residues constituting the antigenic site was at best hypothetical. A more precise definition of the antigenic site was therefore desirable.

B. Surface-Simulation Synthesis of the Antigenic Site

Rationale for the design of the surface-simulation peptides

Our introduction and successful application of the 'surface-simulation' synthetic concept for the precise definition of antigenic site 2 (Atassi et al., 1976d; Lee and Atassi, 1977b) and antigenic site 3 (Lee and Atassi, 1976, 1977a) in lysozyme made the reexamination of antigenic site 1 imperative so that the precise picture at the residue level will be formulated for the entire antigenic structure of lysozyme. These studies were completed very recently (Atassi and Lee, 1978a).

The residues previously proposed to constitute the antigenic site describe an imaginary line which circumscribes part of the surface of the molecule. A careful reexamination of a constructed lysozyme model showed that Ala-10 is not very likely to be a part of the antigenic site described by this imaginary line. Therefore, we decided (Atassi and Lee, 1978a) to investigate whether a glycine spacer between Arg-14 and Glu-7 will fulfill the requirement.

```
    6                                14
    Cys-Glu-Leu-Ala-Ala-Ala-Met-Lys-Arg
126  |  128
Gly-Cys-(Arg)
```

Fig. 8. Covalent structure of antigenic site _1_ that we had initially delineated by the classical synthesis of nine disulfide peptides around the disulfide bond 6-127 (see Fig. 7). The residues underlined by a solid line were proposed to be directly involved in the binding with antibody, while the residue underlined by a dotted line may come in contact with antibody. The classical synthetic approach left some uncertainty about the active involvement of Arg-128 in the site. See the text for details (From Atassi _et al_., 1976b).

Similarly, we investigated whether the possible involvement of Cys-6 can be satisfied by a glycine spacer. Finally, synthesis of the site (Fig. 7) by a classical strategy could not adequately differentiate whether the antigenic site required Arg-125 or Arg-128 (Atassi _et al_., 1976b), possibly because the folding of the structure shown in Fig. 8 may conceivably fulfill either requirement. Accordingly the distances between Glu-7 on the one hand and Arg-128 or Arg-125 on the other were measured and are shown in Table 7 (Atassi and Lee, 1978a). The table also gives the number of glycine spacers to be incorporated into the surface-simulation

TABLE 7: Distances Separating Arg-5 from Arg-125 or Arg-128 and Design of Spacers

The distances (in nm) are from C^{α}-to-C^{α}. The number of required glycine spacers in surface-simulation synthesis is based on an ideal C^{α}-to-C^{α} peptide bond distance of 0.362 nm. For details see text.

Separation	Distance C^{α}-to-C^{α} (nm)	Required glycine spacers	No. of spacers used in synthesis
Arg-5 to Arg-125	0.93	2.57	2 and 3
Arg-5 to Gly-126 to Arg-128	1.63	4.50	4

Table from Atassi and Lee (1978a).

RESIDUES COMPRISING THE ANTIGENIC REACTIVE SITE

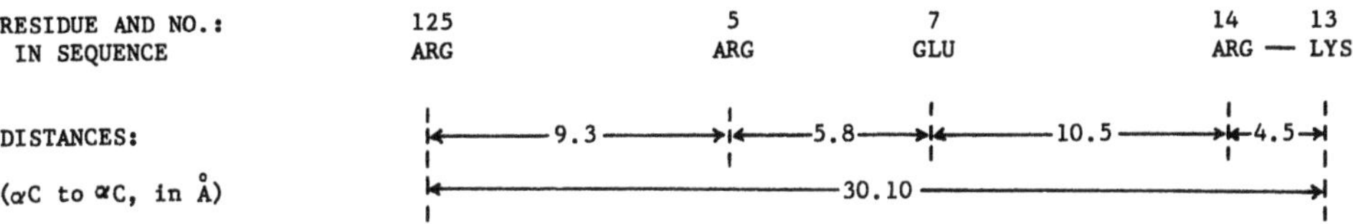

THE SYNTHETIC PEPTIDES

SEQUENCE (I) LYS — ARG — GLY — GLY — GLU — GLY — ARG — GLY — GLY — GLY — ARG

(II) ARG — GLY — GLY — GLY — ARG — GLY — GLU — GLY — GLY — ARG — LYS

(III) ARG — GLY — GLY — GLY — GLY — ARG — GLY — GLU — GLY — GLY — ARG — LYS

(IV) ARG — GLY — GLY — ARG — GLY — GLU — GLY — GLY — ARG — LYS

Fig. 9. Spatially contiguous surface residues constituting antigenic site 1 and their numerical position in the primary structure of lysozyme. The distances (in Å) separating the consecutive residues of the site are given as C^{α}-to-C^{α} distances together with the overall extended dimension of the site. Below, the primary structures of the surface-simulation synthetic peptides that were designed to copy the site and investigate its directional and conformational requirements are given. For the rationale behind the design of the peptides, see the text. (From Atassi and Lee, 1978a).

synthetic peptides if Arg-125, or alternatively Arg-128, is part of the antigenic site. It can be seen that if Arg-125 is part of the site, then about 2 glycine spacers are required. On the other hand, if Gly-126 and Arg-128 are essential parts of the site as we had proposed (Atassi et al., 1976b), then approximately 4 glycine spacers are required. Previously, we had shown (see Sections VII-C and VIII-B) for antigenic sites 2 and 3, that the correct spacing between the residues is critical in the design of surface-simulation synthetic sites (Lee and Atassi, 1977a, 1977b). In addition to this conformational restriction, the synthetic surface-simulation sites exhibited a preferred 'direction'. Accordingly, in order to determine the appropriate synthetic direction, peptides I and II of exactly reverse sequences, were synthesized (Atassi and Lee, 1978a) using three glycine spacers. Three spacers were initially selected, since they represented an average distance situation for the involvement of Arg-125 or Arg-128. The determination of the most favourable direction can then be followed by design and synthesis of peptides having distances of separation corresponding to Arg-125 or Arg-128 and in the correct synthetic direction. This strategy affords the rationale for the peptides that we synthesized and studied (Fig. 9) (Atassi and Lee, 1978a).

Accurate definition and conformational restrictions of the site

The immunochemical findings (Atassi and Lee, 1978a) which are summarized in Table 3 indicated that the surface-simulation synthetic sequence expressed in peptide II (Fig. 9) was immunochemically more reactive with each of the four antisera than the structure of the reverse sequence represented by peptide I. Having thus found the correct 'direction' of the surface-simulation synthetic site, the distance separating the first two arginine residues from the amino end was varied. It is significant that the inclusion of four glycine spacers (peptide III), gave a peptide having a lower immunochemical reactivity than the peptide which carried two glycine spacers between the N-terminal arginine and the residue corresponding to Arg-5 (peptide IV). In fact, rabbit antisera L7 and L21 and goat antiserum G10 were extremely sensitive to the alterations in the spacing between the reactive residues. On the other hand, a smaller but significant difference was exhibited in reaction with antiserum G9. The activity of the site (peptide IV) was greatly improved when reactions were carried out with the IgG fractions of the antisera (Table 8). These findings enabled us to conclude unambiguously (Atassi and Lee, 1978a) that the residue constituting a critical part of the antigenic site is Arg-125 and not Arg-128 and that antigenic site 1, like the other two antigenic sites of lysozyme (Lee and Atassi, 1977a, 1977b), exhibits stringent restrictions on the conformational degrees of freedom.

Obviously, antigenic site 1 has a preferred direction on the surface of the globular protein. Similar directional preferences for antigenic site 2 (Lee and Atassi, 1977b) and antigenic site 3 (Lee and Atassi, 1977a) of lysozyme have been discussed. As mentioned above, the directional sensitivity is a function of side-chain orientations (Lee and Atassi, 1977b).

To determine whether the maximum inhibitory activity of the surface-simulation site expressed its true immunochemical reactivity, we investigated (Atassi and Lee, 1978a) the ability of an immunoadsorbent carrying the most inhibitory synthetic peptide (peptide IV in Fig. 9) to bind radioiodinated antibodies to lysozyme. The amount of antibody from a given antiserum bound by the peptide-Sepharose relative to that bound by lysozyme-Sepharose was similar to the maximum inhibitory activity of the free peptide with the IgG fraction of the antiserum (compare Tables 9 and 10). Thus, as previously concluded for antigenic sites 2 and 3, the inhibition values do in fact provide a faithful measure of the immunochemical reactivity of the peptide.

TABLE 8: Inhibitory Activities of Peptide IV (Fig. 9) with Whole Antisera and with Their IgG Fractions: Comparison with the Expected Reaction of the Site

Results are expressed in maximum percentage inhibition by peptide IV of the precipitin reaction of native lysozyme with a given antiserum or its respective IgG fraction. Each value is the average of six replicate determinations which varied by $\pm$ 0.8% or less. Values in parentheses indicate the peptide/lysozyme molar ratio at 50% of the maximum inhibition. G9 and G10 are goat antisera, L7 and L21 are rabbit antisera, each against native lysozyme.

	Maximum inhibitory activity (%)		
Antiserum	Whole antiserum	IgG fraction of antiserum	Expected reaction of the site
G9	32.5 (90)	n.d.	27.2
G10	33.3 (150)	32.3 (55)	32.1
L7	22.2 (260)	33.4 (80)	n.d.
L21	21.3 (280)	31.4 (85)	n.d.

n.d., not determined

Table is from Atassi and Lee (1978a).

In summary, for the antisera studied (Atassi and Lee, 1978a), antigenic site 1 of native lysozyme is constructed (Fig. 10) precisely by the five spatially adjacent surface residues: Arg-125, Arg-5, Glu-7, Arg-14, Lys-13. The synthetic surface-simulation site (Fig. 10) shows a mono-directional preference (Arg-125 → Lys-13) which appears to be species-independent since it was the same for the two rabbit and the two goat antisera tested. The site is subject to conformational restrictions and requires the correct residue spacing in its synthetic surface-simulation.

X. THE PRECISE AND ENTIRE ANTIGENIC STRUCTURE OF LYSOZYME

With the precise boundary, conformational and directional definitions of the three antigenic sites of lysozyme by surface-simulation synthesis, we have now achieved the precise determination of the entire antigenic structure of the native protein. In this section, a summary of the main features of the antigenic structure of lysozyme will be presented.

TABLE 9: Quantitative Accounting of the Three Surface-Simulation Synthetic Sites for the Total Antigenic Reactivity of Lysozyme

The values are given in maximum percentage inhibition of the quantitative precipitin reaction of lysozyme by each of the synthetic sites independently. The sites were immunochemically independent (see text). The identities of sites 1, 2 and 3 are shown in Fig.10. The IgG fractions accounted for 99-100% of the total immune reaction of the respective parent antisera.

Site	Maximum percentage inhibition			
	Goat antisera		Rabbit antisera	
	G9	G10	L7	L21
(A) Reactions with whole antisera				
Site 1	32.5	33.3	22.2	21.3
Site 2	35.7	32.3	12.7	18.2
Site 3	33.3	28.8	19.2	22.2
TOTAL	101.5	94.4	54.1	61.7
(B) Reactions with the IgG fractions of the antisera				
Site 1		32.3	33.4	31.4
Site 2		34.5	28.6	28.9
Site 3		30.3	33.3	35.2
TOTAL		97.1	95.3	95.5

Table is from Atassi and Lee (1978b).

A. Do the Three Antigenic Sites of Lysozyme Account for Its Total Immune Reaction?

In evaluating whether the antigenic structure elucidated in our laboratory does in fact represent the entire antigenic profile of the protein, a vital piece of evidence is to determine the extent of the lysozyme immune reaction that can be accounted for by the total reactivities of the three antigenic sites. This is most critical in view of the fact that our delineation culminated in the production and synthesis of antigenic sites that are 'unconventional' in character.

A most direct way to answer this question can be derived from the total inhibitory activities of the three sites towards the lysozyme immune reaction. Table 9 summarizes the results from Atassi and Lee (1978b) obtained with rabbit and goat antisera. With goat

TABLE 10: Binding of Radioiodinated Antibodies to Lysozyme by Immunoadsorbents Carrying the Three Surface-Simulation Synthetic Sites*

The specific ^{125}I-labelled antibody fractions from antisera G9 and G10 were isolated on a lysozyme immunoadsorbent prior to use in these studies. The amounts of antibody applied were: G9, 5.21 x 10^4; G10, 7.56 x 10^4 c.p.m. Each value represents the average of four replicate analyses which varied ± 1.3% or less. Results have been corrected for the amount of antibody bound in control experiments using glycine-Sepharose, histidine-Sepharose and myoglobin-Sepharose. Also another set of controls was employed using non-immune goat ^{125}I-labelled IgG. The amount of nonspecific background binding in the various controls ranged 1-3% of the total label applied.

	Antibody from G9		Antibody from G10+	
Immunoadsorbent	Amount Ab bound (c.p.m.)	% Ab bound	Amount Ab bound (c.p.m.)	% Ab bound
Lysozyme*	50,180	100	73,330	100
Site 1*	15,760	31.4	20,335	27.7
Site 2*	18,015	35.9	27,600	37.6
Site 3*	14,950	29.8	22,300	30.0
Total of indep.* binding by three sites	48,725	97.1	70,235	95.8
Binding by** passage through sites serially	49,880	99.4	71,670	97.7

* Results for independent binding were obtained by passage of an aliquot of the antibody solution on only one of the immunoadsorbents indicated.

** Results obtained by serial passage of the same antibody sample on the immunoadsorbent of site 1, then site 2, then site 3.

\+ Results from Atassi and Lee (1978b).

antiserum G9 and the IgG fraction of antiserum G10, the total of immunochemical reactivities of the three sites accounted for 101.5% and 97% respectively. With the IgG fractions from rabbit antisera L7 and L21, the combined inhibitory activities of the three sites were 95.3% and 95.5% respectively. Perhaps it should be noted here that the IgG fractions accounted for 99-100% of the immune reaction of the respective antisera.

Another approach to quantitative accounting of the total immunochemical contribution of the site is to determine the fraction of lysozyme antibodies that can be specifically bound by the synthetic surface-simulation sites. Table 10 summarizes the binding results of ^{125}I-labelled antibodies by immunoadsorbents of the three sites (Atassi and Lee, 1978b). In a single passage of a sample of the labelled antibodies through only one of the site-Sepharose columns, the three sites bound a calculated total of 97% and 96% with antibodies G9 and G10 respectively relative to the amount of antibody bound by lysozyme. Serial passage of the same antibody sample through all three sites (site 1, then site 2, then site 3) removed, from antibodies G9 and G10, 99.4% and 97.7% respectively relative to the amount removed by lysozyme. It is critical to point out that the sites were immunochemically independent, since antibody eluted from one site-immunoadsorbent could not bind with another site-immunoadsorbent, but was adsorbed quantitatively on re-passage on to the site-Sepharose that was initially used for its isolation (Atassi and Lee, 1978b). The correspondence observed (Lee and Atassi, 1977a, 1977b; Atassi and Lee, 1978a, 1978b) between the inhibition values and the amount of total antibody bound by each site is not unusual and has been reported for the synthetic antigenic sites of myoglobin (Atassi and Koketsu, 1975) and for the two inhibitory fragments of bovine serum albumin (Atassi _et al._, 1976a; Habeeb and Atassi, 1976).

The fact that the surface-simulation synthetic sites (Fig. 10) can account for 96-100% of the total immune reaction of native lysozyme provides a most convincing and powerful demonstration of the correctness of the delineation. The impact of these results becomes even more remarkable when it is pointed out that it has been shown (Atassi, 1972; Koketsu and Atassi, 1973, 1974a) that an intact antigenic site with no extraneous amino acids would usually react less than when it is an integral part of a longer peptide. The extraneous residues or segments are frequently important for the correct folding of the site (Atassi, 1972).

It may be relevant to comment here briefly about the binding efficiency of the surface-simulation synthetic antigenic sites. This has been discussed in detail earlier in the papers dealing with the behavior of each of the three surface-simulation synthetic sites (Atassi _et al._, 1976d; Lee and Atassi, 1976, 1977a, 1977b; Atassi and Lee, 1978a) and of the synthetic intact antigenic sites of sperm-whale myoglobin (Koketsu and Atassi, 1973, 1974a, 1974b; Pai and Atassi, 1975; Atassi and Pai, 1975). The large molar excess of peptide required can in part be attributed to conformational factors in view of the fact that, in solution, these peptides will be expected to exist in greatly unfolded conformational states. The immune response to native protein antigens is directed against their native three-dimensional structure (Atassi, 1967b; Atassi and Thomas, 1969). For proper interaction with antibody, an antigenic site must have (at least reasonably approximately) the shape that it has in the native protein (Atassi, 1967a; Atassi and Saplin, 1968; Atassi, 1970; Habeeb and Atassi, 1971a) and antibody is able somewhat to induce its own required conformation on an antigenic site (Atassi, 1975). The probability of finding such a favorable conformational state will improve with increase in peptide concentration (Atassi and Saplin, 1968). It is to be remembered that the peptides studied here do not even exist in native lysozyme but merely attempt to simulate a spatial arrangement of adjacent surface residues most of which are distant in sequence. Furthermore, it is not entirely possible to duplicate in the synthetic peptides the exact distances separating the various side chains of the antigenic site in the native protein. Therefore, the mere reactivity of these peptides is remarkable and the fact that the immunochemical efficiency of the surface-simulation sites resembles those of the synthetic sites of myoglobin (which are in the native protein made up of residues directly linked to one another in the sequence; Atassi, 1975) is indeed startling.

The improvement in the immunochemical efficiency of the peptides when the IgG fractions of the antisera were employed may have been indicative of proteolysis and/or binding of the synthetic sites by serum proteins (Lee and Atassi, 1977a, 1977b). Similar observations have previously been made with fragments of lysozyme (Atassi _et al_., 1973), of bovine serum albumin (Habeeb _et al_., 1974; Atassi _et al_., 1976a; Habeeb and Atassi, 1976) and with the synthetic antigenic sites of myoglobin (Atassi, 1977b).

B. Summary of the Main Features of the Antigenic Structure of Lysozyme

Native lysozyme carries three antigenic sites. The identities of the sites are summarized in Fig. 10, and Plates 1 and 2 show their locations in the three-dimensional structure.

Site 1. This antigenic site is constructed by the side chains of the spatially contiguous five surface residues (Atassi and Lee, 1978a): Arg-125, Arg-5, Glu-7, Arg-14, Lys-13. The dimension of the site, in the extended form, from Arg-125 to Lys-13 is 30 Å (C^{α}-to-C^{α} distance). These residues bind with antibody as if in direct peptide linkage. In fact the reactivity of this site is fully satisfied by the surface-simulation synthetic peptide Arg-Gly-Gly-Arg-Gly-Glu-Gly-Gly-Arg-Lys, which does not exist in native lysozyme. The surface-simulation synthetic site exhibits a directional preference (Arg-125 to Lys-13), which appears to be independent of the species of the immunized animal (at least with the rabbits and goats so far tested) and possesses a restricted conformational freedom, as demonstrated by its sensitivity to

THE ANTIGENIC SITES OF LYSOZYME AND THEIR
SYNTHETIC SURFACE-SIMULATIONS
SITE 1
CONSTITUANT RESIDUES:
125 ARG
5 ARG
7 GLU
14 ARG
13 LYS
DISTANCES:
(αC-to-αC, in nm)
0.93
0.58
1.05
0.45
3.01
THE SYNTHETIC SITE:
ARG — GLY — GLY — ARG — GLY — GLU — GLY — GLY — ARG — LYS
DISTANCES:
(αC-to-αC, in nm)
3.26
SITE 2
CONSTITUANT RESIDUES:
62 TRP
97 LYS
96 LYS
93 ASN
89 THR
87 ASP
DISTANCES:
(αC-to-αC, in nm)
0.71
0.41
0.56
0.51
0.54
2.73
THE SYNTHETIC SITE:
PHE — GLY — LYS — LYS — ASN — THR — ASP
DISTANCES:
(αC-to-αC, in nm)
2.16
SITE 3
CONSTITUANT RESIDUES:
116 LYS
113 ASN — 114 ARG
34 PHE
33 LYS
DISTANCES:
(αC-to-αC, in nm)
0.5
0.4
0.8
0.4
2.1
THE SYNTHETIC SITE:
LYS — ASN — ARG — GLY — PHE — LYS
DISTANCES:
(αC-to-αC, in nm)
1.8

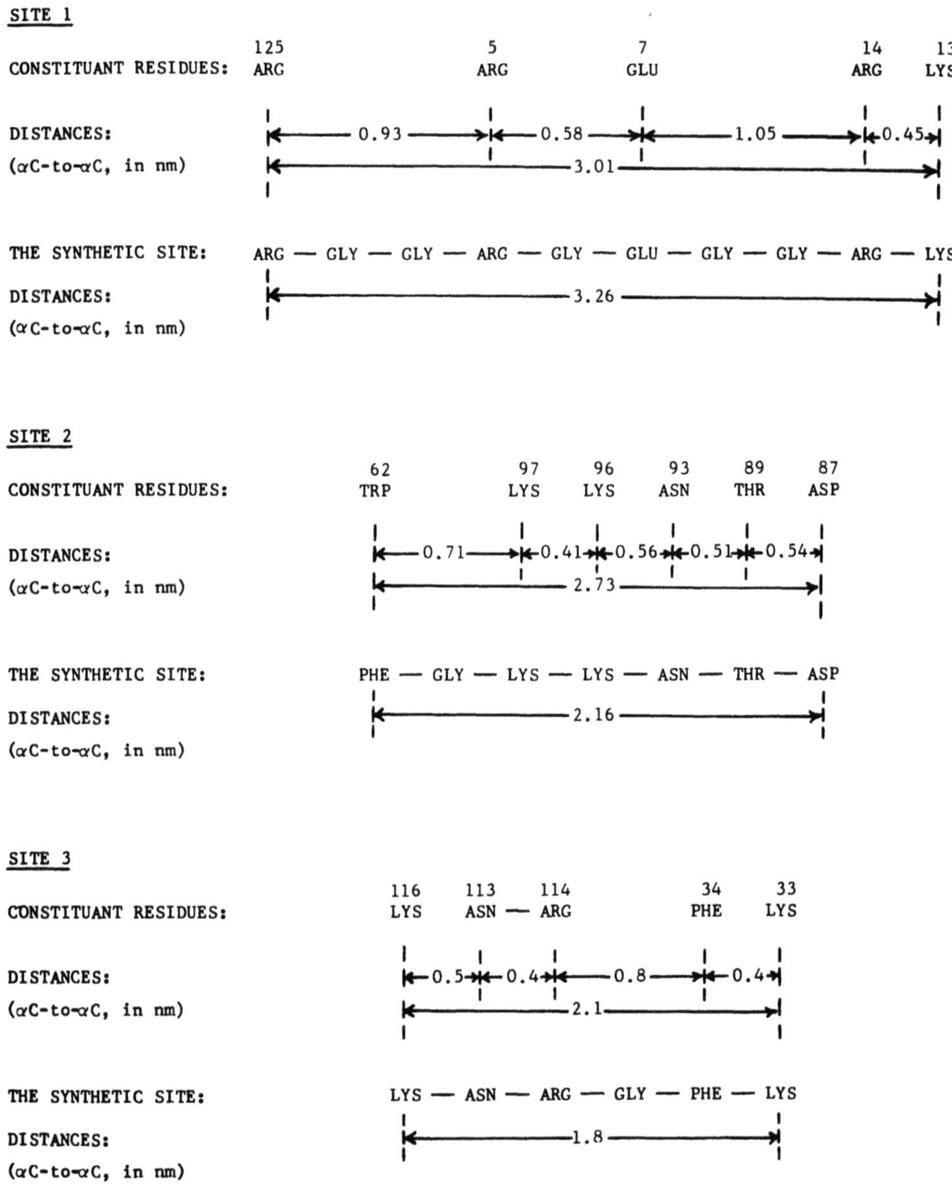

Figure 10

Fig. 10. The three antigenic sites representing the entire antigenic structure of lysozyme. The diagram shows the spatially contiguous residues constituting each antigenic site and their numerical positions in the primary structure. The distances (in nm) separating the consecutive residues and the overall dimension of each site (in its extended form) are given, together with the dimension of each surface-simulation synthetic site. The latter assumes an ideal C^{α}-to-C^{α} distance of 0.362 nm. The precise boundary, conformational and directional definitions of sites 3 and 2 and 1 were described earlier (Lee and Atassi, 1977a, 1977b; Atassi and Lee, 1978a respectively). The three sites account quantitatively for the entire (96-100%) antigenic reactivity of lysozyme (see the text for details). (From Atassi and Lee, 1978b).

---

variation of the residue spacing in surface-simulation synthesis (Atassi and Lee, 1978a). The intactness of the disulfide bond 6-127 in native lysozyme is critical for the integrity of this site (Atassi *et al.*, 1973, 1976b).

Site 2. This site consists of the spatially adjacent surface residues: Trp-62, Lys-97, Lys-96, Asn-93, Thr-89, Asp-87 (Atassi *et al.*, 1976a). As with site 1, site 2 also forms an imaginary line circumscribing part of the surface topography of the protein (Atassi *et al.*, 1976d). This line, which has an overall extended length (from Trp-62 to Asp-87 in C^{α}-to-C^{α} distance) of 27.3 Å, passes through the residues forming the site which bind with antibody as if in direct peptide bond linkage (Atassi *et al.*, 1976d). Thus the surface-simulation synthetic peptide Phe-Gly-Lys-Lys-Asn-Thr-Asp, which does not exist in lysozyme, carries the full reactivity of the site (Atassi *et al.*, 1976d; Lee and Atassi, 1977b). With the antisera so far studied, the antigenic site exhibits a preferred 'direction' in surface-simulation synthesis (Trp-62 to Asp-87) towards the goat antisera and none towards the rabbit antisera (Lee and Atassi, 1977b). The antigenic site is subject to conformational restrictions indicated by spacing-between-residues requirements (Lee and Atassi, 1977b). The intactness of the disulfide bonds 64-80 and 76-94 is critical to bring together the various constituent residues of the site (Atassi *et al.*, 1976c). This antigenic site overlaps with the enzymic active site because they both share Trp-62 (Lee and Atassi, 1975; Atassi *et al.*, 1976c).

Site 3. Like sites 1 and 2, this site is also constructed of conformationally adjacent surface residues. The antigenic site comprises five residues which are: Lys-116, Asn-113, Arg-114, Phe-34, Lys-33 (Lee and Atassi, 1977a). These residues describe an imaginary line which circumscribes part (21 Å in C^{α}-to-C^{α} extended distance from Lys-116 to Lys-33) of the surface of the molecule.

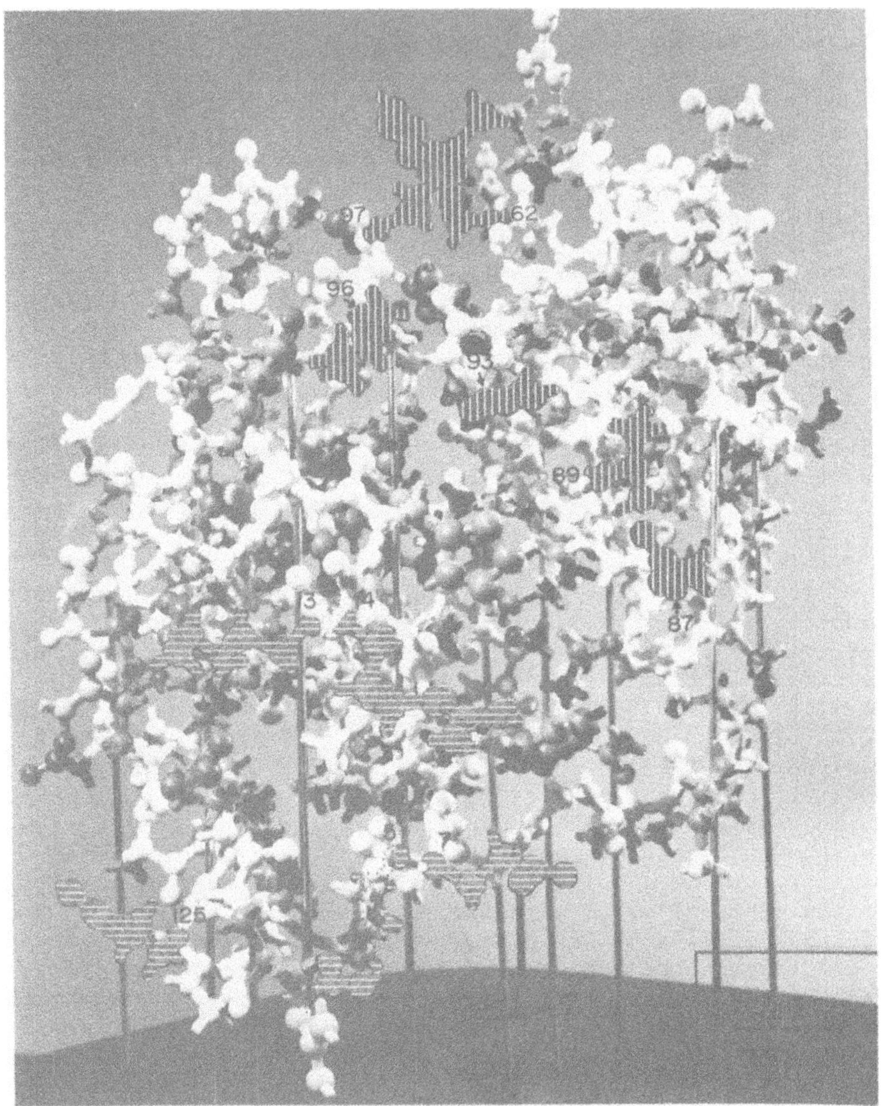

Plate 1. Photograph of a lysozyme model showing the relative positions of the residues constituting antigenic sites 1 and 2. The side chains of the residues in the sites are outlined, those making up site 1 with horizontal bars and those constituting site 2 with vertical bars, to avoid confusion. The preferred 'direction' of site 1 (at least by surface-simulation synthesis) is Arg-125 to Lys-13. Site 2 had a preferred 'direction' only with goat antisera (Trp-62 to Asp-87), but exhibited no directional preference with rabbit antisera. (From Atassi and Lee, 1978b.)

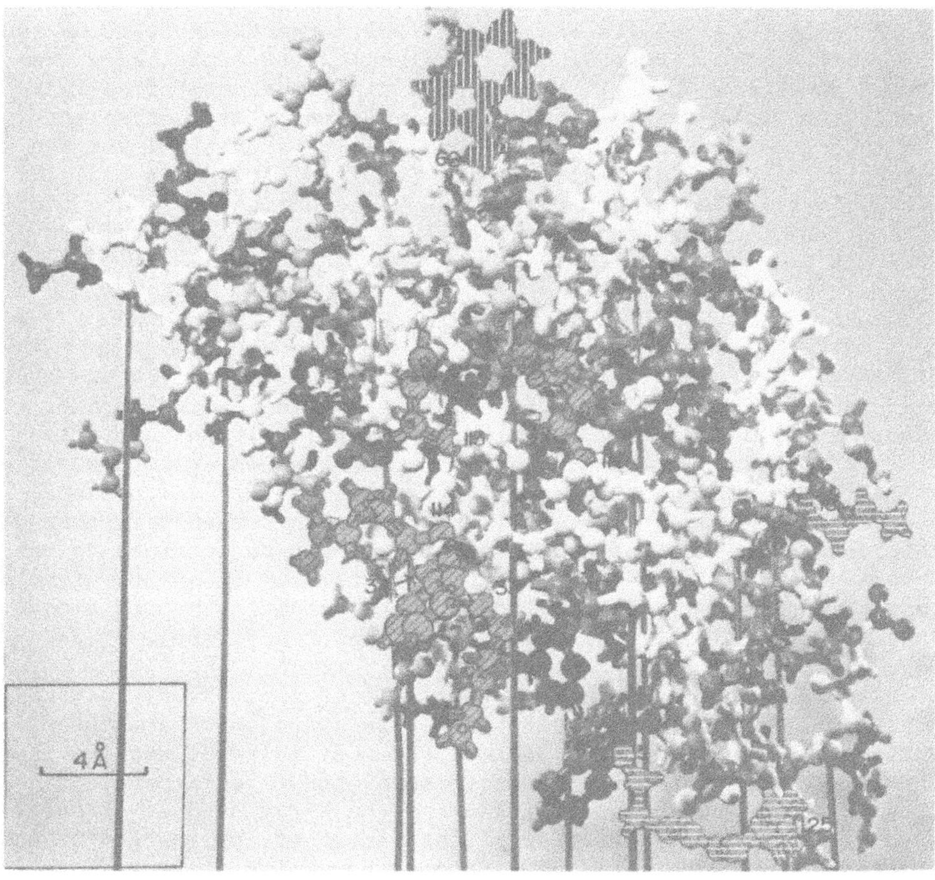

Plate 2. Photograph of a lysozyme model showing the position of antigenic site 3 on the molecule relative to sites 1 and 2. The side chains of the residues comprising the sites are outlined. The residues constituting site 3 have diagonal bars. This view is taken by rotating the model 125° anticlockwise on the vertical axis relative to the view shown in Plate 1. From this perspective only parts of site 1 can be seen which are the residues Lys-13, Arg-5 and Arg-125 (horizontal bars). Of site 2, only Trp-62 can be seen (vertical bars). Site 3 showed the same directional preference (Lys-116 to Lys-33) towards rabbit and goat antisera. (From Atassi and Lee, 1978b.)

They act functionally towards the antibody as if they are in direct peptide bond linkage. Accordingly, the surface-simulation synthetic peptide (which does not exist in lysozyme) having the structure Lys-Asn-Arg-Gly-Phe-Lys carries the full immunochemical reactivity of the site (Lee and Atassi, 1977a). With the two rabbit and two goat antisera so far studied the antigenic site exhibited a preferred direction (Lys-116 to Lys-33), since the reverse surface-simulation synthetic sequence was immunochemically inefficient. The intactness of the disulfide bond 30-115 is critical for the integrity of this antigenic site in lysozyme (Atassi et al., 1973). Antigenic site 3 overlaps with the hexasaccharide substrate binding site at the carbonyl group of Phe-34 and the side chain of Arg-114 (Lee and Atassi, 1977a).

XI. THE POTENTIAL OF THE SURFACE-SIMULATION CONCEPT

From the foregoing short treatment, it is quite obvious that the precise determination of the entire antigenic structure of lysozyme would have been totally unattainable without our introduction of the "surface-simulation" synthesis concept. However, it has already been pointed out (Atassi et al., 1976d; Lee and Atassi, 1976; Atassi and Lee, 1978b) that the remarkable power of this unorthodox concept should not in any way be confined to the determination of protein antigenic structures. It may be of value to mention here very briefly some of its potential applications that we have recently outlined (Atassi and Lee, 1978b).

We have already pointed out (Atassi et al., 1976d; Lee and Atassi, 1976) that the results from this approach on the three antigenic sites of lysozyme afford the most powerful and convincing chemical evidence for the correctness of the three-dimensional structure of lysozyme as derived from the X-ray studies of the crystalline protein. In view of the fact that application of this strategy reports on the conformational proximity of several surface residues simultaneously, it will be enormously more informative and precise than studying the availability of certain side chains to chemical modification or physicochemical studies on the protein solution which afford overall shape or conformational parameters. Thus, for example, the three antigenic sites of lysozyme (Fig. 10) report on the spatial interrelationships of a total of sixteen surface residues.

It is relevant to note that the utility of the immunochemical application of this concept should not be limited to exploitation of antigenic sites. Other parts of the surface could be copied into appropriate surface-simulation synthetic peptides linking conformationally contiguous residues. Then, these synthetic surface-simulations can be coupled to a suitable carrier and the conjugate used for immunization. This will enable the preparation of antibodies against the surface-simulation peptides. The antibodies thus prepared will recognize and react with those regions in the native protein, even though the regions are not antigenic sites when the native protein is used as an immunogen. Several surface-simulation peptides could thus be made at will and the antibodies to these could be employed as conformational scanners to double-check the three-dimensional structure of a protein. The approach could also be used as a probe to monitor the acquisition of correct residue alignments by various preselected parts of the surface of a protein molecule (or a fragment thereof) upon renaturation of a denatured protein or refolding of a derivative having previously reduced disulfide bonds. This should find wide application by those interested in the mechanism of protein refolding as it gives a unique and direct region-by-region readout of the surface. Furthermore, should methods for predicting protein conformation from its sequence ever become more reliable then the predicted three-dimensional structure could be readily double-checked by antibodies to surface-simulation synthetic peptides designed from the predicted structure. Since we have shown the immunochemistry of surface-simulation peptides to be quite sensitive to the distance separating the constituent residues as well as to the direction of synthesis (i.e. side chain orientations) (Lee and Atassi, 1977a, 1977b; Atassi and Lee, 1978a), this approach is eminently suited for the aforementioned investigations.

The concept should also find application in studies on subunit interactions in oligomeric proteins. Surface-simulation synthesis of an ineracting face of a subunit should interfere with and enable understanding of the molecular mechanism of such interactions. A related application of this concept will be in protein-receptor interactions, where the binding site on the protein can be copied by surface-simulation synthesis. This should open up untapped avenues leading to a molecular elucidation of such matters as the mode of hormone action, allergic reactions, soluble factors in immunology and indeed the basis of the immune response.

However, the concept should be applicable in principle to other interactions involving proteins. For example, it should be possible in certain cases to reconstruct a substrate-binding site of an enzyme by surface-simulation synthesis. It should also be applicable in studying the interactions of some proteins with lipids, carbohydrates and other prosthetic groups.

It ought to be emphasized that in all these aspects, the three-dimensional structure of the protein under study must be known in detail. Furthermore, surface-simulation synthesis can only be applied after all the chemical groundwork has been done implicating various residues and parts of the molecule in binding of a protein with the receptor, antibody or other protein interactions.

The most intriguing question is whether an antibody combining site can be mimicked by surface-simulation synthesis. Ability to perform this task will have far-reaching implications in immunology. Recent findings from our laboratory (described in the next section) indicate that this may have indeed been accomplished by synthesizing two surface-simulation synthetic peptides that were complementary to antigenic sites 2 and 3 (Fig. 10) of lysozyme. Thus, by mimicking the antibody combining site, at least in terms of binding function, the surface-simulation concept has scored a climax in protein immunochemistry. Although the concept came as a by-product of our determination of the antigenic structure of lysozyme, it should present a major new asset in protein chemistry.

XII. THE POSSIBLE SURFACE-SIMULATION SYNTHESIS OF ANTIBODY-COMBINING SITES TO LYSOZYME ANTIGENIC SITES

The remarkable success of the surface-simulation synthesis concept in reconstructing antigenic sites of spatially contiguous surface residues has suggested to us its usefulness to investigate the feasibility of mimicking the antibody-combining site (Atassi and Zablocki, 1977). It is evident from the preceding sections that the proper application of surface-simulation synthesis requires the detailed knowledge of the three-dimensional structure of the protein under study and a full chemical identification of the residues constituting a binding site as well as their accurate conformational spacing and directional requirements. Obviously, these requirements are not known for the antibody-combining sites directed against lysozyme. However, we indicated (Atassi and Zablocki, 1977) that the situation is not entirely hopeless since, in all likelihood, the antibody-combining site will be expected to comprise residues (presumably in the hypervariable regions of both the heavy and light chains and not necessarily in direct peptide bond linkage) that are complementary to those in the corresponding antigenic sites. Furthermore, the spacings between the residues of the antigenic site and those of its complementary antibody-combining site must be equivalent or comparable in order for appropriate binding to take place. Thus by the precise knowledge of all the parameters of an antigenic site it should be possible to create a reasonable design of its corresponding antibody-combining site. This was done (Atassi and Zablocki, 1977) for two antigenic sites in native lysozyme. Fig. 11 shows the residues and spacings constituting each of antigenic sites 2 and 3 of native lysozyme and the corresponding surface-simulation synthetic antigenic sites.

The peptides CS-2 and CS-3 were designed (Atassi and Zablocki, 1977) on the basis of complementarity to antigenic sites 2 and 3 respectively in ionic, hydrophobic, hydrophilic and side-chain length of the constituent amino acids. Each of the two complementary peptides exhibited an appreciable inhibitory activity (Table

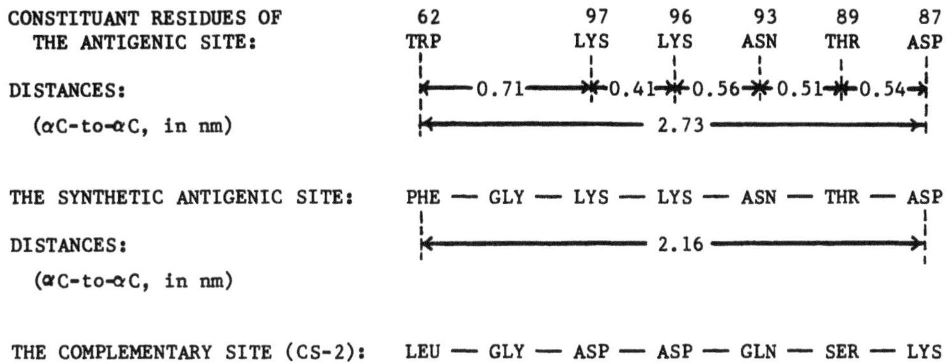

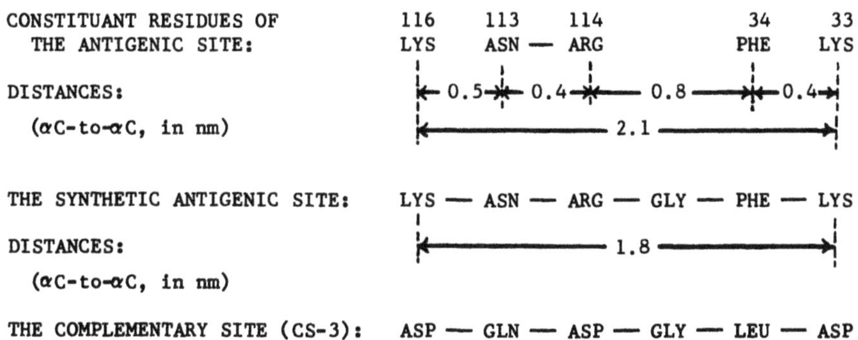

Fig. 11. A diagram showing antigenic sites 2 and 3 of hen egg-white lysozyme and their predicted complementary 'antibody-combining' sites. The spatially contiguous surface residues constituting each antigenic site and the numerical positions of these residues in the primary structure of lysozyme are shown. The distances (in nm) separating the consecutive residues and the overall dimension of each site are given, together with the dimension of the respective surface-simulation synthetic antigenic site. Below each antigenic site is given the structure of the respective complementary surface-simulation peptide which was predicted to mimic the antibody-combining site directed against that antigenic site. (From Atassi and Zablocki, 1977).

11) towards the reaction of lysozyme with its antisera and these activities were additive when the peptides were used in combination. Peptide immunoadsorbents bound only lysozyme and not antibody or

TABLE 11: Inhibitory Activities by the Pure Synthetic Complementary Sites (Fig. 11) and Comparison with Activities of the Respective Antigenic Sites

	Complementary site CS-2		Antigenic site 2		Complementary site CS-3		Antigenic site 3	
Anti-serum*	Max. inhibit. act. (%)+	Molar ratio at ½ max. inhibn.‡	Max. inhibit. act. (%)+	Molar ratio at ½ max. inhibn.‡	Max. inhibit. act. (%)+	Molar ratio at ½ max. inhibn.‡	Max. inhibit. act. (%)+	Molar ratio at ½ max. inhibn.‡
G9	23.9	165	35.7	170	19.5	103	33.3	40
G10	19.3	70	34.5	170	26.0	73	30.3	200

* G9 and G10 are goat antisera, each against native lysozyme. Reactions were carried out with the IgG fractions of the antisera which accounted for 99-100% of the immune reaction of the respective parent antiserum.

+ Maximum percentage inhibition of the precipitin reaction of native lysozyme. Each value is the average of six replicate determinations which varied ± 0.8% or less.

‡ Indicate the peptide/lysozyme molar ratio at 50% of the maximum inhibition.

Table from Atassi and Zablocki (1977).

myoglobin. Neither of the two peptides had any immunochemical activity in the myoglobin or bovine serum albumin immune systems. Furthermore, it was shown that three control synthetic peptides of myoglobin, of similar charge but different sequence, had no inhibitory effect on the lysozyme immune reaction (Atassi and Zablocki, 1977). The evidence indicated that the antibody-combining sites against antigenic sites 2 and 3 of native lysozyme were successfully mimicked synthetically, at least in terms of binding function.

We have already stressed (Atassi and Zablocki, 1977) that the residues deduced in peptides CS-2 and CS-3 are in no way implied to be the actual residues brought together in the binding sites of the antibodies by the three-dimensional folding of the latter. This is difficult to know. Also, it should be emphasized that the functional success of the peptides designed here does not imply a unique antibody site to each of the lysozyme antigenic sites. Other complementary amino acids may serve equally as well in the antibody molecule. For example, the role of leucine may be satisfied by isoleucine, valine, phenylalanine, etc., but we have not tested that yet. By employing related alternatives to each residue, it will not be difficult to rationalize antibody heterogeneity and differences in affinity. We are now making antibodies to these synthetic surface-simulations of antibody-combining sites by immunization after coupling to appropriate carriers. These antibodies will serve to reveal whether or not the antibody-combining site and the idiotypic determinants incorporate the same residues on the antibody molecule. The results will be reported in detail elsewhere.

To test whether or not the success of the present approach represents a special situation, we are now studying complementary peptides to antigenic site 1 of lysozyme (Atassi and Lee, 1978a), the antigenic sites of myoglobin (Atassi, 1975), as well as the surface-simulations of the binding sites in two myeloma proteins towards phosphorylcholine (Padlan *et al.*, 1973) and a hydroxyl derivative of vitamin K_1 (Poljak *et al.*, 1973; Amzel *et al.*, 1974) which are known from X-ray crystallographic studies.

XIII. CONCLUSIONS

This is the second antigenic structure of a protein to be precisely defined. Very recently, the entire antigenic structure of sperm-whale myoglobin was elucidated (Atassi, 1975; or in more detail Atassi, 1977b). However, it is critical to note that the antigenic structure of lysozyme (like that of myoglobin) was determined with early-course (3-4 weeks after the first immunization) antisera raised only in goats and in rabbits. The primary antibody response to a globular protein is directed against its native three-dimensional structure (Atassi and Thomas, 1969), and proteolytic fragmentation of the protein may play a relatively more significant role in the antigenic expression in late-course antisera (Atassi and Thomas, 1969). We are now studying the changes, if any, of the antigenic structures of both myoglobin and lysozyme over an extended period of immunization (up to a year) in goats and in rabbits and then in other species using the elucidated antigenic structures as valuable reference models.

Many general conclusions relating to antigenic structures of proteins were derived from our accurate mapping out of the antigenic structure of myoglobin (Atassi, 1972, 1975, 1977b). All of these conclusions are applicable to lysozyme equally as well. These include: the small size and sharp boundaries of the antigenic sites, their presence only in a limited number, their surface locations(see Plates 1 and 2), their sensitivity to conformational changes and many other features which, for lack of space, cannot be rediscussed here. The reader may consult the pertinent references (Atassi, 1975, 1977b).

The five antigenic sites of myoglobin are made up of residues in direct peptide-bond linkage, whereas the three sites of lysozyme each constitutes conformationally contiguous residues that were frequently very distant in sequence. Even though we had previously suggested (Atassi and Saplin, 1968) the existence of such antigenic sites in proteins, their identification and precise definition in lysozyme (Atassi et al., 1976d; Lee and Atassi, 1976, 1977a, 1977b; Atassi and Lee, 1978a) is the first such example in protein immunochemistry. However, it should be stressed that the antigenic sites both in myoglobin and in lysozyme are sensitive to conformational changes in the respective proteins, with those of lysozyme showing as expected a much higher sensitivity. Accordingly, it is totally inadequate to identify the antigenic sites of myoglobin by the terms 'linear', 'sequential', or 'pirmary' or some such terms, while identifying the antigenic sites of lysozyme by the terms 'spacial', 'conformational', etc. A common feature to these two types of antigenic sites is that they occupy exposed regions on the surface topography of the respective protein (Atassi et al., 1976d) and this will most likely be the situation with all antigenic sites in native proteins. I would like to propose that antigenic sites of the type seen in myoglobin (Atassi, 1975) and hemoglobin (Kazim and Atassi, 1977b) be named "continuous sites" which implies that they consist of conformationally-distinct continuous surface portions of the polypeptide chain. For antigenic sites of the type seen in lysozyme, the term "discontinuous sites" will be appropriate. A "discontinuous site" is made up of conformationally (or spatially) contiguous surface residues that are totally or partially not in direct peptide bond linkage. Whether the antigenic sites in a protein will belong to one type or another or a mixture of both will obviously depend on the protein, and may be determined to a great extent by the presence of internal cross-links (Lee and Atassi, 1976). In this regard, it is pertinent to caution that immunization with a protein that had been chemically cross-linked is likely to alter its antigenic expression.

It should be relevant to comment here on the antibody combining site that will be complementary to the antigenic sites of lysozyme. The sizes of the lysozyme antigenic sites in their extended forms are 30, 27 and 21 Å respectively. This is quite similar to the dimensions of the extended antigenic sites of sperm-whale myoglobin (Atassi, 1975, 1977b) which range between 22.3 and 26.7 Å. Since the antigenic sites on the protein are not in the extended form, the actual dimensions of the sites will be smaller than the values given. Nevertheless, the size of the antibody combining sites required for the two proteins will be somewhat larger than the combining site for haptens as determined by X-ray crystallography. This is seen in the combining site of the Fab' fragment of protein New (a human IgG) towards a hydroxyl derivative of vitamin K_1 (Poljak *et al.*, 1973; Amzel *et al.*, 1974); of the Fab' fragment of a myeloma protein from mouse (McPc 603) towards phosphorylcholine (Padlan *et al.*, 1973) and a bence-Jones protein (λ chain) dimer (Ely *et al.*, 1973; Schiffer *et al.*, 1973). The latter revealed a conical cavity 10 Å deep with an opening of 15 Å connected to a pocket of 17 Å and the part of the combining site involved in binding depended on the size and structure of the bound hapten. Therefore, the antibody combining site can vary to provide maximum complementarity to the antigenic site with which it binds. With proteins, unlike haptens, the antigenic site will be expected to fill the entire combining site (Atassi and Lee, 1978b). Thus, the above dimensions found for antibody combining sites accommodating haptens may represent an artifical situation and the combining sites towards protein antigenic sites will be larger (Atassi and Lee, 1978b). This should be readily achieved by the flexibility of the hypervariable region.

Examination of the antigenic sites of lysozyme (Fig. 10) shows that they are very rich in basic amino acids. This was also seen in myoglobin, but we caution against premature generalizations. Obviously, interactions with antibody are predominantly polar in nature with considerable stabilizing effects being contributed by hydrophobic interactions and some hydrogen bonding, especially with site 2. However, it should be emphasized that the basicity of the sites cannot be the only rationalization for their antigenicity because other alignments of basic conformationally contiguous residues, which are non-antigenic, can be generated on the surface. Clearly, the arrangement of the residues in the imaginary surface-encircling line bearing the aligned residues is highly critical. It is well to caution here that the sequence and three-dimensional features that confer immunogenicity on given parts or surface areas of a protein molecule are still not too clear (Atassi, 1975). Undue speculation is inadvisable at this stage.

Significantly, both rabbits and goats make antibodies to native lysozyme with identical specificities for the same three antigenic sites. Also, antibodies produced in both rabbits and goats to sperm-whale myoglobin recognized the same antigenic sites on myoglobin (Atassi, 1975, 1977b). In myoglobin, it has recently been shown (Kazim and Atassi, 1977a) that the antigenicity of its sites is inherent in their three-dimensional locations and is independent of any sequence identities between the immunogen myoglobin and the myoglobin of the immunized host. In fact, we have recently predicted and confirmed by synthesis two antigenic regions of human hemoglobin (one each on the α and β chains) by extrapolation of the three-dimensional location of an antigenic site of sperm-whale myoglobin (Kazim and Atassi, 1977b). Furthermore, rabbits immunized with rabbit myoglobin produced autoantibodies against this protein (Kazim and Atassi, 1977c). These findings strongly demonstrated that the conformational uniqueness of certain parts of a protein molecule, plays a most critical role in the antigenic expression of the protein (Kazim and Atassi, 1977c).

Finally, it may be of interest to provide some time perspectives. It took us eleven years of intensive research to determine the entire antigenic structure of myoglobin. With lysozyme, a ten-year period was needed. Thus the determination of the entire antigenic structure of a protein is not likely to be a routine endeavour in the foreseeable future. It will continue to be a complex task of immense proportions that demands a unique blend of imagination, chemical expertise and sustained long-term determination. This concludes the antigenic structure of hen egg-white lysozyme.

XIV. ACKNOWLEDGEMENTS

The work was supported by a grant (AI 13181) from the National Institute of Allergy and Infectious Diseases, and in part by a grant (AM 18920) from the Institute of Arthritis and Metabolic Diseases, National Institutes of Health, U.S. Public Health Service. The early stages of the work were sponsored by a grant (71-910) from the American Heart Association and carried out during the tenure to the author of an Established Investigatorship of the American Heart Association.

REFERENCES

Amzel, L.M., Poljak, R.J., Saul, F., Varga, J.M. and Richards, F.F. (1974) Proc. Natl. Acad. Sci. U.S. 71:1427.

Arnon, R. and Sela, M. (1969) Proc. Natl. Acad. Sci. U.S. 62:163.

Arnon, R., Maron, E., Sela, M. and Anfinsen, C.B. (1971) Proc. Natl. Acad. Sci. U.S. 63:1450.

Atassi, M.Z. (1967a) Biochem. J. 102:488.

Atassi, M.Z. (1967b) Biochem. J. 103:29.

Atassi, M.Z. (1968) Biochemistry 7:3078.

Atassi, M.Z. (1969) Immunochemistry 6:801.

Atassi, M.Z. (1970) Biochim. Biophys. Acta 221:612.

Atassi, M.Z. (1972) Specific Receptors of Antibodies, Antigens and Cells, 118-136. 3rd International Convocation of Immunology, June 12-15, S. Karger.

Atassi, M.Z. (1975) Immunochemistry 12:423.

Atassi, M.Z. (1977a) Immunochemistry of Proteins (Atassi, M.Z., Ed.), Volume 1, p. 1-161, Plenum, New York.

Atassi, M.Z. (1977b) Immunochemistry of Proteins (Atassi, M.Z., Ed.), Volume 2, p. 77-176, Plenum, New York.

Atassi, M.Z. (1977c) Adv. in Exp. Med. and Biol. Volume 86 A, p. 89-139, Plenum, New York.

Atassi, M.Z. and Habeeb, A.F.S.A. (1969) Biochemistry 8:1385.

Atassi, M.Z. and Habeeb, A.F.S.A. (1972) Methods in Enzymology 25B:546.

Atassi, M.Z. and Habeeb, A.F.S.A. (1977) Immunochemistry of Proteins (Atassi, M.Z., Ed.), Volume 2, p. 177-264, Plenum, New York.

Atassi, M.Z. and Koketsu, J. (1975) Immunochemistry 12:741.

Atassi, M.Z. and Lee, C.-L. (1978a) Biochem. J., in press.

Atassi, M.Z. and Lee, C.-L. (1978b) Biochem. J., in press.

Atassi, M.Z. and Pai, R.C. (1975) Immunochemistry 12:735.

Atassi, M.Z. and Rosemblatt, M.C. (1974) J. Biol. Chem. 249:482.

Atassi, M.Z. and Saplin, B.J. (1968) Biochemistry 7:688.

Atassi, M.Z. and Thomas, A.V. (1969) Biochemistry 8:3385.

Atassi, M.Z. and Zablocki, W. (1975) Biochim. Biophys. Acta 386:233.

Atassi, M.Z. and Zablocki, W. (1976) J. Biol. Chem. 251:1653.

Atassi, M.Z. and Zablocki, W. (1977) J. Biol. Chem., 252:8784.

Atassi, M.Z., Habeeb, A.F.S.A. and Rydstedt, L. (1970a) Biochim. Biophys. Acta 200:184.

Atassi, M.Z., Tarlowski, D.P. and Paull, J.H. (1970b) Biochim. Biophys. Acta 221:623.

Atassi, M.Z., Perlstein, M.T. and Habeeb, A.F.S.A. (1971) J. Biol. Chem. 246:4291.

Atassi, M.Z., Suliman, A.M. and Habeeb, A.F.S.A. (1972) Immunochemistry 9:907.

Atassi, M.Z., Habeeb, A.F.S.A. and Ando, K. (1973) Biochim. Biophys. Acta 303:203.

Atassi, M.Z., Rosemblatt, M.C. and Habeeb, A.F.S.A. (1974) Immunochemistry 11:495.

Atassi, M.Z., Suliman, A.M. and Habeeb, A.F.S.A (1975a) Biochim. Biophys. Acta 405:452.

Atassi, M.Z., Litowich, M.T. and Andres, S.F. (1975b) Immunochemistry 12:727.

Atassi, M.Z., Habeeb, A.F.S.A. and Lee, C.-L. (1976a) Immunochemistry 13:547.

Atassi, M.Z., Koketsu, J. and Habeeb, A.F.S.A. (1976b) Biochim. Biophys. Acta 420:358.

Atassi, M.Z., Lee, C.-L. and Habeeb, A.F.S.A. (1976c) Immunochemistry 13:7.

Atassi, M.Z., Lee, C.-L. and Pai, R.C. (1976d) Biochim. Biophys. Acta 427:745.

Blake, C.C.F., Koenig, D.F., Mair, G.A., North, A.C.T., Phillips, D.C. and Sarma, V.R. (1965) Nature (Lond) 206:757.

Blake, C.C.F., Mair, G.A., North, A.C.T., Phillips, D.C. and Sarma, V.R. (1967) Proc. Roy. Soc. (London) Ser. B167:365.

Brown, R.K. (1962) J. Biol. Chem. 238:1162.

Brown, R.K., Durieux, J., Delaney, R., Leikem, E. and Clark, B.J. (1959) Ann. N.Y. Acad. Sci. 81:524.

Canfield, R.E. (1963a) J. Biol. Chem. 238:2691.

Canfield, R.E. (1963b) J. Biol. Chem. 238:2698.

Canfield, R.E. and Liu, A.K. (1965) J. Biol. Chem. 240:1997.

Ely, K.R., Girling, R.L., Schiffer, M., Cunningham, D.E. and Edmundson, A.B. (1973) Biochemistry 12:4233.

Fujio, H., Imanishi, M., Nishioka, K. and Amano, T. (1968a) Biken. J. 11:207.

Fujio, H., Imanishi, M., Nishioka, K. and Amano, T. (1968b) Biken. J. 11:219.

Geiger, B. and Arnon, R. (1974) Eur. J. Immunol. 4:632.

Gerwing, J. and Thompson, K. (1968) Biochemistry 7:3888.

Ha, Y.M., Fujio, H., Sakato, N. and Amano, T. (1975) Biken. J. 18:47.

Habeeb, A.F.S.A. and Atassi, M.Z. (1969) Immunochemistry 6:555.

Habeeb, A.F.S.A. and Atassi, M.Z. (1970) Biochemistry 9:4939.

Habeeb, A.F.S.A. and Atassi, M.Z. (1971a) Biochim. Biophys. Acta 236:131.

Habeeb, A.F.S.A. and Atassi, M.Z. (1971b) Immunochemistry 8:1047.

Habeeb, A.F.S.A. and Atassi, M.Z. (1976) J. Biol. Chem. 251:4616.

Habeeb, A.F.S.A., Atassi, M.Z.,and Lee, C.-L. (1974) Biochim. Biophys. Acta 342:389.

Imoto, T., Johnson, L.N., North, A.C.T., Phillips, D.C. and Rupley, J.A. (1972) The Enzymes (Boyer, P.D., Ed.) 7:665. Academic Press, N.Y.

Johnson, E.R., Anderson, W.L., Wetlaufer, D.B., Lee, C-L. and Atassi, M.Z. (1978) J. Biol. Chem., in press.

Jollès, J., Jauregui-Adell, J., Bernier, I. and Jollès, P. (1963) Biochim. Biophys. Acta 78:668.

Jollès, J., Sportono, G. and Jollès, P. (1965) Nature (Lond) 208:1204.

Kazim, A.L. and Atassi, M.Z. (1977a) Biochim. Biophys. Acta 494:277.

Kazim, A.L. and Atassi, M.Z. (1977b) Biochem. J. 167:275.

Kazim, A.L. and Atassi, M.Z. (1977c) Immunochemistry, in press.

Koketsu, J. and Atassi, M.Z. (1973) Biochim. Biophys. Acta 328:289.

Koketsu, J. and Atassi, M.Z. (1974a) Immunochemistry 11:1.

Koketsu, J. and Atassi, M.Z. (1974b) Biochim. Biophys. Acta 342:21.

Komatsu, T., Shinka, S., Dohi, Y. and Amano, T. (1975) Biken. J. 18:61.

Lee, C.-L. and Atassi, M.Z. (1973) Biochemistry 12:2690.

Lee, C.-L. and Atassi, M.Z. (1975) Biochim. Biophys. Acta 405:464.

Lee, C.-L. and Atassi, M.Z. (1976) Biochem. J. 159:89.

Lee, C.-L. and Atassi, M.Z. (1977a) Biochem. J. 167:571.

Lee, C.-L. and Atassi, M.Z. (1977b) Biochim. Biophys. Acta 495:354.

Lee, C.-L., Atassi, M.Z. and Habeeb, A.F.S.A. (1975) Biochim. Biophys. Acta 400:423.

Lee, C.-L, Pai, R.C. and Atassi, M.Z. (1976) Immunochemistry 13:681.

Maron, E., Shiozawa, C., Arnon, R. and Sela, M. (1971) Biochemistry 10:763.

Padlan, E.A., Segal, D.M., Spande, T.F., Davies, D.R., Rudikoff, S. and Potter, M. (1973) Nature New Biol. 245:165.

Pai, R.-C. and Atassi, M.Z. (1975) Immunochemistry 12:285.

Poljak, R.J., Amzel, L.M., Avey, H.P., Chen, B.L., Phizackerly, R.P. and Saul, F. (1973) Proc. Natl. Acad. Sci. U.S. 70:3305.

Sakato, N., Fujio, H. and Amano, T. (1972) Biken J. 15:135.

Schiffer, M., Girling, R.L., Ely, K.R. and Edmundson, A.B. (1973) Biochemistry 12:4620.

Shinka, S., Imanishi, M., Miyagawa, N., Amano, T., Inouye, M. and Tsugita, A. (1967) Biken. J. 10:89.

Sokolovsky, M., Riordan, J.F. and Vallee, B.L. (1967) Biochim. Biophys. Res. Commun. 27:20.

Taubman, M.T. and Atassi, M.Z. (1968) Biochem. J. 106:829.

Young, J.D. and Leung, C.Y. (1970) Biochemistry 9:2755.

IMMUNOCHEMISTRY OF BOVINE SERUM ALBUMIN

A.F.S.A. Habeeb

Department of Biochemistry and Nutrition
Medical Sciences Campus, University of Puerto Rico
G.P.O. Box 5067, San Juan, Puerto Rico 00936

I. INTRODUCTION

A basic question that faces immunochemistry, is what constitutes an antigenic determinant? What are the characteristic features that cause a given arrangement of amino acid residues in a given sequence and conformation to be recognized as antigenic and to elicit the synthesis of antibody. Thus in sperm whale myoglobin, the antigenic reactivity is localized in five regions, each containing 6 - 7 amino acid residues which are adjacent in sequence (Atassi, 1975). On the other hand the antigenic reactivity of lyzozyme resides in three surface regions each consisting of 6 - 7 amino acid residues that are distant in sequence but brought in close proximity by the native folding of the polypeptide chain (Atassi and Habeeb 1977). The present immunochemical studies on bovine serum albumin reveal a novel feature namely that bovine serum albumin (BSA) contains repeating identical or very similar antigenic determinants, this evidence was obtained from studying the immunochemistry of fragments derived from different parts of the molecule. The amino acid sequence of BSA (Brown, 1975) reveals the proteins to consist of three compact regions having some degree of homologies each containing 190 amino acid residues and the compact structure is maintained by 17 disulfide bonds. The disulfide bonds are arranged in nine loops, eight of which contain double cystine bridges and one loop has a single cystine residue. Of the eight loops containing double disulfide bridges, seven loops have adjacent half cystines, each of which is linked to a different half cystine at a different site on the polypeptide chain. The disulfide bonds are important in maintaining the native antigenic determinants since reduction and alkylation which is accompanied by drastic conformational changes abolishes completely the reaction of reduced BSA with anti BSA (Habeeb and Borella, 1966). However on reduction and reoxidation, a stable monomer was recovered whose conformation was significantly different from native BSA yet it reacted as well as BSA with anti BSA (Peters and Goetzl, 1969). This unusual behavior may be due to reformation of mismatched disulfide bonds within the two cystine residues at a loop and not between the disulfides from different loops. Such restriction in the reformation of the disulfide bonds may lead to the generation of the antigenic sites despite the unfolding at regions outside the antigenic reactive sites. At least, in the case of BSA, which is rather unique, the immunochemical reactivity can not be used as a criterion for recovery of the native conformation.

II. FRAGMENTATION OF BOVINE SERUM ALBUMIN

As a prerequisite for localizing the antigenic determinants, immunochemically reactive fragments of BSA were obtained. The first fragment was obtained from native BSA with its intact disulfide bonds after reversible modification of the free amino groups with citraconic anhydride (Habeeb et al., 1974; Atassi et al., 1976). The modification induces conformational changes in BSA which renders it susceptible to tryptic hydrolysis at arginine residues. After deblocking it is possible to effect hydrolysis at lysine residues. However it was found that only fragments obtained by cleavage at arginine residues were immunochemically active while those obtained from cleavage at both lysine and arginine residues were immunochemically inert. After tryptic hydrolysis of citraconylated BSA, a fragment was isolated by gel filtration on Sephadex G 100 in a pure form as shown by disc electrophoresis in SDS gels. From the amino acid analysis and the amino acid sequence of the first 14 amino acid residues it was assigned sequence Phe 11 — Arg 193 (less Arg 143).

The fragment inhibited the reaction of BSA - anti BSA serum by 80 - 83%. By using the IgG fraction of anti BSA, the inhibition was 88%. Performic acid oxidation or cleavage at lysine residues abolished the immunochemical reactivity of the fragment. Thus the intactness of the disulfide bonds is important for constituting the antigenic reactive sites. Moreover scission of polypeptide chain at lysine residues disrupts the antigenic reactive sites leading to complete loss of its ability to inhibit the reaction of BSA - anti BSA.

An immunoabsorbent column of the fragment removed 84 - 88.6% of antibody to BSA from anti BSA serum. Moreover a fluorescein derivative (with fluorescein isothiocyanate) of the fragment was found to co-elute with anti BSA on Sephadex G 100 column and to bind two moles antibody/mole fragment. The fact that one fragment comprising about a third of the albumin molecule can account for almost the entire immunochemical reactivity of the molecule as shown by inhibition and by binding to an immunoabsorbent was significant and was rationalized by advancing the concept that the BSA molecule carries repeating identical or very similar antigenic determinants.

Further support to this concept emerged from the isolation of another immunochemically reactive fragment from tryptic hydrolyzate of native BSA which represented the last third of the molecule.

In studying the susceptibility of BSA to tryptic cleavage, it was observed that different batches from the same manufacturer as well as batches from different suppliers exhibited significant variation in their tryptic hydrolysis (Habeeb, 1977). This variability was considered in part to be the outcome of conformational non-identity and was revealed rather clearly when the availability of the disulfide bonds to reduction at the neutral transition was used as a conformational probe.

Figure 1 shows the availability of the disulfide bonds to reduction of five batches of Cohn fraction V. It is observed that during the neutral transition gradual unfolding of the BSA molecule with concomitant exposure of the disulfide bonds to reduction occurred as the pH was increased from pH 7 - 9.5. Not only was the availability of the disulfide bonds to reduction capable of demonstrating the degree of unfolding of the molecule at the neutral transition but it was also able to discriminate rather effectively between the dif-

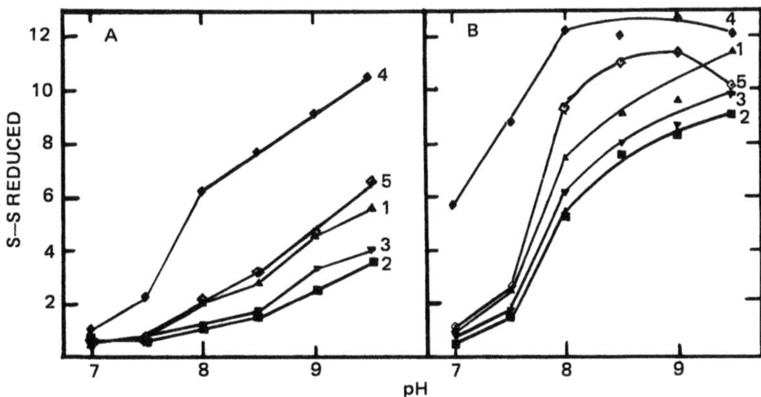

Figure 1. The number of disulfide bonds (S-S) reduced with β-mercaptoethanol as a function of pH in various batches of Cohn fraction V. A, reduction at room temperature; B, reduction at 40°.

ferent conformational states of the different batches at given pH and at a given temperature. The susceptibility to tryptic hydrolysis paralleled the availability of the disulfide bonds to reduction, the latter was a measure of unfolding. Thus with Cohn fraction V only batch #4 was the most susceptible to reduction of its disulfide bonds and was fragmented with trypsin. Batch #1 resisted fragmentation with trypsin but on defatting both the availability of the disulfide bonds to reduction and the susceptibility to tryptic fragmentation were augmented. Similar results are shown for crystalline BSA (Fig. 2), of the three batches examined only batch 1 showed limited exposure of the disulfide bonds to reduction and was relatively resistant to tryptic cleavage. On defatting, all four batches (three were defatted Cohn fraction V) examined showed very similar reducibility and indicated that the variation among the different samples of BSA was due to fatty acid contaminants (Fig. 3).

Fragmentation of BSA was done in 1% solution in 0.01 M phosphate buffer for 1 hr at 40°C pH 8.2 with TPCK-trypsin (Habeeb and Atassi, 1976). The tryptic hydrolyzate was fractionated on Sephadex G 100 or G 75. Fraction 3, was found to be immunochemically reactive and was further purified by chromatography on DEAE-cellulose 0.005 M sodium phosphate pH 6.2 (Fig. 4). Amino acid analysis and sequence determination of the first 20 amino acids as well as the COOH-terminal residue indicated that the fragment corresponds to sequence Hist 377 - Lys 571. The fragment inhibited the reaction of BSA - anti BSA by about 90% and with IgG fraction of anti

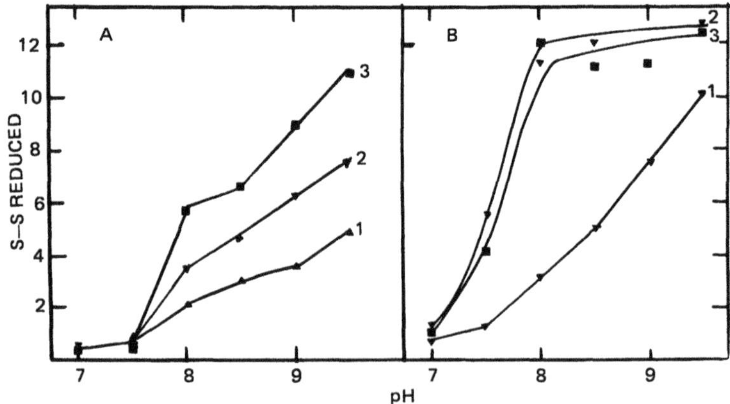

Figure 2. The number of disulfide bonds (S-S) reduced with β-mercaptoethanol as a function of pH in various batches of crystalline BSA. A, reduction at room temperature; B, reduction at 40°.

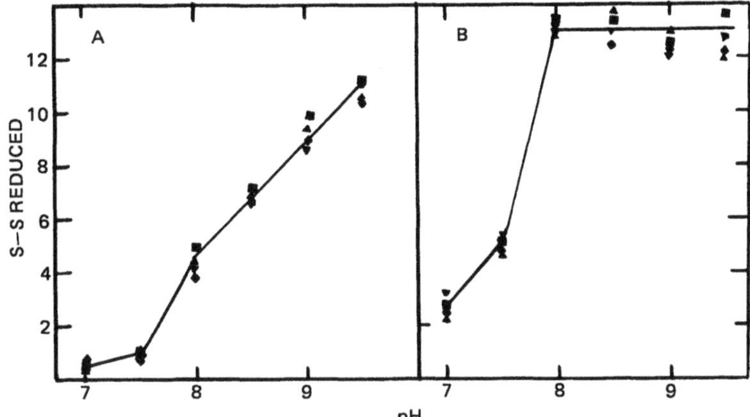

Figure 3. The number of disulfide bonds (S-S) reduced with β-mercaptoethanol as a function of pH in various batches of defatted BSA ▼, ▲, ♦ and ■ represent samples 1, 2, 3 and 4. A, reduction at room temperature; B, reduction at 40°.

BSA, the inhibition was 96% (Fig. 5). The molar excess of fragment required for 50% inhibition was 11. After reduction and alkylation, the immunochemical activity was completely abolished indicating the importance of the disulfide bonds for maintaining the antigenic reactive sites. An immunoabsorbent of the fragment trapped 90 - 95% of anti BSA indicating that the fragment 377 - 571 contains all the antigenic determinants of BSA. A fluorescein derivative of the fragment co-eluted with anti BSA and was found to bind 2 moles antibody/mole fragment (Fig. 6) indicating that it has two antigenic sites. These results are explainable by considering BSA to contain repeating identical or very similar antigenic sites.

III. CHEMICAL MODIFICATION OF FRAGMENT 377 - 571

In order to identify some of the amino acid residues at the antigenic sites chemical modification of tyrosines and methionines was undertaken (Kazim et al., 1977).

Modification of all four tyrosines (residues 399, 408, 449 and 494) of fragment 377 - 571 by tetranitromethane yielded a homogeneous derivative which suffered no conformational alteration as shown by ORD and CD but showed limited conformational changes by S-S availability. The nitrated derivative behaved in an identical manner to unmodified peptide 377 - 571 in precipitin reaction with

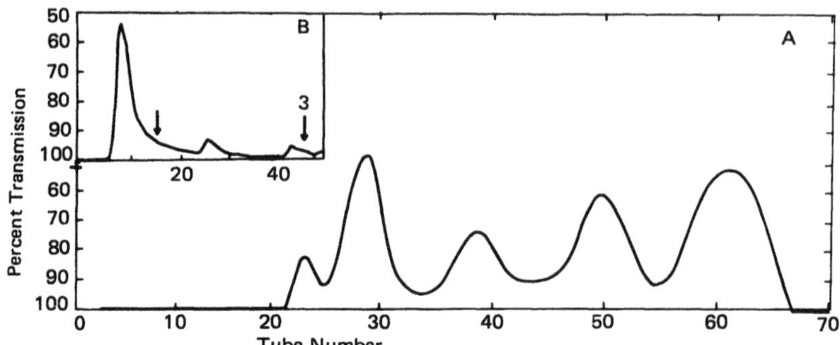

Figure 4. A, gel filtration pattern of a 40° tryptic hydrolyzate (1 hour) of albumin. The hydrolyzate (0.3 g) was applied onto a column (2.7 x 80 cm) of Sephadex G-100 which was eluted with 0.01 M NH_4HCO_3. Fractions (7.5 ml each) were analyzed continuously by an ultraviolet monitor. B, chromatographic pattern on DEAE-cellulose of Peak 3 from A. The material (100 mg) was applied on column (1.5 x 20 cm) which was subjected to stepwise elution. Initial elution was with 0.005 M sodium phosphate buffer at pH 6.2. At Position a the column was eluted with 0.0175 M phosphate, pH 6.2, and at Position b the eluent was changed to 0.0175 M phosphate, pH 6.2, + 0.077 M NaCl. Fractions (3 ml) were read continuously by an ultraviolet monitor.

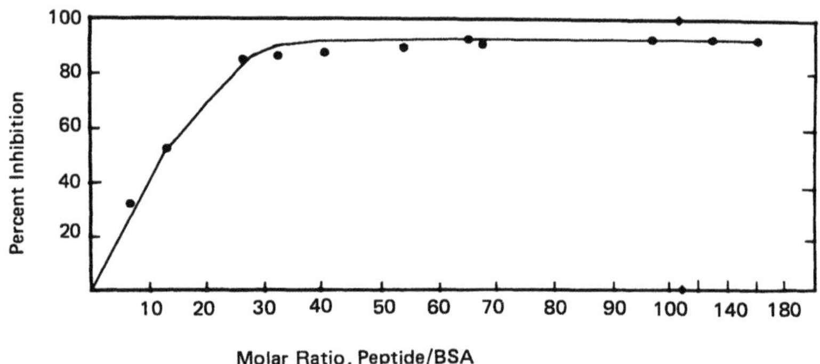

Figure 5. Inhibition of the precipitin reaction of native bovine serum albumin (BSA) with the IgG fraction of its homologous antiserum by fragment 377-571. The IgG fraction accounted for 96% of the total antibody activity in the antiserum.

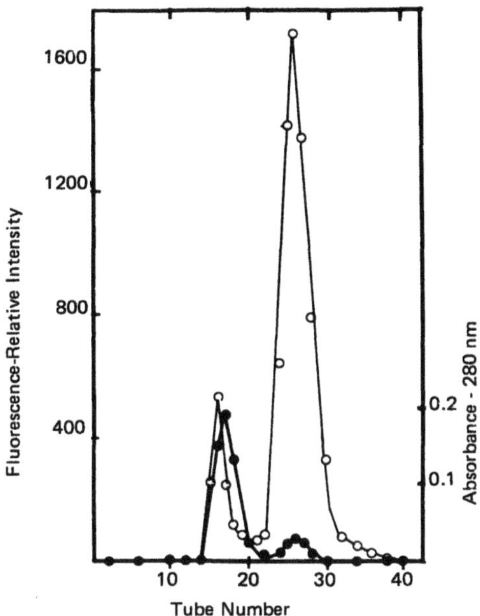

Figure 6. Elution pattern of a mixture of the IgG fraction of anti-albumin and the fluorescent derivative of fragment 377-571 on Sephadex G-100 (1.5 x 86 cm). Fractions (3.3ml) were monitored for absorbance at 280 nm (●), and for fluorescence at 520 nm (O).

antisera to 377 - 571 and was equally as effective in inhibiting the precipitin reaction of BSA with antisera to BSA. Also in immunoabsorbent studies, the derivative and the unmodified peptide absorbed identical amounts of antibodies from antisera to peptide 377-571 and antisera to BSA. The absence of changes in the immunochemical reactivity of this derivative indicates that tyrosines 399, 408, 449 and 494 do not contribute to the antigenic reactivity of this fragment.

When methionine 443 and 545 were modified by β-propiolactone the derivative precipitated 12 - 36% less than unmodified fragment with antisera to peptide 377 - 571. An immunoabsorbent of the methionine-modified fragment bound only 71% of anti fragment compared to unmodified fragment. Moreover the derivative inhibited the reaction of BSA - anti BSA by 59% compared to 92% for the unmodified fragment. This decrease in immunochemical reactivity implicated either one or both of methionine as being at or near an antigenic site.

IV. CROSS REACTIVITY OF FRAGMENTS PHE 11 - ARG 193 AND HIS 377 - LYS 571

Following the isolation of two immunochemically reactive fragments from BSA, the immunochemical cross reactivity of the fragments was examined. Antisera were prepared to each of the fragments (11 - 193 and 377 - 571) and the cross reactions of the two fragments as well as of BSA with these antisera were studied (Habeeb and Atassi, 1977). Fragment 377 - 571 was more antigenic in rabbits than fragment 11 - 193. Considerable cross reaction occurred with anti C-terminal fragment and BSA or N-terminal fragment.

A summary of cross reaction of antisera to C-terminal fragment (377 - 571) with BSA and fragment 11 - 193 is shown (Table I) only results from two rabbits are presented for clarity. Cross reaction of BSA increased with time after immunization and reached 60 - 85%. It was even more remarkable that these antisera which were against the C-terminal fragment exhibited a large cross reaction with the N-terminal piece which amounted to 40-94%. To ascertain that these were true immune reactions, absorption experiments were carried out.

The antisera to the C-terminal fragment were absorbed with BSA and the supernatant was reacted with BSA, N-terminal fragment and C-terminal fragment. With some antisera absorption with BSA removed all the reactivity with fragment 11 - 193 and with other bleedings from rabbits 487 or 489 a small amount of reactivity with fragment 11 - 193 persisted (8 - 15%). In most antisera, the decrease was accounted for quantitatively by the amount of antibody removed by BSA (Table II). Similarly absorption with the N-terminal fragment left little reaction with BSA. The homologous reaction decreased by an amount that is quantitatively accounted for by the antibody removed in the absorption step. Also the total antibody recovery approaches the expected value.

A summary of extensive immunoabsorbent studies with antisera to the C-terminal fragment is shown (Table III). It can be seen that all antibodies can be removed on any of the immunoabsorbents carrying the homologous antigen or BSA or the N-terminal fragment. In addition antibodies isolated on a given heterologous immunoabsorbent did not react best with the antigen used for the isolation, but their reactivity paralleled the behavior of the parent whole antiserum. The finding that an immunoabsorbent carrying BSA or fragment 11 - 193 removed quantitatively all the antibodies in antisera to fragment 377 - 571 clearly demonstrated that no new antigenic specificity was generated when fragment 377 - 571 was injected in rabbits. However the behaviors of the eluted antibody fractions in quantitative precipitin reactions towards BSA or fragment 377 - 571 compared well with those of the respective original antisera. These studies clearly indicate the presence of non precipitating antibodies, the pre-

Table I. Quantitative precipitin reactions with antisera to fragment 377 - 571[a]

Protein or Fragment	Antiserum B7[b]		Antiserum 487[c]		
	18-day bldg	10-wk bldg	7-10 wk pool	11-13 wk pool	14-16 wk pool
377 - 571	100	100	100	100	100
11 - 193	59.0	75.8	17.8	30.9	39.1
BSA	62.5	84.5	24.6	60.0	61.1

[a] Values are given in per cent precipitation at equivalence relative to reaction of fragment 377-571 with the respective antiserum as 100 per cent. Results represent the average of 3 to 6 replicate determinations which varied ± 1.2% or less. The per cent cross-reaction is based on mg of antibody precipitated at equivalence by each antigen as determined by the Folin reaction and comparison with a standard curve of rabbit IgG run simultaneously.

[b] Single bleedings of these antisera, at the indicated periods after the first injections, were studied.

[c] Antisera from weekly bleedings of the indicated periods after the first injection were pooled in groups, and these pools were studied.

Table II. Reactions of antisera to fragment 377-571 after quantitative absorption with BSA

Protein or Fragment	Reactions of absorbed antiserum relative to unabsorbed antiserum[a]				
	Antiserum B7		Antiserum 487		
	18-day bldg	10-wk bldg	7-10 wk pool	11-13 wk pool	14-16 wk pool
BSA	0	0	0	0	0
Fragment 11-193	0	0	8.0	15.2	15.2
Fragment 377-571	33.0	18.5	45.7	32.6	30.9
Ab absorbed by BSA[b]	67.1	83.3	23.9	63.1	61.7
Total Ab recovery[c]	100.1	101.8	69.6	95.7	92.6

[a] Values were determined at equivalence from precipitin curves on each antigen with the antiserum supernatant obtained after absorption of the whole antiserum with BSA at equivalence and removal of the BSA-immune precipitate by centrifugation. Results are given in per cent reaction with the absorbed antiserum relative to reaction of unabsorbed antiserum (similarly diluted) with fragment 377-571 as 100%. Each value is the average of 3 or 6 replicate determinations which varied $\pm$ 1% or less. Per cent reactions were based on mg antibody precipitated, determined as in footnote (a) of Table I.

[b] This represents the amount of antibody removed upon absorption of the whole antiserum by BSA at equivalence.

[c] Total antibody was the sum of antibody removed by BSA and the residual reaction of the supernatant (absorbed antiserum) with fragment 377-571.

Table III. Immunoabsorbent studies on antisera (489) to fragment 377 - 571

		Immunoabsorbent, antibody recovered and its reactions[a]		
	Whole	Immunoabsorbent of fragment 377-571	BSA-immunoabsorbent	Immunoabsorbent of fragment 11-193
Antigen	Antiserum	Ab eluted[c]	Ab eluted[c]	Ab eluted[c]
I. Antiserum of the 7-10 week pool				
Ab recovered (mg)[b]		7.8	7.9	7.7
BSA	39	40	49	29
Fragment 377-571	100	100	100	100
II. Antiserum of the 11-13 week pool				
Ab recovered (mg)[b]		11.7	11.9	11.3
BSA	72	75.4	77	n.d.
Fragment 377-571	100	100	100	n.d.

[a] Values are given in per cent quantitative precipitin reaction at equivalence relative to reaction of fragment 377-571 as 100 per cent. Results represent the average of triplicate analyses which varied $\pm$ 1.5 per cent or less.

[b] Amount of antibody recovered from 1 ml of whole antiserum applied on the immunoabsorbent.

[c] This represents the amount and reactivity of the antibody fraction that was displaced from the immunoabsorbent by 5M guanidine hydrochloride. After dialysis against 0.01 M phosphate buffer at pH 7.4 containing 0.15 M NaCl, its quantitative precipitin reactions with BSA and fragment 377-571 were determined.

cipitating efficiency of which is best with the homologous antigen. Although they do not precipitate efficiently with BSA or fragment 11 - 193 yet they can be removed entirely by their respective immuno-absorbents.

Antisera to one fragment are recognized totally by the other fragment as well as by intact BSA. However, they only showed differences in their abilities to form immune precipitates with the three antigens but not in their ability to bind. The present data strongly establish that BSA has repeating identical or similar antigenic determinants. It is not implied that one site is repeating six times but at least two sites are repeating three times each. Furthermore no particularly unique antigenic specificity that is distinct to the immunogen is generated regardless of whether the immunogen is BSA, the N-terminal fragment or C-terminal fragment.

V. CROSS REACTIVITY OF SERUM ALBUMINS FROM DIFFERENT SPECIES

Immunochemical cross reactivity among serum albumins from various species BSA, goat serum albumin (GSA), pig serum albumin (PSA), horse serum albumin (ESA) and human serum albumin (HSA) has been attributed to the presence of similar rather than identical antigenic sites. Cross reactivity as revealed by immunoabsorbents was shown to be three - to four - fold more than that demonstrated by precipitin reaction. Such a behavior was indicative of the presence of non precipitating antibody which was not revealed by precipitin reaction. That this was the case, was demonstrated by the decreased precipitability of the eluted antibody when reacted with the homologous albumin as that on the immunoabsorbent (Table IV).

It was found possible to obtain immunochemically reactive fragments by fragmentation of the albumins with trypsin under conditions similar to that for BSA. With HSA, it was found necessary to use fatty acid-free HSA to get meaningful fragmentation pattern. The tryptic product was chromatographed on Sephadex G 75 (Fig. 7) and a large fragment was isolated from the hydrolyzates (mol. wt 21,000 - 23,000) which did not precipitate with the homologous antiserum but inhibited the immune precipitation of the homologous system (Table V).

Immunoabsorbents prepared with these fragments were found to trap antibodies against the homologous native protein (Table VI). The fragment isolated from HSA was found to inhibit the reaction of HSA-anti HSA by 91% and to trap 93% of anti HSA indicating that the fragment contains all the antigenic reactive sites, a situation reminiscent of BSA which is considered to contain repeating identical or similar antigenic determinant. From amino acid analysis and sequence studies, the fragment was assigned to sequence Leu 198 - Lys 389 of HSA.

Table IV. Immunochemical cross-reaction of anti-bovine serum albumin and heterologous serum albumins determined on immunoabsorbents

Anti-BSA	Seph-GSA	Seph-ESA	Seph-PSA	Seph-HSA
Absorbed[a]	71%	35.7%	66.4%	39%
Antibody precipitating with BSA	83.7%	51.7%	71.8%	43%
Antibody precipitating with homologous antigens as that of immunoabsorbent	67%	13.9%	24.4%	14.5%
Unabsorbed[b]	29%	64.3%	33.6%	61%
Antibody precipitating with BSA	67.3%	86.8%	88%	92.4%

[a]Antibody absorbed was eluted from immunoabsorbent by 5 M guanidine HCl pH 7 and then dialyzed versus water followed by phosphate saline buffer pH 7.2. The amount of total antibody was computed from absorbance at 280 nm using a factor of 1.38 for absorbance of 1 mg antibody per mil. Precipitin curves were done on the antibody using BSA and also the homologous native antigen as that on immunoabsorbent.

[b]The unabsorbed antibody was absorbed on Sepharose BSA immunoabsorbent and after elution with 5M guanidine HCl and dialysis, its concentration was calculated from its absorbance at 280 nm. Precipitin curves were done using BSA as antigen and per cent of precipitating antibody was estimated.

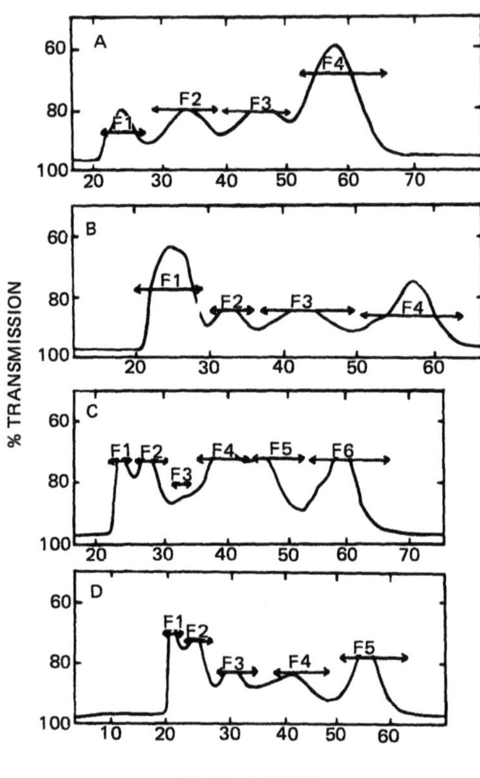

Figure 7. Gel filtration of tryptic hydrolyzates of various serum albumins. The hydrolyzate (0.3 gm) was applied onto a column (2.7 x 80 cm) of Sephadex G-75 which was eluted with 0.01 M NH_4HCO_3. Fractions (7.5 ml) were analyzed continuously by an ultraviolet monitor. Tryptic hydrolyzates of A, GSA; B, ESA; C, PSA and D, HSA.

Table V. Maximum inhibition of the homologous antigen-antibody reaction by serum albumin fragments*

	F2 of GSA	F3 of PSA	F3 of HSA
Anti HSA			
R#155 Pool 1			76%
R#155 Pool 2			79%
R#156 Pool 1			91%
R#156 Pool 2			94%
Anti GSA			
R#157	66%		
R#158	31.6%		
Anti PSA			
G#533		81%	
R#215		79%	
R#216		68%	

*The fragment was incubated with the homologous antiserum for 1 hr at 40°C, then at 4° for 24 hr, after which the homologous serum albumin was added at an equivalence amount, mixed, incubated at 40°C for 1 hr then overnight at 4°. The amount of the immune precipitate was quantitated. The per cent inhibition was calculated from the amount of decrease in immune precipitate in presence of fragment to that in absence of fragment. R-refers to antisera raised in rabbits and G-refers to antiserum raised in a goat.

Table VI. Absorption of anti-albumin on a fragment immunoabsorbent

	Anti GSA R#157	Anti PSA R#215	Anti HSA R#156 Pool 1
Absorbed on Sepharose-fragment[a]	43.3%	56%	93.4%
2nd absorption on Sepharose-fragment[b]	0	0	0
Absorbed on Sepharose-albumin[c]	56.7%	44%	6.6%

[a] Antiserum was applied on an immunoabsorbent prepared with a fragment obtained from homologous albumin. Thus anti GSA was applied on Sepharose-GSA fragment; anti PSA on PSA fragment immunoabsorbent and anti HSA on HSA fragment immunoabsorbent. The antibody absorbed was eluted with 5 M guanidine HCl pH 7 and then dialyzed against water followed by phosphate saline buffer pH 7.2. The amount of total antibody was calculated from absorbance at 280 nm using a value of 1.38 for absorbance of 1 mg antibody per mil.

[b] Unabsorbed serum from previous step was put a second time on the same immunoabsorbent, washed with phosphate saline buffer pH 7.2, and eluted with 5 M guanidine HCl and proceed as above.

[c] The unabsorbed serum was put on an immunoabsorbent prepared with the homologous albumin. The absorbed antibody was eluted with 5 M guanidine HCl, dialyzed and its concentration determined.

VI. SUMMARY

Two fragments were isolated from BSA one was derived from the first terminal third of the molecule and the second from the last third of the molecule. Each fragment inhibited the reaction of BSA-anti BSA by 90% or better. An immunoabsorbent of each bound 90% of anti BSA. Each fragment bound two antibody molecules per mole of fragment. These results are explained by the concept that BSA contains repeating identical or similar antigenic determinants.

Conformational non identity of various batches of BSA was revealed by reactivity of the disulfide bonds at the neutral transition.

Trypsin was found to cleave GSA, PSA, and HSA to yield an immunochemically reactive fragment. At least in the case of HSA, the fragment exhibited all the immunochemical reactivity of the native protein.

REFERENCES

Atassi, M.Z. (1975) Immunochemistry 12, 423.

Atassi, M.Z., Habeeb, A.F.S.A., and Lee, C.-L. (1976) Immunochemistry 13, 547.

Atassi, M.Z. and Habeeb, A.F.S.A. (1977) in Immunochemistry of Proteins (M.Z. Atassi, ed.) Vol II pp 177-264.

Brown, J.R. (1975) Fed. Proc. 34, 2105 Abst.

Habeeb, A.F.S.A. (1977) Fed. Proc. 36, 838 Abst.

Habeeb, A.F.S.A. and Atassi, M.Z. (1976) J. Biol. Chem. 251, 4616.

Habeeb, A.F.S.A. and Atassi, M.Z. (1977) Immunochemistry 14, 449.

Habeeb, A.F.S.A. and Borella, L. (1966) J. Immun. 97, 951.

Habeeb, A.F.S.A., Atassi, M.Z. and Lee, C.-L. (1974) Biochim. Biophys. Acta 324, 389.

Kazim, A.L., Habeeb, A.F.S.A. and Atassi, M.Z. (1977) Fed. Proc. 36, 742 Abst.

Peters, J.H., and Goetzl, E. (1969) J. Biol. Chem. 244, 2068.

ANALYSIS OF A COMPLEX ANTIGENIC SITE ON HORSE CYTOCHROME *c*[*]

Ronald Jemmerson and E. Margoliash

Department of Biochemistry and Molecular Biology

Northwestern University, Evanston, Illinois 60201

Abstract

Of the antigenic determinants so far identified for cytochrome *c*, only one involves more than a single amino acid substitution between the immunogen and host proteins. Both a threonine at position 89 and a glutamic acid at position 92 control one of the three antigenic sites identified in horse cytochrome *c*, as expressed in rabbits. Three antibody subpopulations, all directed against this region of the molecule, were isolated from the serum of a single rabbit by adsorption on a series of insolubilized cytochromes *c*. Antibody fluorescence quenching titrations with a variety of cytochromes *c* were used to confirm the identification of the antigenic determinant and to examine the subtle differences in the specificities of the three subpopulations. The determinant in the region of Residues 89-92 is affected by amino acid substitutions at positions 88 and 96. Since all these residues are in an α-helix the farthest distance between them is only 12 Å and therefore, the Residues 88-96 can all be accommodated in the antibody binding site. The ability to identify and describe the antigenic determinant, as well as separate subpopulations directed against this site, demonstrates the resolution possible using a series of homologous protein antigens.

[*]Supported by Grants AI-12001 and GM-19121 from the National Institutes of Health.

Antigenic Determinants Controlled By Single Amino Acid Residues

The cytochromes *c* constitute a homologous series of naturally occurring protein derivatives, for which the amino acid sequences of more than 85 of these proteins from different eukaryotes are known (Dayhoff, 1972, Borden and Margoliash, 1976). Their polypeptide-backbone spatial structures are the same (Dickerson and Timkovich, 1975), so that an immune response evoked by one such protein but not another must be due to antigenic determinants on the immunogen that are local changes in amino acid side chains at the surface of the protein corresponding to the sequence differences between the cytochromes *c* examined. Such determinants have been described as *topographic* (Urbanski and Margoliash, 1976, 1977).

Table I

Antigenic Determinants That Have Been Identified in Cytochrome c

Amino Acid Sequence Comparison

Cytochrome *c*	11111 12345	4 4	44445 67890	55666 89012	8 3	88999 89012
Rabbit	VQKCA	V	FSYTD	TWGED	A	KDERA
Mouse	VQKCA	A	FSYTD	TWGED	A	KGERA
Guanaco	VQKCA	V	FSYTD	TWGEE	A	KGERA
Horse	VQKCA	P	FTYTD	TWKEE	A	KTERE
Human	IMKCS	P	YSYTA	IWGED	V	KEERA

Residues not listed are identical for the cytochromes *c* compared. The residue positions are given vertically, e.g. 1 1 referring to Residue 11, etc.

Cytochrome *c*	Host	Variant Residue in Antigenic Determinants
Mouse	Rabbit	[Ala,44][Asp,62][Gly,89]
Rabbit	Mouse	[Val,44][Asp,62][Asp,89]
Guanaco	Rabbit	[Glu,62][Gly,89]
Guanaco	Mouse	[Val,44][Glu,62]
Horse*	Rabbit	[Pro,44][Lys,60][Thr,89-Glu,92]
Human*	Rabbit	[Ile,58]

*Incompletely characterized antigenic structure

Topographic determinants have been identified for mouse and guanaco cytochromes *c* as manifested in rabbits, and rabbit and guanaco cytochromes *c* as manifested in mice (Urbanski and Margoliash, 1977). One of at least four antigenic determinants has so far been identified for human cytochrome *c* (Nisonoff et al., 1970) and three for the horse protein as manifested in rabbits (Eng and Reichlin, 1977, Jemmerson, Brautigan, and Margoliash, 1977). Each of these identified determinants appears in one of three regions of the cytochrome *c* molecule: Residue 44; Residues 58-62; and Residues 89-92 (Table I).

Most of these determinants result from single amino acid residue replacements between the immunizing and host proteins. An exception is the autoimmune-type of response elicited against the region of Residue 62 in rabbit and mouse cytochromes *c* when rabbits and mice are immunized with the other's protein. Both cytochromes *c* have an aspartyl residue at position 62 and are identical elsewhere throughout that region of the molecule. Cytochromes *c* that carry a glutamyl residue at position 62, but are otherwise identical in the region, bind the antibodies with an increased affinity (Urbanski and Margoliash, 1977). It appears that B-cells that recognize a glutamyl residue at position 62 respond to an aspartic acid at that position when the host is presented with such a determinant under immunizing conditions. Thus, even this autoimmune-type of determinant can be classified as a site involving a single amino acid replacement.

When variations of more than one residue between immunizing and host proteins occur in spatial proximity on the molecule, one can no longer rely on the stoichiometry of the antigen-antibody reaction to establish whether these sequence differences represent one or more than one antigenic determinant. Indeed, an antibody binding to one residue may well hinder the binding of a different antibody to another close by, without being affected by the presence of the second variant residue. If the residue differences all affect the antibodies elicited by this region, one may consider it to constitute a complex site. If some antibody populations bind to one variant residue and are unaffected by the others, while other populations bind to the latter and not the former, then one must regard the region as containing more than one independant determinant. The only case in cytochrome *c* examined to date is that of Residues 89 and 92, in the horse protein, which, as described below, were found to constitute a complex site rather than two independant determinants. (Jemmerson and Margoliash, 1977).

A Determinant Controlled by Two Amino Acid Residues

We have been able to fractionate from a single rabbit anti-horse cytochrome *c* serum three antibody populations in approximately equal amounts (9mg/100ml serum) directed against both amino acid residues 89 and 92. The antibody isolation scheme is shown in Figure 1 along with a comparison of the amino acid sequences of the cytochromes *c* used in the isolation.

Amino Acid Sequence Comparison

Cytochrome c	3	5	33	44	47	58	60	62	89	92	96	100	103	104
Horse	V	K	H	P	T	T	K	E	T	E	A	K	N	E
Rabbit	V	K	H	V	S	T	G	D	D	A	A	K	N	E
Guanaco	V	K	H	V	S	T	G	E	G	A	A	K	N	E
Beef	V	K	H	P	S	T	G	E	G	E	A	K	N	E
Mouse c_t	A	A	W	P	S	V	S	E	S	E	K	Q	S	S

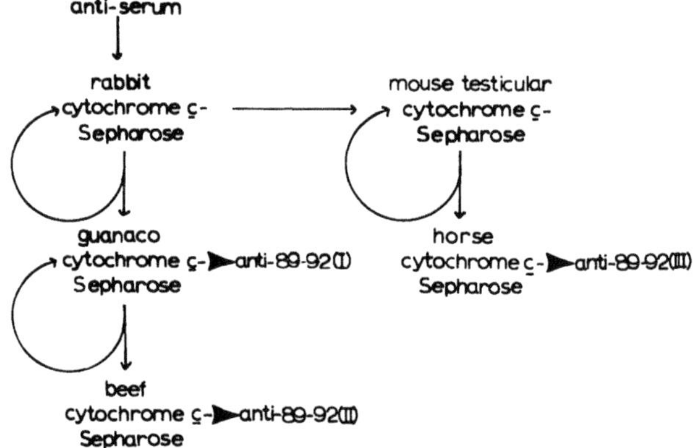

Figure 1: *Isolation of Rabbit Antibody Populations Directed Against the Region of Residues 89 and 92 in Horse Cytochrome c. The Table* at the top of the figure lists the sequence differences between the cytochromes *c* employed. The residue positions are numbered vertically. *The Figure* is a flow diagram of the successive adsorptions on columns of insolubilized cytochrome *c* used for the fractionation of the antiserum (Rabbit 2007). The vertical arrows refer to non-adsorbed material, while the horizontal arrows refer to adsorbed antibodies. Circular arrows indicate that the adsorption was repeated until no additional antibody could be removed.

Antiresidues 89-92 (Subpopulation I). Insolubilized rabbit cytochrome *c* adsorbs approximately 50% of the rabbit anti-horse cytochrome *c* antibodies. The Sepharose-bound guanaco protein is capable of adsorbing some of the antibody material not adsorbed to the rabbit protein. Since guanaco and rabbit cytochromes *c* differ at only two positions, 62 and 89, the antibodies isolated on the guanaco protein must be directed against one of these two regions. At position 62 guanaco and horse cytochromes *c* carry a glutamyl residue while the rabbit protein has aspartic acid. Antibodies directed against the glutamic acid at this position in guanaco cytochrome *c* have been shown to bind to insolubilized rabbit cytochrome *c* (Urbanski and Margoliash, 1977); antibodies directed against horse cytochrome *c* in the region of Residue 62 likewise should not discriminate between the insolubilized guanaco and rabbit proteins. Hence, from this information alone, it appears that the antibody population directed against horse cytochrome binds in the region of Residue 89 where the horse protein carries a threonyl residue, the rabbit protein an aspartic acid, and guanaco cytochrome *c* a glycine. In addition to the charge change, the added bulk of the aspartic acid residue prevents the antibody from binding, whereas the antibody can be accommodated by a neutral residue with a smaller side chain, in this case a hydrogen atom.

Final demonstration of the specificity of this population was obtained from determinations of the stoichoimetry of its reactions with various cytochromes *c*. Indeed, the purified antibody populations (Fab') denoted anti-89-92 (I) yields a 1:1 stoichiometry with horse cytochrome *c* in fluorescence quenching titrations, using the procedure of Noble et al. (1969). The antigen binding fragment of this population was also titrated with other cytochromes *c* having one or more amino acid sequence differences from the horse protein in the region around Residue 89 as shown in Figure 2.

Dog cytochrome *c*, which is identical to the beef protein through Residue 87, does not bind these antibodies while the beef protein quenches about 50% of the fluorescence quenched by the immunogen, horse cytochrome. Since the above isolation scheme demonstrates that this population is directed toward either the region of Residue 62 or of Residue 89, the latter area must represent the effective binding site. Mouse testicular cytochrome *c* (c_t), like the beef and horse proteins, carries a glutamic acid at position 92, while Residue 89, for these proteins, is serine, glycine and threonine respectively, and mouse c_t approximates the fluorescence quenched by the beef protein. None of the other proteins tested (Figure 2) has a glutamic acid at position 92, but all show less fluorescence quenching. Hence, Residue 92 represents an important segment of this site.

Cytochrome c	position 88	position 89	position 92
rabbit	Lys $-CH_2-CH_2-CH_2-CH_2-NH_3^+$	Asp $-CH_2-COO^-$	Ala $-CH_3$
horse	Lys	Thr $-CH(OH)-CH_3$	Glu $-CH_2-CH_2-COO^-$
beef	Lys	Gly $-H$	Glu
guanaco	Lys	Gly	Ala
duck	Lys	Ser $-CH_2OH$	Ala
pigeon	Lys	Ala $-CH_3$	Ala
dog	Thr $-CH(OH)-CH_3$	Gly	Ala
mouse c_t	Lys	Ser	Glu

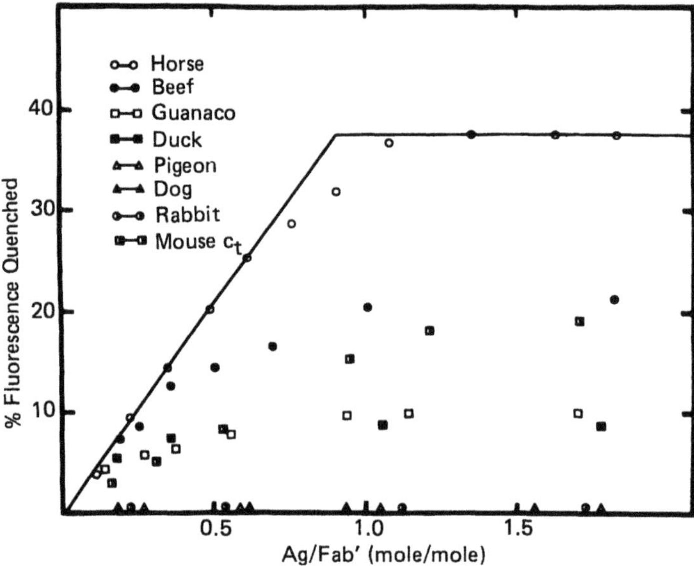

Figure 2: *Cross Reactivities of Rabbit Anti-horse Cytochrome c Residues 89-92 (Subpopulation I).* Antibody fluorescence quenching titrations with the cytochromes *c* listed. The top of the figure gives the sequence differences in the region of Residues 89-92 between the cytochromes *c* tested.

Evidence for the involvement of threonine 89 in the antibody binding, aside from failure of the antibodies to bind to rabbit cytochrome *c*, which contains aspartic acid at that position, is given by the fact that duck cytochrome *c* binds better than the pigeon protein, although the only difference between the two in the region of 89-92 is at position 89 where a serine is carried by the duck protein and alanine by pigeon cytochrome *c*.

Even though Residues 89 and 92 appear to be the major controlling side chains in this determinant, it is also influenced by Residues 88 and 96. Thus, dog cytochrome *c* which does not bind this population and guanaco cytochrome *c* which does, differ in this region only at position 88, where the dog protein carries a threonine and the guanaco, as well as all other proteins tested, has a lysine. Similarily, at the lower cytochrome concentrations, mouse c_t quenches less fluorescence than does the beef protein. This difference must be due to either Residue 89, serine in mouse c_t and glycine in beef cytochrome, or the nearby Residue 96, lysine in mouse c_t and alanine in the beef protein. However, the difference at position 89 is the same as that between the duck and guanaco proteins, which react identically. Hence, it must be the lysyl residue at position 96 in mouse c_t that interferes with the binding.

The region of the cytochrome *c* molecule against which these antibodies are directed is an α-helix. Because of this structure, the side chains (β carbons) of Residues 88, 89, 92 and 96 are all within 12 Å of each other and can surely be accommodated within the antibody binding site.

Residues 89-92 (Subpopulation II). Some of the antibodies in the rabbit anti-horse cytochrome *c* serum that do not adsorb the insolubilized rabbit or guanaco proteins, are nevertheless adsorbed by beef cytochrome *c* bound to Sepharose. This antibody population is denoted anti-89-92 (II). The corresponding antigen binding fragments give a 1:1 stoichiometry with horse cytochrome *c* and must be directed against one of two regions of the molecule. The guanaco and beef proteins differ at only two amino acid positions, 44, where beef has proline and guanaco carries valine, and 92, where beef has glutamic acid and guanaco has alanine. Although the dog protein is identical to beef cytochrome *c* in the region of Residue 44, these antibodies were not adsorbed on the insolubilized dog protein. Clearly then, they are directed against the region of Residue 92.

Fluorescence quenching titrations of the Fab' derived from this subpopulation with several cytochromes *c* is shown in Figure 3. Glutamic acid at position 92 is a requirement for antibody binding. This is demonstrated by the fact that beef and mouse c_t proteins (glutamic acid at position 92) quench the fluorescence, while the

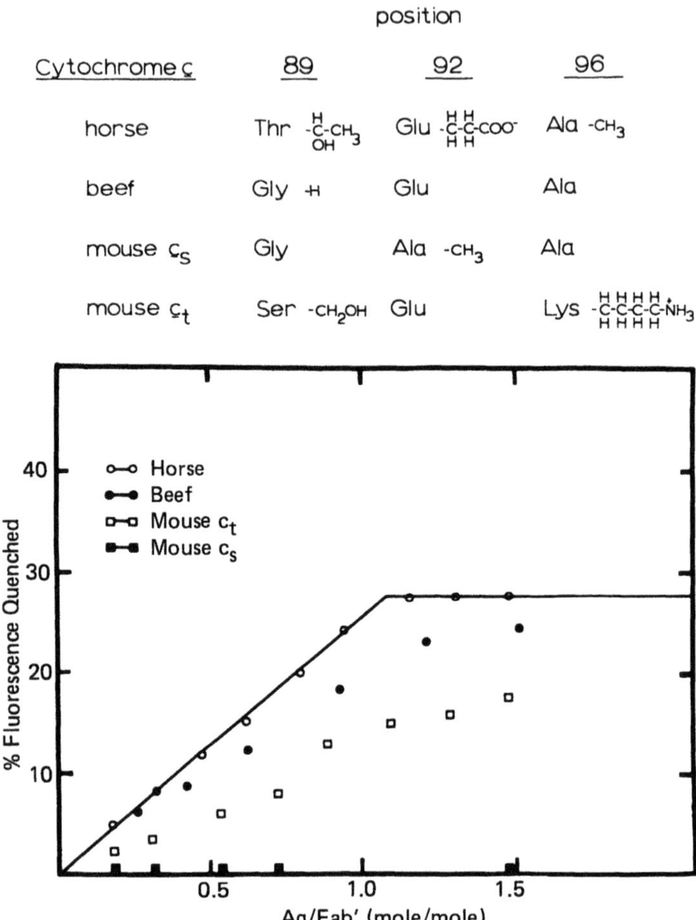

Figure 3: *Cross Reactivities of Rabbit Anti-horse Cytochrome c Residues 89-92 (Subpopulation II).* Antibody fluorescence quenching titrations with the cytochromes *c* listed. The top of the figure gives the sequence differences in the region of Residues 89-92 between the cytochromes *c* tested.

mouse somatic protein (c_s) does not react at all, even though it is identical throughout this region with the beef protein, except for an alanine at position 92. Residue 89 is also involved in the antibody binding since horse cytochrome *c*, which differs from the beef and mouse c_t proteins at that position, quenches the fluorescence more effectively. The difference in binding between the beef and mouse c_t proteins is probably due to the lysyl residue at position 96 in the mouse c_t protein, located next to Residue 92 in the α-helix.

Residues 89-92 (Subpopulation III). The third antibody population directed against the region of Residues 89-92 and denoted anti-89-92 (III) was isolated from the same serum as anti-89-92 (I) and (II). From the antibodies adsorbed on Sepharose-bound rabbit cytochrome *c* was obtained a population that subsequently failed to bind to the insolubilized mouse testicular protein. Antigen-binding fragments were prepared from this material and show a 1:1 stoichiometry with horse cytochrome *c* (Figure 4). Since the

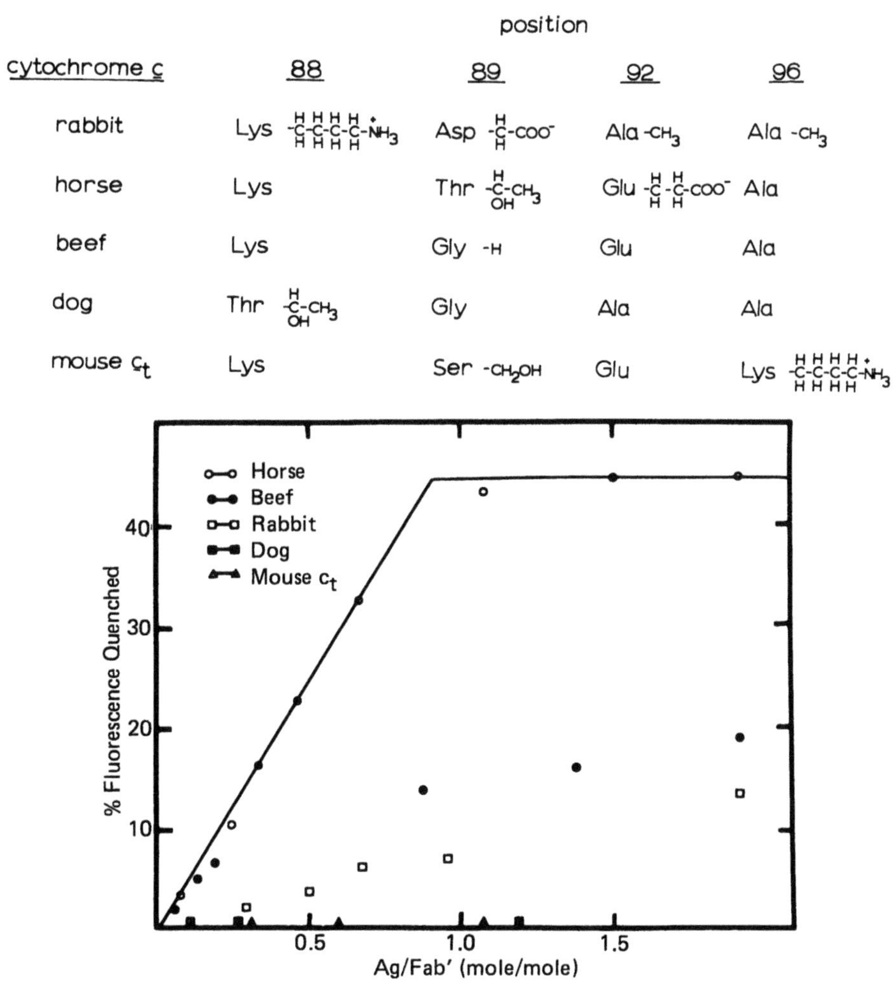

Figure 4: *Cross Reactivities of Rabbit Anti-horse Cytochrome c Residues 89-92 (Subpopulation III).* Antibody fluorescence quenching titrations with the cytochromes *c* listed. The top of the figure gives the sequence differences in the region of Residues 89-92 between the cytochromes *c* tested.

Fab' bind better to the horse than to the rabbit protein, this antibody population must be directed against a region of the molecule where the amino acid sequence differs between these two proteins, namely at Residues 44, 47, 60, 62, 89 and 92 (See sequence comparison in Figure 1). Furthermore, the binding site must be in a region where the beef and rabbit proteins differ from mouse c_t, since this last cytochrome does not bind the antibody while the other two proteins do (Figure 4). This requirement eliminates Residues 44, 47 and 62 as possible sites. Finally, the failure of the dog protein to bind the Fab', although the beef and dog cytochromes are identical at position 60, again implicates Residues 89 and 92 in the antigenic determinant.

Although mouse c_t is as similar to the horse protein as is the beef in the region of Residues 89-92, the lysyl residue at position 96, which is present only in the mouse c_t protein and positioned in the α-helix next to Residue 92, interferes with the binding of the antibody. Again Residue 89 must also be involved in the binding, since the horse protein binds far better than does beef cytochrome *c*, and these two proteins differ in this region only at position 89.

Conclusions

The present observations demonstrate that the region on the surface of cytochrome *c* which influences the binding of the anti-residue 89-92 antibodies is the same for all three subpopulations. The site of binding encompasses Residues 88 and 96 as well as the more centrally located and dominant Residues 89 and 92, all on the C-terminal α-helix of cytochrome *c*, and within a distance of 12 Å from each other. There are subtle differences in the specificities which made possible the separation of the subpopulations, even though they are directed towards a single complex site rather than two different antigenic sites.

It is important to note that the above results emphasize that one cannot conclude that antibody populations isolated by successive adsorptions on homologous insolubilized proteins necessarily represent different antigenic determinants.

The differing abilities among the proteins examined to quench the antibody fluorescence is clearly due to differences in binding. In those cases where an antibody did not bind to a cytochrome *c*, as shown by the failure of the antibody to adsorb to the insolubilized protein, no fluorescence quenching was observed. In other situations where the antibody can be adsorbed to a protein, the fluorescence quenched is often significantly less than that quenched by the immunogen, horse cytochrome *c*. An example is antiresidues 89-92 (subpopulation I) which was isolated on the basis of its ability to bind to guanaco cytochrome *c*, yet the fluorescence quenched by the guanaco protein is markedly less than that quenched by horse cytochrome *c* in the antigen concentration range examined. This results from differences in affinities or, less likely, in the relative spatial positions of the cytochrome and the antibody in the antigen-antibody complex. In either case, the data show that in addition to determining the stoichiometry of the reaction, the fluorescence quenching technique can be employed for examining the specificity of the antibody combining site.

References

Borden, D., and Margoliash, E. (1976) In Handbook of Biochemistry and Molecular Biology, 3rd ed. Proteins, Vol. 3. G. D. Fasman, ed. Chemical Rubber Co., Cleveland, Ohio.

Dayhoff, M. O. (1972) Atlas of Protein Sequence and Structure, Vol. 5 and Supplements 1 and 2, National Biomedical Research Foundation, Silver Spring, Maryland.

Dickerson, R. E., and Timkovich, R. (1975) In The Enzymes, 3rd ed. Vol. 11, P. D. Boyer, ed. Academic Press, New York. P. 397.

Eng, J., and Reichlin, M. (1977) Federation Proc., 36, 2474.

Jemmerson, R., Brautigan, D. L., and Margoliash, E. (1977) Div. of Biol. Chem., 174th American Chemical Society Meeting. Chicago, Ill., Abstract 81.

Jemmerson, R., and Margoliash, E. (1977) unpublished results.

Nisonoff, A., Reichlin, M., and Margoliash, E. (1970) J. Biol. Chem. 254, 940.

Noble, R. W., Reichlin, M., and Gibson, Q. H. (1969) J. Biol. Chem. 244, 2403.

Urbanski, G. J., and Margoliash, E. (1976) In Immunochemistry of Enzymes and Their Antibodies. M. Salton, ed. J. Wiley and Sons, New York, P. 203.

Urbanski, G. J. and Margoliash, E. (1977) J. Immunol. 118, 1170.

A MODEL IMPLICATING ALTERED MACROPHAGE FUNCTION IN H-2 LINKED NONRESPONSIVENESS TO HEN LYSOZYME

Alexander Miller

Department of Bacteriology, University of California
Los Angeles, California 90024

ABSTRACT

Studies on the basis of differential responsiveness of $H\text{-}2^b$ mice to gallinaceous lysozymes suggest T cell involvement and active T cell suppression with those lysozymes not responded to. Results from other laboratories suggesting a directive role for macrophages through limited presentation are summarized. A model is presented proposing that suppressors (recognizing a determinant only on lysozymes not responded to) are present in all strains; that suppression requires antigen bridging between suppressor determinant and positive T determinant; that this bridge is disrupted in all strains but $H\text{-}2^b$; and that this failure to disrupt the antigen bridge is a result of a genetically (Ia) controlled loss of a normal macrophage processing step.

The following abbreviations are used: CFA, complete Freund's adjuvant; GRF, macrophage derived genetically related factor forming adduct with processed antigen; HEL, chicken (hen) egg white lysozyme; (H,G)-A-L, branched copolymer of the general structure (His, Glu)-Ala-Lys; Ir, immune response; KLH, keyhole limpet hemocyanin; L_I, L_{II}, L_{III}, the three CNBr peptides of HEL comprising positions 1-12, 13-105, and 106-129, respectively; LPS, *E. coli* lipopolysaccharide; PETLES, peritoneal exudate, T lymphocyte enriched cells; RBC, red blood cells; RCM-X, the reduced carboxymethylated derivative of X; REL, ringed-neck pheasant egg white lysozyme; TNP-HEL, guanidinylated HEL trinitrophenylated at the N-terminal amino group; (T-G)-A-L, branched copolymer of the general structure (Tyr, Glu)-Ala-Lys.

It was found in our laboratory (Hill and Sercarz, 1975; Sercarz, et al. 1978) that in mice there is an H-2-linked genetic control of the ability to differentially respond to a set of closely related gallinaceous egg-white lysozymes. In H-2^b animals, no response is found with lysozymes from chicken (HEL)[1], bobwhite, Gambol or Valley quail and guinea hen; a good response obtained with lysozymes from Japanese Quail and ring-neck pheasant (REL); and a limited response with turkey and peafowl lysozymes. Using mice with other H-2 haplotypes essentially equal responsiveness is obtained with all the above lysozymes. Comparison of the sequences of these lysozymes, indicates that the only consistent difference is the presence of tyrosine at position 3 in those lysozymes responded to by H-2^b mice, with phenylalanine being present at position 3 in other lysozymes. Because of the limited response to turkey and peafowl, it would appear that in addition to the dominant effect of tyrosine-3, other substituents can have a modifying influence.

Responsiveness has been assayed in several ways: primary or secondary production of anti-lysozyme plaques; production of anti-lysozyme serum antibody; provision of help for an anti-TNP response; and through generation of T cells showing a proliferative response to antigen.

Evidence for T Cell Involvement in H-2^b Lesion

In H-2^b as well as non-H-2^b mice, a response, measured by serum antibody or plaque-forming cells, is obtained when HEL is presented conjugated to red blood cells (HEL-RBC) or as an adduct with *E. coli* lipopolysaccharide (HEL-LPS) (Hill, et al. 1975). In both cases, it is likely that the need for HEL-specific T helper cells is being circumvented either through the provision of other T helper cells (RBC-specific) or through a signal which bypasses the need for T help (LPS). Thus, it appeared failure to respond to HEL in H-2^b mice could be attributed to failure to generate HEL-specific T helper cells.

Evidence for Suppression

Several lines of experimentation strongly support the idea that failure of T helper function in H-2^b mice is a result of active suppression rather than lack of T helper precursors.

In our laboratory, Adorini has developed an *in vitro* system in which TNP-HEL stimulates either B10 (H-2^b) or B10.A (congenic with B10 but of H-2^a haplotype) unprimed spleen cells to produce anti-TNP as measured in a plaque assay. When B10.A cells from mice primed three weeks previously with HEL in CFA are used, about the same or at most a slightly increased response to TNP is observed. However, when cells from similarly immunized B10 mice are used, essentially complete inhibition of the anti-TNP response is observed. By combining such primed cells with unprimed ones, evidence was obtained for active suppression. The suppressing cells are sensitive to anti-T sera and are relatively radiosensitive, both properties associated with T suppressor cells. A preliminary report has been published (Sercarz, et al. 1978).

Using another approach, Yowell, in our laboratory, has also obtained evidence for active suppression in H-2^b mice. Using the PETLES system (Schwartz, et al. 1975), priming of T cells for antigen-specific stimulation of *in vitro* proliferation has been studied. Either B10 or B10.A mice are immunized in the footpads with REL, and after three weeks, stimulated by thioglycollate to induce peritoneal exudate cells. PETLES from such animals show a high degree of proliferation upon incubation with REL *in vitro*. Both such B10 and B10A PETLES are strongly cross-stimulated by HEL as well. B10A mice also yield active PETLES when immunization is with HEL and challenge with either HEL or REL. PETLES from B10 mice immunized with HEL show only a low degree of proliferation when incubated with HEL. However, it has been a fairly consistent finding that use of REL for *in vitro* stimulation of HEL-primed PETLES from B10 mice leads to more proliferation than does use of the original priming antigen, HEL. Such a result is compatible with the idea that HEL-induced proliferation in B10 is limited by a suppressor population specific for HEL which does not recognize REL.

It has been well established that at the T cell level, HEL and its reduced, carboxymethylated derivative, RCM-HEL are highly cross-reactive. As might be predicted, with the PETLES system, immunization with RCM-HEL leads to a response in B10.A but not B10 mice. When RCM-HEL is treated with cyanogen bromide, it is cleaved at the two methionines of HEL to yield three peptides: RCM-L_I (Pos. 1-12), RCM-L_{II} (Pos. 13-105) and RCM-L_{III} (Pos. 106-129). Immunization of B10 mice with RCM-L_{II}, unlike that with RCM-HEL, leads to a proliferative PETLES response comparable to that found with REL. Furthermore, *in vitro* stimulation is as good with RCM-HEL as with RCM-L_{II}. These results are consistent with the idea that the activity of RCM-L_{II} in B10 mice is a result of "amputation" of a suppressor determinant.

Paradox of Recessive Suppression

As with other H-2 linked Ir genes, non-responsiveness to HEL is recessive, i.e., F1 offspring of responders and nonresponders are phenotypically indistinguishable from responders. Nevertheless, the evidence presented above clearly indicates the failure of $H\text{-}2^b$ mice to respond is due to active suppression (several other H-2 linked Ir genes seem to function in a similar manner). Thus, an apparent paradox exists in that an active process is not expressed in heterozygotes.

Requirements for Suppression

If suppression occurs through the mediation of T suppressor cells, it is a necessary but not sufficient condition that there be a suppressor determinant on the molecule, the response to which is being suppressed. In the present instance, such a determinant would be on HEL and RCM-HEL but not on REL or $RCM\text{-}L_{II}$, and thus there would be response to the latter two antigens. Presence of a receptor determinant is, however, not sufficient in itself to account for suppression. In addition, it is necessary that a mechanism exist for interaction of suppressor (or suppressor factor) and a target T cell. It appears likely that with a monomeric protein antigen such as HEL, the mechanism for interaction is by means of an antigen bridge which allows the suppressor to act on a T cell with specificity for a determinant other than that recognized by the suppressor. Given the fact that two determinants exist, the persistance of a bridge between them would depend on the manner in which antigen were processed by macrophages prior to presentation to T cells. Some evidence suggesting a key role for macrophage processing in determining the course of T cell activation is summarized below.

Restrictions on Macrophage Function

It is reasonable to assume that there is extreme genetic selection in animals for non-destruction of self by macrophages. That is, macrophage functions must be specifically limited in that there is, in general, no phagocytosis nor destruction of body constituents. In the context of the following argument, non-destruction of normal serum constituents is of particular interest. In contrast, processing of protein immunogens by macrophages appears to be a prerequisite for presentation to T cells. At the very least, it would seem from the work of Erb and Feldman (1975a), that a protein antigen must be "adapted" for presentation to T helper precursors. Adaptation is through attachment to a so-called "genetically related factor" or GRF, the nature of which is unknown but which reacts with anti-Ia sera of appropriate haplotype. The mode of attachment of antigen to GRF is totally unknown at present. However, it can be argued that there are severe limitations with regard to what structures are recognized on protein antigens since "foreignness" must be recognized in a veritable ocean of self proteins. Since it would be expected that there would be rather strong twin selection against recognition of self and toward maximum recognition of foreignness within a limited genetic library, rather rapid divergence within a species might well be expected. That is, there may be rather striking differences between strains in recognition of the same antigen.

There is a large literature detailing the rather extensive degradation of proteins which is brought about by peritoneal exudate cells. However, the relevance of such breakdown to activation of T cells is completely unknown. Erb and Feldman did obtain evidence that in the course of formation of KLH-GRF, the rather high molecular weight protein, KLH was extensively reduced in size. However, their results were still compatible with the KLH fragment which formed an adduct with GRF being of the order of 10^4 daltons. The extensive cross-reaction at the T cell level observed with several proteins and their denatured congeners and, in particular, that between HEL and its reduced, carboxymethylated derivative, RCM-HEL (reviewed by R. Scibienski, this volume) suggests presentation of antigen fragments to T cells. We have made an extensive search for cross-reaction at the antibody level between HEL and RCM-HEL. With neither anti-HEL nor anti-RCM-HEL was any cross-reaction found, even when the technique of isoelectric focussing was used. With this technique, a single cross-reactive clone can easily be detected in a highly multiclonal antiserum. This result suggests little conformational identity between HEL and RCM-HEL. Since HEL is a typical "tight" globular protein, and, therefore, of rather fixed conformation, the observed cross-reactivity between HEL and RCM-HEL at the T cell level suggests that HEL is broken down to some extent, i.e., HEL is broken down sufficiently to change conformation and now share at least one determinant with RCM-HEL. Limited breakdown of antigen by macrophages would be subject to a similar restriction as binding of antigen to GRF. Self proteins must be recognized and _not_ broken down. Again, rapid divergence of genes controlling such a process might be expected.

Both selective processes - limited bonding to GRF and limited degradation - could operate independently. However, the existence of a selective degradation mechanism would negate the need for high selectivity at level of GRF complex function. That is, selection in the latter case could be for determinants on fragmented, and, hence, "denatured," protein. Obvious candidates for selectivity would be exposed hydrophobic amino acids.

Directive Role of Macrophages

There has recently been a spate of papers indicating that macrophages do indeed play an important role in selection of T cell subsets for activation. The prototype experiment is to prime F1(AxB) T cells with antigen on either of the parental macrophages (A or B). Depending on the specific protocol and system, different but consistent effects were observed. Pierce and coworkers (summarized in this volume) and Kappler and Marrack (1976), using mouse strains were able to observe memory for the primary macrophage. For example, F1 T cells from animals primed with A macrophages were restimulated much more strongly by antigen presented on A macrophages (or F1 macrophages) than by antigen on B macrophages. Reciprocal effects were observed with primary B macrophage priming and restimulation. A possible interpretation is on the basis of Ia differences in the GRFs delivering antigen to the T cells. Erb and Feldman (1976b) have shown that GRF not only contains Ia antigens but react effectively only with Ia-matched T cells. To explain the above results, it is necessary to postulate, in addition, that F1 T cells are heterogeneous with respect to Ia antigens, some containing Ia antigens of one parental type and others of the second parental type. Such a result may be the natural consequence of T cells differentiating with respect to specificity of receptors.

Rosenthal and coworkers (work summarized in this volume) have carried out similar experiments in strain (2 x 13) F1 guinea pigs, using pork insulin as an antigen. To briefly summarize their elegant experiments, they found that when pork insulin was presented on strain 13 macrophages, a B-chain determinant was recognized by a subset of F1 T cells. In contrast, when pork insulin was presented on strain 2 macrophages, an A-chain loop region determinant was recognized by a different subset of F1 T cells. These non-overlapping T cell specificities are precisely those found in strain 13 and strain 2 animals, respectively, and shown to be under the control of Ir genes linked to the major histocompatibility complex of guinea pigs.

In a similar vein, Singer, et al. (1977), have shown that in an *in vitro* system, an anti-TNP response can be obtained in (B10.A x B10) F1 mice after stimulation with either TNP-(T,G)-A-L or TNP-(H,G)-A-L. However, if the F1 cells are depleted of macrophages, addition of B10.A ($H-2^a$) macrophages allows a response TNP-(H,G)-A-L but not TNP-(T,G)-A,L. Conversely, addition of B10($H-2^b$) macrophages allows an anti-TNP response to TNP-(T,G)-A-L but not TNP-(H,G)-A-L. This pattern of response is consistent with the fact that $H-2^a$ respond to (H,G)-A-L and not (T,G)-A-L, while with $H-2^b$ mice, high response is found to (T,G)-A-L and not (H,G)-A-L.

Scheme for Antigen Processing

In view of the results summarized above, a hypothetical scheme can be suggested for limited antigen processing by macrophages. In the primary interaction antigen loosely adheres to (or is possibly taken up by) macrophages. This is followed by a "recognition" event:

because there has been no selection for resistance to macrophage protease activity, the "foreign" protein begins to undergo proteolysis. This limited digestion leads to, at least, partial unfolding of the protein revealing hydrophobic amino acid side chains normally not exposed. (With denatured proteins, such as RCM-HEL, this preliminary digestion might well be unnecessary). These hydrophobic entities, singly or in combination, are now recognized and bound by one of the relatively small library of GRFs. (This library might be comparable in size to the library of amino acid activating enzymes present in all cells.) Binding to a specific GRF (GRF_1) would serve to protect a limited part of the antigen from further degradation. Binding to GRF_1, rather than GRF_2, GRF_3, etc., would be assured by the rather limited susceptibility of native antigen to proteolytic attack, and, therefore, rather specific mode of uncovering of internal groups. Most of the antigen would still be subject to degradation by the large array of proteases assumed to be associated with macrophages. In fact, it is imagined that in general degradation would proceed to such a degree as to pare all suppressor determinants from the determinant protected by GRF. Only occasionally would a large fragment containing a suppressor determinant be the ultimate antigenic moiety left in association with a GRF.

Finally, fragmented antigen in association with GRF is presented to the appropriate primary T cell. The work of Erb and Fedlmann (1975a,b) indicates that antigen-GRF can act as a soluble factor with the proviso that IA matching is necessary. This could lead to the idea of dual recognition by the T cell: for antigenic determinant and for IA-related portion of GRF. However, in light of recent studies with helper factors (M. Feldmann, this volume) in which helper factor-antigen adducts act through formation of a complex with macrophages, an alternative explanation may be considered. Namely, that the need for IA matching is a reflection of the need for antigen-GRF to be rebound by macrophage before interaction with T cells IA recognition would then be a property of receptors on macrophages and quite apart from antigen recognition by T cells.

Model for Ir Gene Control

Alteration in antigen processing by macrophages provides a means of explaining Ir gene control which avoids the problems associated with trying to link Ir genes control directly to the lymphoid system. In particular, the problem of redundancy in lymphoid recognition is avoided. It seems to be a general finding that there are multiple molecular solutions at the receptor level to the problem of recognition of a single epitope, much less a determinant region. Also, there is no evidence for clustering of genes controlling any particular V-region specificity. Hence, the straight-forward Mendelian inheritance of Ir genes is difficult to explain in terms of changes in lymphoid cell specificity.

Secondly, the existence of "recessive suppression" in those Ir gene systems where a suppression mechanism has been implicated is difficult to explain at the lymphoid cell level. However, the recessive character of nonresponsiveness follows directly from a model in which the nonresponders lack a function necessary for effective antigen processing. In those cases where suppression is found, failure in the nonresponder to disrupt an antigen bridge between positive and recessive determinants would lead to a dominant phenotype for responsiveness in F_1 animals (see below). Similar dominance of responsiveness would be found if nonresponders (1) lacked ability to degrade antigen in such a way as to form an antigen-GRF adduct; or (2) lacked the proper GRF to form a functional antigen-GRF complex.

Thirdly, the almost total linkage of Ir genes to the H2 complex of mice would be explained in terms of regulation of surface constituents of cells, and, in particular, macrophages. Here, it is postulated that an important function of the Ia complex is to determine the amount and relative distribution of GRF and other surface constituents such as proteolytic enzymes, on the surface of macrophages.

Model for H-2^b Differential Responsiveness to Lysozymes

In the specific case of H-2^b mice, there is no response to HEL, while there is normal response to REL. It is supposed that all mouse strains contain suppressor cells which recognize a determinant on HEL which is absent on REL (and RCM-L_{II}). This could, for example, be a determinant on a major self constituent. In all strains but H-2^b, the connection between the suppressor determinant and positive determinant(s) is destroyed during processing and formation of GRF and a fragment of HEL. In H-2^b animals, however, there is a deficiency in processing and an antigen bridge is maintained between positive determinant and suppressor determinant. This allows effective delivery of a suppressor signal to those T cells which otherwise would give a positive response upon recognition of a particular HEL determinant.

ACKNOWLEDGEMENTS

This work was supported in part by NIH grant AI-08198 and NCI contract CB-43972. It is a pleasure to thank my associates and, in particular, Jessica Clarke, Dale Kipp and Sven Britton for their helpful criticism.

REFERENCES

Erb, P. and Feldmann, M. (1975a) Eur. J. Immunol. 5, 759.

Erb, P. and Feldmann, M. (1975b) J. Exp. Med. 142, 460.

Hill, S.W. and Sercarz, E.E. (1975) Eur. J. Immunol. 5, 317.

Hill, S.W., Yowell, R.L., Kipp, D.E., Scibienski, R.S., Miller, A. and Sercarz, E.E. (1975) in "Advances in Experimental Medicine and Biology," M. Feldmann and A. Globerson, Eds., Plenum Press, New York, London.

Kappler, J.N. and Marrack, D.C. (1976) Nature 262, 797

Schwartz, R.H., Jackson, L. and Paul, W.E. (1975) J. Immunol. 115, 1330.

Sercarz, E.E., Yowell, R.L., Turkin, D., Miller, A., Araneo, B.A. and Adorini, L. (1978) Immunol. Reviews, in press.

Singer, A., Cowing, C., Pickler, H.B. and Hodes, R.J. (1977) Manuscript submitted.

Immunobiology of Proteins and Peptides

T-LYMPHOCYTE ACTIVATION BY IMMUNOGENIC DETERMINANTS

Joel W. Goodman, Sherman Fong, George K. Lewis, Roberta Kamin, Danute E. Nitecki and Georges Der Balian

Department of Microbiology, University of California, San Francisco, San Francisco, California 94143

ABSTRACT

Synthetic antigens have been of great value in elucidating the relationships between antigen structure and lymphocyte activation. The compound RAT behaves as a monofunctional antigen in guinea pigs and mice, inducing T-lymphocyte responses without appreciable circulating antibody, although the ABA-specific B cell population is expanded by immunization with the monovalent molecule. On the other hand, bifunctional antigens composed of one RAT moiety serving as a carrier and a second chemical group, either identical to or different from RAT, serving as a hapten,induced antibody responses. In such responses, T cell specificity was always directed against the RAT component. Using symmetrical bifunctional antigens with rigid or flexible spacers between the two determinants, marked differences in structural requirements for cell triggering, assessed by antigen-induced lymphocyte proliferation, and for cell cooperation, determined by antibody formation, were found. Rigidly spaced bifunctional antigens serve admirably for cooperation but poorly for T cell activation, underscoring the advantage of two-point binding for the latter.

Abbreviations: ABA, azobenzenearsonate; anti-id, rabbit antiserum to CRI; BSA, bovine serum albumin; CFA, complete Freund's adjuvant; CRI, cross-reactive idiotype; DNP, dinitrophenyl; IFA, incomplete Freund's adjuvant; KLH, keyhole limpet hemocyanin; LNC, lymph node cells; PEC, peritoneal exudate cells; RAH, L-histidine-azobenzene-arsonate; RAN, p-hydroxyphenyl-propane-azobenzene-p'-arsonate; RAT, L-tyrosine-p-azobenzenearsonate; SAC, 6-aminocaproic acid; TAT, L-tyrosine-p-azobenzenetrimethylammonium chloride; RFC, rosette-forming cell

Immunization of strain A/J mice with RAT induced a 30-fold increase in antigen-binding B and T cells, assayed by formation of specific rosettes between lymphocytes and haptenated erythrocytes. Although mice did not make significant PFC responses to bifunctional RAT compounds, it was discovered that ABA derivatives of L-histidine engendered appreciable helper activity. Cell transfer experiments with carrier-primed and hapten-primed spleen cell populations established the existence of helper T cells with specificity for the arsanilate epitope.

The occurrence of a major idiotype on a portion of anti-ABA antibodies from all A/J mice prompted a search for this idiotype on antigen-binding T cells. Using inhibition of rosette formation by anti-id to detect the CRI, it was found that a substantial part of the Thy-1-positive rosetting lymphocytes from immune A/J mice were CRI positive. The capacity to form rosettes was abrogated by treating cells with trypsin, but recovered following culture for 16-24 hours, suggesting resynthesis of receptors. Although these preliminary findings are encouraging, the evidence for T cell receptors which bear the idiotypic marker characteristic of anti-ABA specificity is still incomplete. If more exhaustive efforts are confirmatory, then a promising means of delineating the fine structure of the T cell antigen receptor and its relationship to antibodies which share the same idiotype will be at hand.

INTRODUCTION

The fundamental concept that T cells and B cells may recognize and respond to different regions (determinants) of an antigen molecule, initially proposed by Mitchison (1969), has received sufficient experimental support in recent years to place it among immunologic dogma. Using conventional haptenated proteins, it was shown that recognition of at least two determinants - presumably one by each cell type - was required for an antibody response (Rajewsky et al. 1969), but the most conclusive evidence has derived from studies using relatively simple, structurally defined antigens (reviewed by Goodman 1975). As one example, glucagon, a polypeptide of 29 amino acids, is immunogenic in guinea pigs and could be dissected by tryptic digestion along functional lines into an amino-terminal portion which housed the major haptenic determinant against which antibody specificity was directed, and a carboxy-terminal region which carried a determinant that induced T cell responses (Senyk et al. 1971).

Synthetic antigens provide greater flexibility for delineating relationships between antigen structure and lymphocyte activation, since it is possible to fabricate antigens which are tailored to address specific questions. The prototype we have attempted to exploit for this purpose is the compound L-tyrosine-p-azobenzenearsonate

(RAT), which induces cellular immunity in guinea pigs without appreciable antibody formation when administered with Freund's complete adjuvant (CFA) (Leskowitz et al. 1966, Alkan et al, 1971, Nauciel and Raynaud 1971). This result is consistent with the idea that a unideterminant antigen, though capable of interacting with T and B lymphocytes, should be unable to mediate cooperation between them. However, an increase in RAT-binding B cells was found in such immunized animals (Goodman et al. 1974), consistent with other findings indicating that antigen itself is capable of inducing B cell proliferation, the T cell signal being required for differentiation to terminal antibody production (Dutton 1974, Schimpl 1974).

On the other hand, it would be anticipated that bifunctional antigens composed of one RAT moiety serving as a carrier and a second chemical group serving as a hapten should behave as complete antigens and induce antibody responses. This proved to be the case whether the haptenic component was multivalent poly-D-glutamic acid, with an average molecular weight of 35,000 (Alkan et al. 1971), or a single dinitrophenyl (DNP) group (Alkan et al. 1972a). In either case, antibody specific for the hapten was produced; but T cell specificity, as minifested by delayed hypersensitivity, *in vitro* antigen-induced lymphocyte transformation and carrier-induced helper activity, was confined to RAT.

Separating the RAT carrier determinant and DNP haptenic determinant of bifunctional molecules with spacers of varying size permitted an assessment of the spatial requirements between hapten and carrier for an anti-hapten response (Alkan et al. 1972a). The spacer used for this purpose was 6-aminocaproic acid (SAC), a flexible chain of six carbon atoms with an extended span of 8A. One or more spacers could be coupled in stepwise fashion to tyrosine, leaving the amino group of the terminal spacer available for substitution with DNP. The magnitude of the anti-DNP response was similar whether the determinants were separated by one or three SAC spacers, but was significantly weaker when the determinants were joined without a spacer. Thus, cooperation could apparently be implemented by an antigen in which the carrier and haptenic moieties were separated by less than 8A.

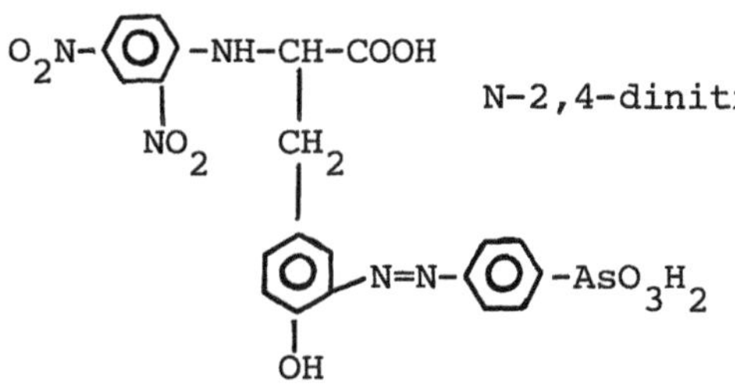

O_2N-(ring)-NH-CH-COOH
(ring)–NO_2; CH–CH_2
CH_2–(ring)-N=N-(ring)-AsO_3H_2
(ring)–OH

N-2,4-dinitrophenyl-L-tyrosine azobenzene-p-arsonate

DNP-RAT

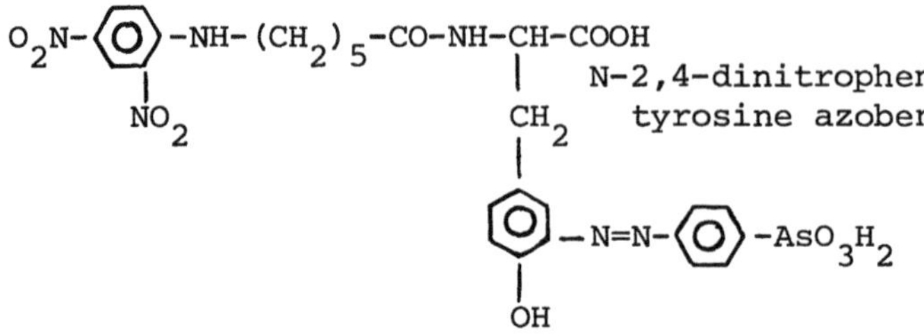

$O_2N-C_6H_3(NO_2)-NH-(CH_2)_5-CO-NH-CH(CH_2-C_6H_3(OH)-N=N-C_6H_4-AsO_3H_2)-COOH$

N-2,4-dinitrophenyl-6-amino-caproyl-L-tyrosine azobenzene-p-arsonate

DNP-SAC-RAT

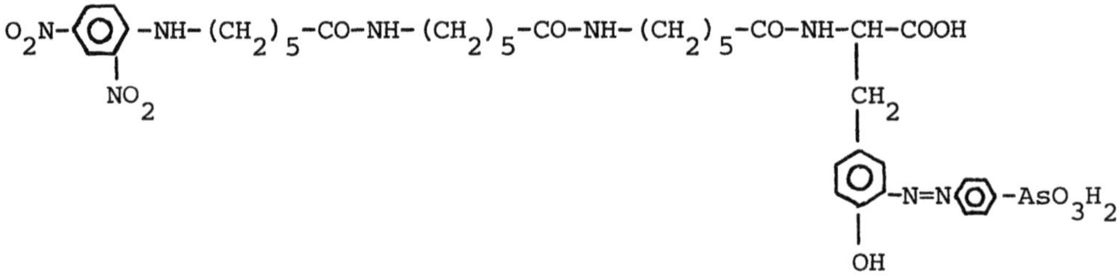

$O_2N-C_6H_3(NO_2)-NH-(CH_2)_5-CO-NH-(CH_2)_5-CO-NH-(CH_2)_5-CO-NH-CH(CH_2-C_6H_3(OH)-N=N-C_6H_4-AsO_3H_2)-COOH$

N-2,4-dinitrophenyl-(6-amino-caproyl)$_3$-L-tyrosine azobenzene-p-arsonate

DNP-SAC$_3$-RAT

STRUCTURAL FEATURES OF AZOBENZENOID DERIVATIVES RESPONSIBLE FOR IMMUNOGENICITY AND FOR SPECIFICITY

Two series of RAT analogs were prepared, one in which other chemical groups were substituted for arsonate (Table I) and the other in which the tyrosine side chain was modified (Table II). These compounds were used to explore the structural requirements for immunogenicity of RAT in guinea pigs. Immunization with the compounds in Table I revealed that other charged moieties (sulfonate and trimethyl-ammonium) could substitute for arsonate without loss of immunogenicity, but modification at the arsonate position yielded compounds with distinctive specificities. Thus, the arsonate group is not essential for immunogenicity of molecules with a tyrosine-azobenzene core, but a charged substituent, either anionic or cationic, appears to be required (Alkan et al. 1972a).

Assessment of the contribution of the side chain of tyrosine to the immunogenicity of RAT by immunization with the compounds in Table II revealed that removal of either the carboxyl or amino group did not markedly affect immunogenicity, measured by delayed cutaneous sensitivity, whereas deletion of both completely abolished it (Alkan et al. 1972b). However, a charged group was not required since side chains containing a polar hydroxyl group could substitute for chains

TABLE I

Monofunctional Antigens with Substitutions at Arsonate Position

Structure		Name	Abbreviation
Derivatives of L-tyrosine azobenzene	R		
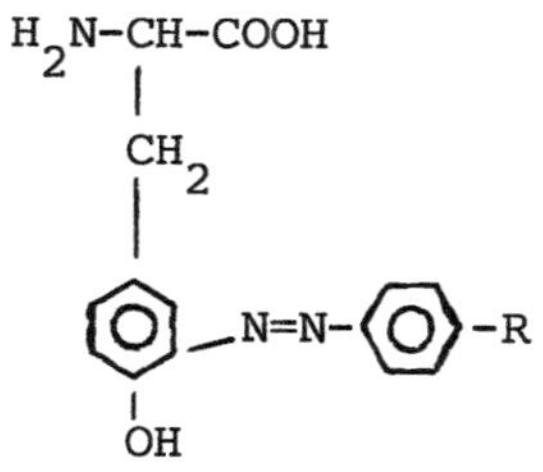 $H_2N-CH-COOH$	$-AsO_3H_2$	-p-arsonate	RAT
CH_2	-COOH	-p-carboxylate	CAT
	$-SO_3H$	-p-sulfonate	SAT
(benzene ring)-N=N-(benzene ring)-R	$-NH-CO-CH_3$	-p-acetamide	AAT
OH	$-SO_2NH_2$	-p-sulfonamide	SNAT
	$-NO_2$	-p-nitro	NAT
	$-N(CH_3)_3Cl$	-p-trimethylammonium chloride	TAT

TABLE II

Monofunctional Antigens with Substitutions in Side Chain of Tyrosine

Core compound: (phenol ring bearing OH, with R ortho to OH and Y para to OH)

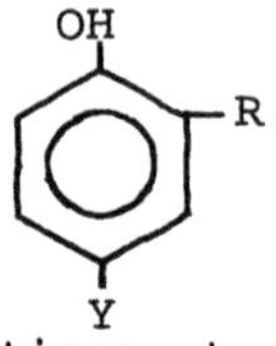

Series of compounds with variations at position Y as follows:

$-N = N-\emptyset-p-AsO_3H_2 = R$

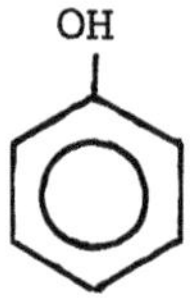

(phenol ring, OH) = A

Y	
$-CH_2-CHNH_2-COOH$	= T
$-CH_2-CH_2-COOH$	= O
$-CH_2-COOH$	= A
$-COOH$	= B
$-CH_2-CH_2NH_2$	= M
$-CH_2-CH_2-CH_3$	= N
$-CH_2-CH_3$	= E
$-CH_3$	= P
$-CH_2-CH_2OH$	= L
$-CH_2OH$	= H

bearing an amino or carboxyl group. The size of the side chain exerted a pronounced influence; the charged or polar substituent had to be extended from the phenolic ring by at least two carbon atoms in order to confer immunogenicity.

CLONAL RESTRICTION OF THE ANTI-HAPTEN ANTIBODY RESPONSE TO BIFUNCTIONAL ANTIGENS

DNP-SAC-RAT induced in guinea pigs a more restricted anti-DNP response than did DNP-proteins, both in terms of the number of DNP-specific B cell clones expressed and the amplitude of anti-DNP titers (Roelants & Goodman 1974). All antisera to the bifunctional antigen analyzed by isoelectric focusing were much more restricted in the number of anti-DNP bands than antisera to the protein conjugates.

Half were probably the products of fewer than three clones, assuming that each clone produces a family of three to four protein bands as ascertained by focusing myeloma proteins (Awdeh et al. 1967), but an unequivocally monoclonal response was not observed. It was noted during the course of the response that once a clone (or several clones) became dominant, it remained so throughout the primary response and was the only one to reappear after a booster injection. This expression of "clonal dominance" during conventional immunization is analogous to the results of Askonas and Williamson (1972), who transferred a single anti-DNP clone to syngeneic, irradiated recipient mice and found that the transferred clone dominated the anti-DNP response.

Relatively homogeneous antibody responses to simple antigens have also been reported by others (Haber 1967, Schlossman 1972). The uncomplicated response to bifunctional molecules may be useful in analyzing regulatory mechanisms governing the immune response as well as in generating relatively homogeneous antibody.

CELL COOPERATION MEDIATED BY SYMMETRICAL BIFUNCTIONAL ANTIGEN MOLECULES

Determining the feasibility of "self-help" - cooperation mediated by identical determinants on an antigen molecule - was approached by employing symmetrical bifunctional antigens with different spacers (Bush et al. 1972, Goodman et al. 1974). RAT or bifunctional RAT compounds with SAC spacers were unable to provoke primary or secondary anti-RAT antibody responses. Molecular models show that the flexible SAC spacers permit association of the two determinants; and since RAT contains electropositive (azo) and electronegative (arsonate) centers, it is likely that these complementary charged groups align in solution in a "deck of cards" geometry. Such intramolecular stacking might easily compromise the effective bifunctionality of the molecule. A predictable consequence of the stacking of aromatic rings is spectral hypochromism, which was observed experimentally with RAT-$(SAC)_3$-RAT (Alkan et al. 1972a). There were two ways out of this dilemma. One involved the deployment of a rigid decaproline spacer in place of SAC, to prevent stacking. Ten proline residues provide a separation of about 22A, similar to the extended span of three SAC groups; DNP-$(SAC)_3$-RAT induces strong antibody responses. The maneuver worked, RAT-$(PRO)_{10}$-RAT stimulating anti-ABA antibody formation (Alkan et al. 1972a). The other involved the manufacture of bifunctional antigens with SAC spacers in which the electronegative arsonate group is replaced by an electropositive trimethylammonium moiety, the immunogenic determinant now being L-tyrosine-p-azotrimethylammonium chloride (TAT), which does not cross-react with RAT (Alkan et al. 1972a). Bifunctional TAT molecules should not stack and, indeed, display no hypochromic effect, although some end-to-end association might occur between the electropositive centers and the single free carboxyl group. The degree of this end-to-end association can be influenced by using different flexible spacers which alter the charge distribution within the molecule. Symmetrical TAT bifunctionals with adipic acid and 1,6-diaminohexane spacers were synthesized. In the former, the spacer is joined to the amino groups of each tyrosyl residue, leaving two carboxyl groups free in the side chains, whereas in the latter the connection is with the carboxyls, leaving the amino groups free. Based strictly on chemical considerations, $(-CH_2-CH_2-CO-TAT-COOH)_2$ (adipic acid spacer) should be a poorer bifunctional antigen than TAT-SAC-TAT, whereas $[NH_2-TAT-NH-(CH_2)_3-]_2$ (diaminohexane spacer), which has only positive charges and should exhibit end-to-end repulsion, should be better. This predicted order of effectiveness was confirmed by the antibody responses to the compounds (Goodman et al. 1974), $[NH_2-TAT-NH-(CH_2)_3-]_2$ giving responses comparable to rigidly spaced $TAT-(PRO)_{10}-TAT$ (Table III).

These findings provide compelling evidence for a correlation between helper activity and the steric availability of determinants, reinforcing the thesis that at least two determinants, which may be identical, must be accessible to obtain an antibody response. They also strengthen the plausibility of antigen-bridging models of cell cooperation, which are summarized in Figure 1 without the role played by macrophages in activating antigen-specific lymphocytes.

TABLE III

Antibody Responses to Symmetrical Bifunctional Antigens

Immunizing Antigen[1]	Ppting Antibody[2]
	μg/ml
RAT	<2
$Ac-RAT-(SAC)_3-RAT$	<2
$Ac-RAT-(PRO)_{10}-RAT$	135 ± 18
$Ac-(PRO)_{10}-RAT$	<2
TAT	<2
Ac-TAT-SAC-TAT	55 ± 10
$[-CH_2-CH_2-CO-TAT-COOH]_2$	7 ± 2
$[NH_2-TAT-NH-(CH_2)_3-]_2$	156 ± 23
$Ac-TAT-(PRO)_{10}-TAT$	189 ± 32

[1] 4-7 guinea pigs immunized with 1 μmole of antigen

[2] $(RAT)_{11}$-BSA and $(TAT)_5$-BSA used in precipitin assays

A

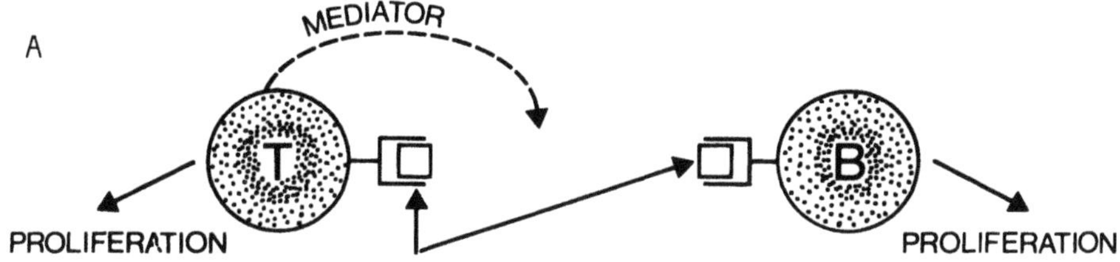

B

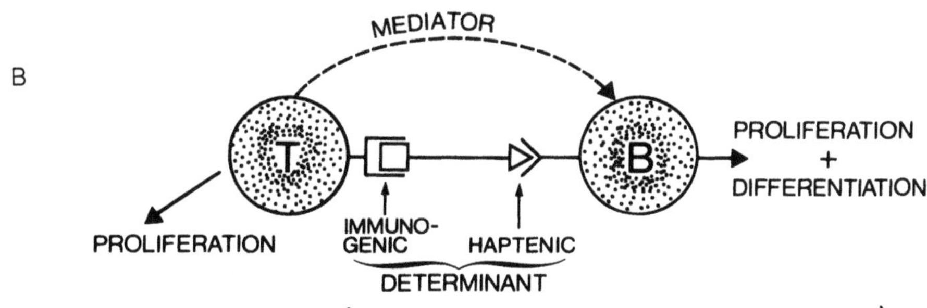

C

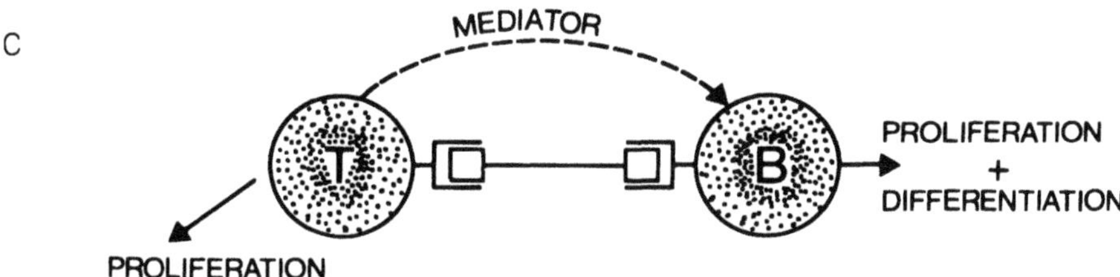

FIGURE 1. Models of cooperation between T and B cells in response to: A) a monofunctional antigen such as RAT or TAT; B) an asymmetric bifunctional antigen such as DNP-SAC-RAT; C) symmetrical bifunctional antigens such as RAT-$(PRO)_{10}$-RAT or TAT-SAC-TAT. The role of macrophages has been omitted.

ANTIGEN STRUCTURAL REQUIREMENTS FOR LYMPHOCYTE ACTIVATION

The series of bifunctional TAT antigens used to assess "self-help" were also ideally suited for comparing the efficiency of single-point and two-point antigen binding in triggering lymphocyte proliferation. Monofunctional antigens elicit proliferative responses in cultures of lymphoid cells (Alkan et al. 1972a), or enriched T cells (Goodman et al. 1974), from sensitized guinea pigs. In view of the greater stability of two-point versus single-point binding, it might be anticipated that symmetrical bivalent antigens would surpass their unideterminant counterparts in triggering DNA synthesis. However, in order for this advantage to be manifested, both determinants must bind to receptors on the same cell surface. For this purpose, bifunctional antigens with rigid spacers, so effective in mediating intercellular responses (B-T cooperation), should offer little, if any, advantage over monofunctionals since the spacer would restrict the mobility of the second determinant. On the other hand, flexible spacers might permit the binding of both determinants to receptors on the same cell. Comparison of the "proliferative efficiency" or dose-response curves of the antigens disclosed the advantage of two-point binding; all the bifunctional TAT compounds were superior to monofunctional TAT (Goodman et al. 1974). The compounds functioned in accordance with their predicted bifunctionality, $[NH_2\text{-TAT-NH-}(CH_2)_3\text{-}]_2$ being the most effective and markedly more efficient than $\text{TAT-}(PRO)_{10}\text{-TAT}$ (Table IV). Thus, structural requirements for cell triggering and for cell cooperation differ dramatically. Rigidly spaced bifunctional antigens serve admirably for cooperation but relatively poorly for antigen-induced proliferative responses.

THE MURINE RESPONSE TO THE AZOBENZENEARSONATE DETERMINANT

While it has been relatively easy to demonstrate the immunogenicity of azobenzenearsonate compounds in the guinea pig and the rat (Becker & Mäkelä 1975), the mouse has clear advantages in terms of T cell identification and the characterization of idiotypic markers associated with anti-ABA specificity (Nisonoff et al. 1977). Therefore, a concerted effort was made to seek evidence for T cell responses to ABA compounds in mice, primarily using strain A/J animals, which manifest a major idiotypic marker found on 20% to 70% of anti-ABA antibodies produced by individual mice (Nisonoff et al. 1977).

A significant response to immunization with RAT itself could be shown only by an increase in antigen-binding lymphocytes; no significant delayed hypersensitivity by footpad swelling or lymphocyte transformation *in vitro* was observed. Antigen-binding cells were assayed by formation of rosettes between lymphocytes and haptenated sheep erythrocytes (ABA-SRBC) (Lewis et al. 1976). The number of rosette forming cells increases about 30-fold following immunization with RAT in CFA (Table V). These rosettes are inhibitable by soluble RAT and about 40% of the antigen-binding lymphocytes are T cells on the basis of indirect fluorescence for the Thy-1 marker. This agrees very closely with the estimated ratio of B and T cells binding the ABA epitope in guinea pigs immunized with RAT (Goodman et al. 1974). Anti-ABA PFC were not found in the mice. The distribution of rosettes on the basis of size is shown in Figure 2. Lymphocytes binding fewer than four RBC were considered negative. Passage of spleen cells through nylon wool columns prior to rosetting removed those lymphocytes which formed the largest rosettes (18 RBC or more) (Figure 2B), whereas treatment with anti-thy-1 serum and complement removed the population of cells which formed smaller rosettes (data not shown). Thus, it can be concluded that immunization of A/J mice with RAT induces an increase in antigen-binding B and T cells, with B cells exhibiting a greater capacity for binding antigen than T cells. Since no PFC are seen and no circulating antibody can be detected by conventional techniques, it is unlikely that T cell rosettes are due to passive acquisition of antibody.

TABLE IV

Proliferative Response to TAT Antigens of LNC from Guinea Pigs Immunized with Monofunctional TAT

Test Antigen	Proliferative Index[1]	Proliferative Efficiency[2]
		μmoles ± S.E.
TAT	3.2 ± 0.46	
$[-CH_2-CH_2-CO-TAT-COOH]_2$	3.3 ± 0.57	0.083 ± 0.010
Ac-TAT-SAC-TAT	5.2 ± 0.69	0.036 ± 0.004
$[NH_2-TAT-NH-(CH_2)_3-]_2$	9.1 ± 2.26	0.004 ± 0.001
$Ac-TAT-(PRO)_{10}-TAT$	3.2 ± 0.66	0.058 ± 0.021

[1] Ratio of ^{14}C-thymidine incorporation in cultures of 2 x 10^6 LNC containing 0.10 μmole of antigen relative to cultures without antigen from the same animal. Values represent mean of 6 animals.

[2] μmoles of antigen required for level of lymphocyte stimulation given by 0.10 μmole of TAT.

[3] The maximum quantity used was 0.05 μmoles.

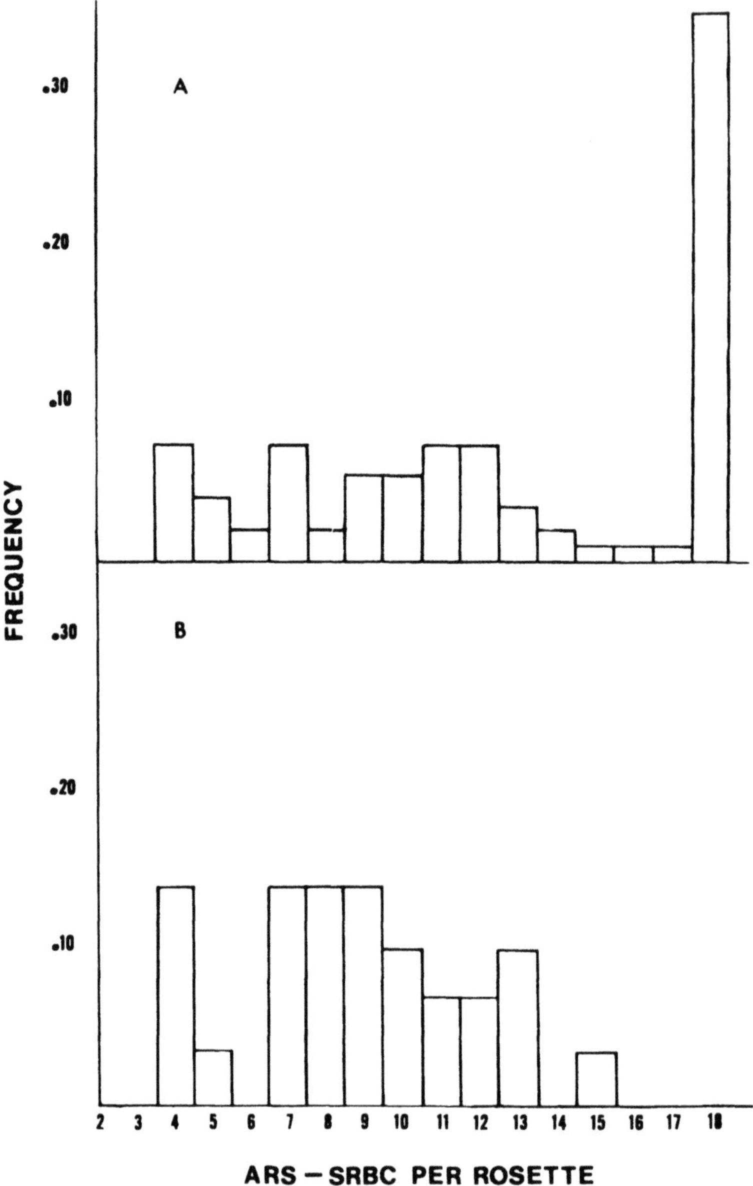

FIGURE 2. The frequency of spleen cells from A/J mice immunized with RAT forming rosettes of varying size with azobenzenearsonate-substituted SRBC: A) unfractionated spleen cells; B) nylon wool-passed spleen cells. The rosettes were more than 95% inhibitable by soluble RAT. Figures on the ordinate are % x 10.

TABLE V

Anti-ABA Rosette-forming Cells in A/J Mice Immunized with RAT

Antigen	$\log_{10}$ RFC/10^6 Spleen Cells	ABA PFC/ Spleen	%T[2]
CFA	1.60 ± 1.12	< 100	ND
RAT[1]	3.09 ± 0.13	< 100	43 ± 7

[1] A/J mice immunized with 500 μg of RAT in CFA intraperitoneally and assayed 9 days later for ABA specific RFC

[2] Determined by first reacting ABA-RFC with DNP-conjugated $(Fab')_2$ fragments of anti-thy-1 followed by Fluorescein-conjugated $(Fab')_2$ fragments of anti-DNP antibody

The response of A/J mice to ABA-KLH conjugates did engender delayed hypersensitivity elicitable by free RAT. This T cell reaction was assayed by footpad swelling 24 hours after local challenge with RAT. Barely detectable 1 week after injfection of ABA-KLH, it reached a peak increase in footpad size of 33% at 6 weeks, declining rapidly thereafter. This was a weaker response than the 59% swelling elicited by the homologous antigen, not unexpected in view of the small size of RAT, which would diffuse from the site of injection more rapidly, and the probable response to the protein carrier. In addition, Arthus reactions were seen in response to skin tests with the conjugate, but not with RAT. The reactions were specific, since swellings were not seen in normal animals skin tested with RAT.

Mice did not make anti-DNP PFC responses to bifunctional DNP-SAC-RAT compounds, tested in a number of inbred strains. However, it was found that azobenzenearsonate derivatives of L-histidine (RAH) engendered stronger helper activity than RAT. Bifunctional RAH compounds were prepared by first reacting N-dinitrophenyl-6-aminocaproic acid (Alkan et al. 1972a) with L-histidine methyl ester, using 1-ethyl-3-(3'dimethyl-aminopropyl) carbodiimide as coupling agent, to obtain N-DNP-6-aminocaproyl-L-histidine methyl ester. The methyl ester group was saponified and the resulting DNP-SAC-L-His-OH was reacted with the diazonium salt of arsanilic acid. The imidazole side chain of histidine yields three diazonium coupling products:

im-2-azo, im-4-azo and im-2,4-bis-azo derivatives. The three products were resolved and purified by repeated passage through LH-20 Sephadex columns in water. Identification of the 2-azo and 4-azo compounds was made possible by characteristic UV spectra for each. The monoazo bifunctional compounds were designated DNP-SAC-2-RAH and DNP-SAC-4-RAH, respectively. The positions of azo substitution in the imidazole ring are shown below.

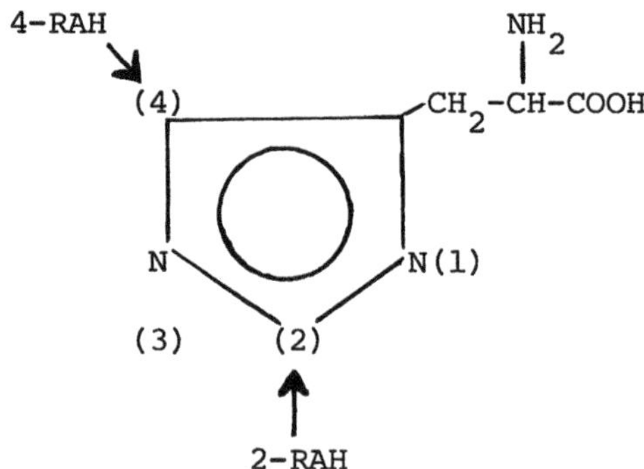

Immunization of A/J mice with each of the two bifunctional compounds led to significant anti-DNP PFC responses which peaked on day 8 (Figures 3 and 4). No anti-ABA PFC responses were detected, indicating that the RAH determinant provided help for the anti-DNP response, but not vice versa.

In order to confirm that T lymphocytes specific for RAH serve as helper cells in the anti-DNP response to the bifunctional compounds, cell transfer experiments were carried out in which irradiated mice were reconstituted with spleen cells from hapten-primed and carrier-primed donors. For this purpose, donor A/J mice were primed with either DNP-KLH to provide anti-DNP memory cells, or with 2-RAH to serve as a source of helper cells. One month later, spleen cells were transferred into irradiated (600r) A/J recipients, which received 0.1 mg of DNP-SAC-2-RAH the following day. Anti-DNP PFC were assayed 7 days later. It can be seen in Table VI that small but distinct PFC responses were obtained when both hapten-primed and carrier-primed spleen cells were transferred. The response was best when carrier-primed cells were passed through nylon wool prior to transfer, a procedure that removes more than 90% of the B lymphocytes (Julius et al. 1973). Transfer of only one of the two cell populations did not result in responses above those given by normal cells. These results indicate that helper T cells are generated by immunization with arsanilate-histidine conjugates. The combined evidence from antigen-binding studies, delayed hypersensitivity and helper effects strongly supports the existence of murine T cells with specificity for the arsanilate determinant.

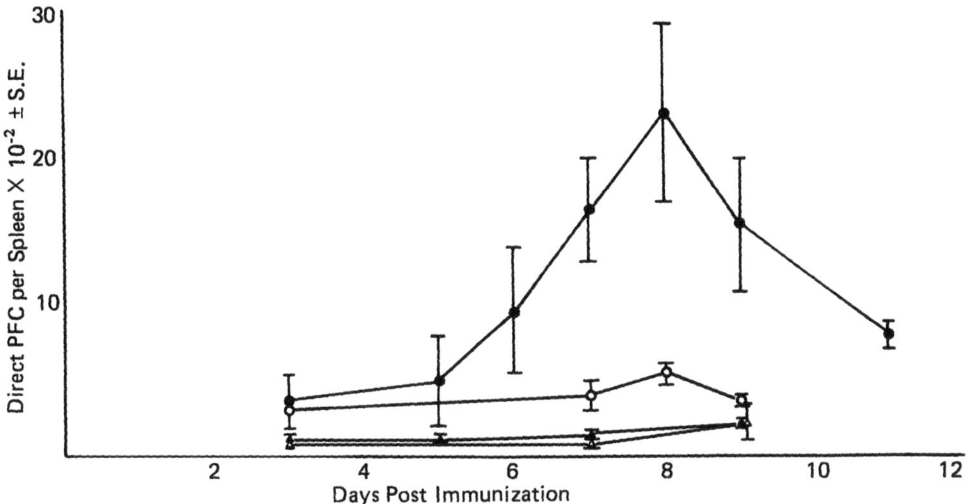

FIGURE 3. The direct PFC responses of A/J mice to DNP-SAC-2-RAH. Animals received 0.1 mg of antigen or an equivalent volume of saline in CFA. ● and ▲ represent anti-DNP and anti-ABA PFC, respectively, from antigen-immunized mice. ○ and △ represent the corresponding responses from saline-injected mice.

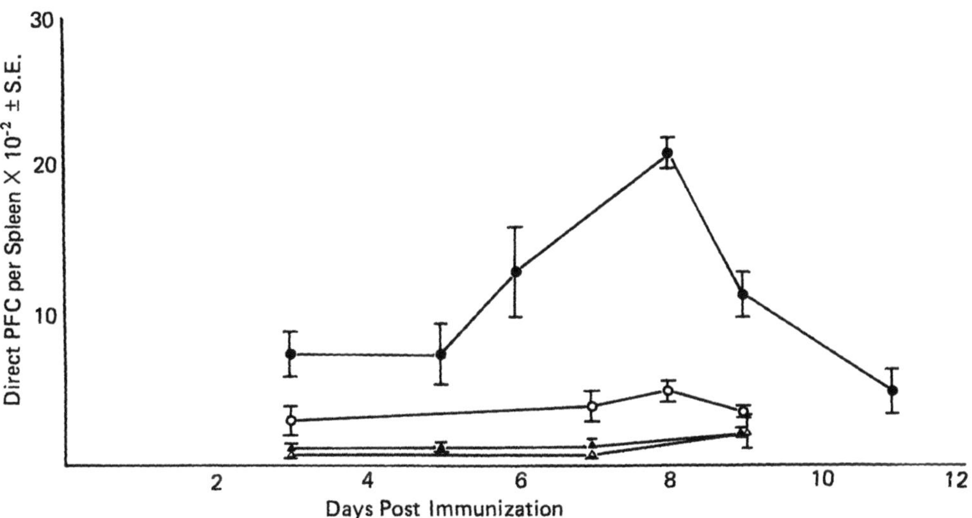

FIGURE 4. Direct PFC responses of A/J mice to DNP-SAC-4-RAH. See legend of Figure 3 for explanation of symbols.

TABLE VI

Reconstitution of Irradiated A/J Mice with Hapten- and Carrier-primed Spleen Cells for PFC Responses to DNP-SAC-2-RAH

Cells transferred[1] Type	Number	Direct PFC[2]/Spleen
DNP-KLH-primed + 2-RAH-primed	2.5×10^7 + 2.5×10^7	1479 ± 410[3]
DNP-KLH-primed + 2-RAH-primed (nylon wool passed)	2.5×10^7 + 2.5×10^7	2649 ± 205
2-RAH primed	2.5×10^7	390 ± 62
DNP-KLH primed	2.5×10^7	333 ± 17
Normal	5×10^7	522 ± 70
None		0

[1] Spleen cells were taken from mice primed 1 month earlier with 0.1 mg of antigen in CFA and transferred into recipients given 600r of x-irradiation.

[2] Recipients given 0.1 mg of DNP-SAC-2-RAH 1 day after cell transfer and assayed for PFC 7 days later.

[3] PFC numbers ± S.E.

A MAJOR IDIOTYPE ON T CELLS WHICH BIND THE ABA DETERMINANT IN A/J MICE

As mentioned earlier, all A/J mice immunized with ABA-KLH conjugates produce anti-hapten antibodies, 20 to 70% of which share a cross-reactive idiotype (CRI) (Nisonoff et al. 1977). The occurrence of this major idiotype on antibodies from all non-suppressed A/J mice and the demonstration of ABA-binding T cells in that strain, even following sensitization by RAT, which does not result in significant circulating antibody formation, raised the possibility that the idiotype might also be found on T cell antigen receptors. Shared idiotypic determinants on B cells and T cells have now been reported in several instances (Binz and Wigzell 1975, Krawinkel et al. 1977,

Ramseier et al. 1977), lending credence to this expectation. Another attractive feature of the ABA-A/J system is the extensive structural work on the idiotype-bearing antibodies being undertaken by Nisonoff and his collaborators (Nisonoff et al. 1977). Should the CRI also be associated with T cell receptors, then fascinating structural comparisons between T and B cell molecules with extremely similar or identical specificity might be feasible. For these reasons, it was clearly of interest to determine if the CRI was present on ABA-binding T cells. In the exploration of this question, rabbit anti-CRI antiserum (anti-id), generously provided by Dr. A. Nisonoff, was used as a probe for the CRI.

After some experimentation with immunization schedules, it was found that priming mice with 0.05 mg of ABA-KLH conjugates in CFA, followed one month later by boosting with the same quantity of antigen in saline, gave maximum numbers of spleen cells, and particularly splenic T cells, which rosetted 3-4 days later with SRBC substituted with ABA groups (ABA-SRBC). Five different experiments yielded a mean of 0.49 ± 0.11% (Table VII) of splenic lymphocytes which were rosette positive, meaning that they bound four or more ABA-SRBC. Virtually all of the rosettes were inhibitable by ABA-bovine IgG conjugates, demonstrating a specificity for the ABA group. In these experiments, 10^4 - 10^5 spleen cells were scanned in duplicate or triplicate from each mouse in order to compile antigen-binding data. To estimate the proportion of antigen-binding cells which carried the CRI, rosettes were counted in the absence and presence of 0.32 μg/ml of anti-id, a concentration well within the maximum inhibition plateau. In these experiments, 62 ± 5% of the rosetting cells were inhibitable by anti-id (Table VII), indicating the presence of CRI on the inhibited population. This figure falls within the 20 to 70% range of circulating anti-ABA antibodies bearing the CRI, reported by Nisonoff. The anti-id had no effect on the formation of rosettes between SRBC and spleen cells from mice immunized with SRBC.

The proportion of rosetting cells which were T cells was estimated by two methods. One utilized fluorescein-conjugated rabbit-anti-mouse Ig antibodies to identify putative B cell rosettes; non-fluorescent rosetting cells were assumed to be T cells. Staining and rosetting were performed under conditions which did not permit capping of membrane components. The second procedure, aimed at positive identification of T cells, employed the indirect fluorescence assay for the Thy-1 antigen described earlier. Anti-mouse Thy-1 antiserum was generated in rabbits using mouse brain as antigen and rendered specific as described previously (Golub 1971). The absorbed antiserum was cytotoxic for 100% of thymocytes, about 40% of splenic lymphocytes and more than 95% of nylon wool-passed splenic lymphocytes. $(Fab')_2$ fragments from this anti-Thy-1 antibody were substituted with DNP groups to a level which did not curtail antigen binding and the DNP-$(Fab')_2$ conjugates were reacted with spleen cells. The cells were washed and then reacted with fluorescein-conjugated rabbit $(Fab')_2$ fragments from antibody prepared against DNP-ovalbumin conjugates. The immunoglobulin reagents used in this procedure were $(Fab')_2$ fragments rather than intact molecules to avoid complications introduced by F_c receptors on lymphocytes, which could result in anomalous binding of the reagents. This indirect immunofluorescent assay for Thy-1 stained the appropriate proportions of thymic cells, spleen cells and nylon wool passed spleen cells. When applied to the rosette assay, it was found that about 40% of the total rosetting spleen cells were Thy-1 positive and 63% of the Thy-1 positive rosettes were CRI positive (Table VII).

The discrepancy between the figures for antigen-binding T cells derived from the two methods (5% versus 40%) is an obvious cause for concern and is part of the more general question concerning the biosynthetic origin of T cell antigen receptors detected in this type of experiment. Immunization with ABA-KLH induces anti-ABA antibody formation as well as cellular immunity, and this antibody may be passively acquired by T cells bearing Fc receptors. Such a mechanism could account for a smaller number of Ig-negative than of Thy-1-positive rosettes, since a proportion of Thy-1-positive cells would express the passively acquired antibody. A plausible way to deal with this difficulty might be to immunize with RAT or RAH instead of with ABA-KLH. The monofunctional antigens raise rosetting B and T cells, as described earlier, but little or no circulating antibody, minimizing the possibility that T cells which bind antigen in such responses do so passively. The disadvantage of this solution is that the monofunctional compounds are relatively weak immunogens, typically yielding only about 10% of the antigen-binding cells seen in response to ABA-KLH.

An alternate approach is to establish the biosynthetic origin of the receptor by enzymatic removal of existing receptors, followed by determination of their reappearance after sufficient time in culture. Ideally, this stripping-resynthesis procedure should be done in the absence of B cells, but because the recovery of rosetting T cells from nylon wool has been poor in our hands, preliminary experiments have been carried out with unfractionated spleen cells. Trypsinization was carried out as described by Prange et al. (1977), and cells were cultured for 16-24 hours to allow resynthesis to take place.

Trypsin treatment for 45 minutes completely abrogated the capacity of both B and T cells to form rosettes, but RFC numbers returned to near control values following culture (Table VIII). This recovery applied equally to T and B cells, the former comprising about 30% of the RFC in these experiments. Although these preliminary findings are encouraging, we have not yet shown recovery of the specific idiotype following enzymatic removal and, of paramount importance, the reappearance of receptors on T cells in the absence of B lymphocytes. Efforts to solidify the evidence for endogenous T cell receptors bearing the CRI are in progress.

TABLE VII

ABA-Binding Spleen Cells from A/J Mice[1]

	Spleen cell rosettes[2] Total	CRI+	T cell rosettes Total	CRI+
	0.43 ± 0.11[3]	62 ± 5[4]		
Ig(-)			5.1 ± 1.2[5]	56 ± 18[6]
Thy-1(+)			40 ±11[5]	63 ± 11[6]

[1] Immunized with ABA-KLH conjugates as described in the text.

[2] Spleen cells from immunized mice which form rosettes with ABA-SRBC.

[3] Expressed as percent of total spleen cells scanned (10^4-10^5 per mouse in triplicate) which are rosette positive. Mean values ± S.E. are given.

[4] Expressed as percent of total rosetting spleen cells which are inhibitable by anti-id.

[5] Expressed as percent of rosetting spleen cells which are T cells by either of two criteria: negative for Ig staining or positive for Thy-1.

[6] Expressed as percent of T rosettes inhibitable by anti-id.

TABLE VIII

Tryptic Removal and Reappearance of Lymphocyte Surface Receptors for ABA

Treatment[1] of A/J Spleen Cells	RFC/10^6 Total	% T	% Loss of RFC
None	5500 ± 451	33 ± 8	--
Culture 16-24 hours	5500 ± 850	30 ± 0	0
Trypsin 45 minutes	53 ± 53	--	99
Trypsin + culture	4400 ± 630	28 ± 2	20

[1] As described by Prange et al. (1977)

CONCLUSION

Mono- and bifunctional antigen molecules of the kind described in this review have been useful probes for studying mechanisms of lymphocyte activation and interaction. They should continue to be of assistance in understanding the nature of antigen presentation by macrophages, parameters of T cell-B cell cooperation, and the comparative structures of B cell and T cell receptors for the same epitope. For example, it should be feasible to obtain an estimate of the maximum permissible distance between T and B cells for delivery of the second signal by fabricating bifunctional antigens with a specified size range of rigid polyproline spacers between the haptenic and immunogenic determinants. This question is currently under investigation.

The demonstration in A/J mice of T cells specific for the ABA epitope offers a promising means of delineating the fine structure of the T cell antigen receptor and its relationship to antibodies which share the same idiotype. The preliminary experiments described here suggest that T cells bear the CRI characteristic of anti-ABA specificity, but fall short of unequivocal proof. The only completely convincing argument must, perforce, entail a demonstration of biosynthesis, preferably by internal radiolabelling, in the essential absence of B lymphocytes. Following this, it should be possible to isolate the idiotype-bearing T cell population with the aid of anti-id antibody and grow cells which express the CRI in continuous culture - perhaps through cell fusion - to provide receptor in quantities sufficient for detailed structural analysis.

ACKNOWLEDGEMENTS

The skilled technical assistance of Ms. Inge M. Stoltenberg is gratefully acknowledged. This work was supported by U.S. Public Health Service Grants AI 05664 and AI 11983 and National Science Foundation Grant GB 27591. Dr. Fong and Dr. Lewis were recipients of United States Public Health Service Postdoctoral Fellowships.

REFERENCES

Alkan, S.S., Nitecki, D.E., and Goodman, J.W. (1971) J. Immunol. 107, 353.

Alkan, S.S., Williams, E.B., Nitecki, D.E., and Goodman, J.W. (1972a) J. Exp. Med. 135, 1228.

Alkan, S.S., Bush, M.E., Nitecki, D.E., and Goodman, J.W. (1972b) J. Exp. Med. 136, 387.

Askonas, B.A.,and Williamson, A. (1972) Nature 238, 339.

Awdeh, Z.L., Askonas, B.A., and Williamson, A. (1967) Biochem. J. 102, 548.

Becker, M., and Mäkelä, O. (1975) Immunochemistry 12, 329.

Binz, H., and Wigzell, H. (1975) J. Exp. Med. 142, 197.

Bush, M.E., Alkan, S.S., Nitecki, D.E., and Goodman, J.W. (1972) J. Exp. Med. 136, 1478.

Dutton, R.W. (1974) In: The Immune Response: Genes, Receptors, Signals. Eds.: Sercarz, E., Williamson, A.R. & Fox, C.F., pp. 485-496. Academic Press, New York.

Golub, E.S. (1971) Cell. Immunol. 2, 353.

Goodman, J.W., Bellone, C.J., Hanes, D., and Nitecki, D.E. (1974) In: Progress in Immunology II, Vol. 2. Eds.: Brent, L. & Holborow, J., pp. 27-37. North Holland Publishing Co., Amsterdam.

Goodman, J.W. (1975) In: The Antigens. III., Ed.: Sela, M., pp. 127-187. Academic Press, New York.

Haber, E. (1967) Ann. Rev. Biochem. 37, 487.

Julius, M.H., Simpson, E., and Herzenberg, L.A. (1973) Eur. J. Immunol. 3, 645.

Krawinkel, U., Cramer, M., Berek, C., Hammerling, G., Black, S.J., Rajewsky, K., and Eichmann, K. (1976) Cold Spring Harbor Symposia on Quantitative Biology 41, 285.

Leskowitz, S., Jones, V., and Zak, S.J. (1966) J. Exp. Med. 123, 229.

Lewis, G.K., Ranken, R., Nitecki, D.E., and Goodman, J.W. (1976) J. Exp. Med. 144, 382.

Mitchison, N.A. (1969) In: Mediators of Cellular Immunity. Eds.: Lawrence, H.S. & Landy, M., pp. 71-80. Academic Press, New York.

Nauciel, C., and Raynaud, M. (1971) Eur. J. Immunol. 1, 257.

Nisonoff, A., Ju, S.-T., and Owen, F.L. (1977) Immunological Rev. 34, 89.

Prange, C.A., Green, C., Nitecki, D.E., and Bellone, C.J. (1977) J. Immunol. 118, 1311.

Rajewsky, K., Schirrmacher, V., Nase, S., and Jerne, N.K. (1969) J. Exp. Med. 129, 1131.

Ramseier, H., Aguet, M., and Lindenmann, J. (1977) Immunological Rev. 34, 50.

Roelants, G.E., and Goodman, J.W. (1974) J. Immunol. 112, 883.

Schimpl, A., Hünig, T.H., and Wecker, E. (1974) In: Progress in Immunology II, Vol. 2. Eds.: Brent, L. & Holborow, J., pp. 135-144. North Holland Publishing Co., Amsterdam.

Schlossman, S.F. (1972) In: Genetic Control of Immune Responsiveness. Eds.: McDevitt, H.O. & Landy, M., p. 54. Academic Press, London.

Senyk, G., Williams, E.B., Nitecki, D.E., and Goodman, J.W. (1971) J. Exp. Med. 133, 1294.

IMMUNOCHEMICAL STUDIES ON THE TOBACCO MOSAIC VIRUS PROTEIN

Eli Benjamini, Cherry Y. Leung, and Donna M. Rennick

Department of Medical Microbiology, School of Medicine
University of California, Davis, California

ABSTRACT

The decapeptide having the amino acid sequence Thr-Thr-Ala-Glu-Thr-Leu-Asp-Ala-Thr-Arg has been shown to be a major antigenic determinant of the tobacco mosaic virus protein in rabbits, mice and guinea pigs. The antigenic specificity of the decapeptide is attributed to its C-terminal tripeptide Ala-Thr-Arg. Although this tripeptide has no demonstrable binding with antibodies to the protein, its N-octanoylated derivative exhibits specific binding with antibodies as well as the capacity to elicit delayed skin reactions in guinea pigs immunized with the protein. The latter results suggest that both B cells and T cells have antigen receptors of identical specificities.

Although all mouse strains tested responded equally to TMVP, with the production of anti-protein, the response to the decapeptide was shown to be correlated (albeit not absolutely) with Ig allotype Ig^a exhibiting generally high responsiveness while Ig^b exhibiting generally low responsiveness. The low responsiveness could not be attributed to suppression of the secondary immune response.

INTRODUCTION

The tobacco mosaic virus protein (TMVP), has been characterized physicochemically and its amino acid sequence has been determined (Anderer et al., 1960; Tsugita et al., 1960; Knight, 1975). Consequently it has served as a model antigen for studying the immune response to protein antigens. Many of the immunochemical studies with TMVP have been performed in collaboration with Dr. Janis D. Young, Dr. William D. Peterson, Mr. Mike Shimizu and Dr. John M. Stewart.

These studies have been the subject of numerous publications and of a recent review (Benjamini, 1977). In this symposium we will present a summary of past and present findings of our immunochemical studies on TMVP with the aim of focusing the findings in the context of contemporary immunological concepts, of correlating our findings with those of our colleagues utilizing other protein antigen systems, and with the hope of identifying new directions for future immunochemical investigations. We will summarize our investigations on the relationship between antigenic structure and several immunological parameters, using an isolated, well characterized antigenic determinant of the protein. The immunological parameters include binding with antibodies, elicitation of delayed hypersensitivity, and immunogenicity. Moreover, we will summarize our up to date studies on what appears to be an allotype linked segregation of immune responsiveness to the determinant. Findings which have not yet been published will be described in detail; other findings will be summarized and reference given to previous publications.

RELATIONSHIP BETWEEN ANTIGENIC STRUCTURE AND BINDING WITH ANTIBODIES

Immunization of rabbits with TMVP induces the formation of antibodies capable of binding with an eicosapeptide representing residues 93-112 of the protein. This has been established by the finding that the complement fixation by the protein and anti-protein could be inhibited to a large extent by this eicosapeptide (Benjamini et al., 1964). Moreover, it has been shown that the [^{14}C]-N-acetyl eicosapeptide exhibited direct binding with rabbit anti-TMVP (Benjamini et al., 1965). In an attempt to localize the antigenic determinant of the eicosapeptide, its C-terminal decapeptide having the amino acid sequence Thr-Thr-Ala-Glu-Thr-Leu-Asp-Ala-Thr-Arg (henceforth called decapeptide) was synthesized by the Merrifield solid phase peptide synthesis (Merrifield, 1964). The binding of the decapeptide with anti-TMVP was ascertained by the ability of the [^{14}C]-N-acetyl decapeptide to exhibit binding with anti-TMVP (Stewart et al., 1966) and by the ability of the decapeptide to inhibit the binding between anti-TMVP and the [^{14}C]-N-acetyl-eicosapeptide (Benjamini et al., 1968a). Moreover, the finding that the above reaction could be completely inhibited by the decapeptide indicated that the latter constituted the entire antigenic determinant of the eicosapeptide. Further studies with synthetic C-terminal portions of the decapeptide revealed that the C-terminal pentapeptide portion having the sequence Leu-Asp-Ala-Thr-Arg (henceforth referred to as pentapeptide) exhibited binding with anti-TMVP (Young et al., 1967) and that the binding between anti-TMVP and [^{14}C]-N-acetyl decapeptide could be completely inhibited by the pentapeptide (Benjamini et al., 1968a). Since the pentapeptide could inhibit completely the reaction between anti-TMVP and the decapeptide, and since the decapeptide could inhibit completely the reaction between anti-TMVP and the eicosapeptide, it can be concluded that the pentapeptide contains the entire antigenic determinant of the eicosapeptide. However, the reaction between anti-TMVP and a given [^{14}C] acetyl peptide was inhibited by the homologous (nonacetylated peptide) to the extent of 50% at a ratio of inhibitor to radioactive antigen of 1:1 and to the extent of 90-100% at a ratio of approximately 5:1. In contrast, the inhibition by shorter C-terminal peptides required large excesses of inhibitor to radioactive test antigen. These findings indicate that although the entire antigenic specificity of the eicosapeptide is contained in the C-terminal pentapeptide, the binding affinities were in the order of eicosapeptide > decapeptide > pentapeptide. These findings imply that sequences N-terminally to the pentapeptide Leu-Asp-Ala-Thr-Arg contribute in a nonspecific manner to the binding of the peptide with anti-TMVP. This conclusion is corroborated by the findings that a synthetic decapeptide having the sequence Ala-Ala-Ala-Ala-Ala-Leu-Asp-Ala-Thr-Arg exhibited binding with anti-TMVP similar in magnitude to that exhibited by the native decapeptide (Benjamini et al., 1968a). Moreover, it has been demonstrated that the shortest peptide which exhibited binding with anti-TMVP was the pentapeptide Leu-Asp-Ala-Thr-Arg; its C-terminal tetrapeptide or shorter peptides did not exhibit binding (Young et al., 1967). However, N-octanoyl-Ala-Thr-Arg (henceforth referred to as the Octanoyl-tripeptide) exhibited specific binding with anti-TMVP similar in magnitude to that exhibited by the decapeptide (Benjamini et al., 1968b). It is important to note that N-octanoyl-Thr-Arg exhibited no binding. These findings indicate that the antigenic specificity of the pentapeptide resides in its C-terminal tripeptide. However, for demonstrable binding with rabbit anti-protein antibodies it was required to attach a hydrophobic group N-terminally. It was shown that demonstrable binding with anti-TMVP begins with the pentapeptide and increases with N-terminal increase in peptide size (Young et al., 1967) and that the entire determinant of the eicosapeptide resides in the pentapeptide. Accordingly it may be postulated that the increase in peptide size brings forth the contribution of auxiliary binding forces and that these forces are largely hydrophobic. It has been proposed (Karush, 1962; Metzger et al., 1963; Singer, 1965; Benjamini et al., 1969) that hydrophobic areas of antigen enhance the binding with antibodies through hydrophobic interaction with complementary hydrophobic areas of the antibody. This implies that, that, in the case of rabbit anti-TMVP, in addition to having an area complementary to the antigenic specificity Ala-Thr-Arg, the antibody combining site may contain hydrophobic area(s) which react with the hydrophobic area N-terminally to this tripeptide. Since experiments have shown that the hydrophobic area of the antigen did not have rigid structural restrictions (it could consist of leucine, isoleucine, D-leucine, tryosine, pentaalanine or octanoic acid) (Benjamini et al., 1968b; Young et al., 1968), it is conceivable that the interaction with the hydrophobic area on the antibody is essentially nonspecific and that it serves as an important auxiliary force in the binding between the specific sterically complementary area of the antigen (Ala-Thr-Arg) and the antibody site.

However, there is a restriction imposed on the hydrophobic interaction in that the participating hydrophobic groups on the antigen and antibody must be present in the correct position for interaction. This restriction is dictated by the juxtaposition of the antigenic sequence and the complementary antibody area. Thus, at least in the case of the antigenic TMVP peptide, the antigenic area is composed of two functionally distinct areas, one which plays a decisive role in conferring antigenic specificity but which by itself has nonmeasurable binding with the antibody, and another area which dramatically increases this binding. This implies that the complimentary antibody site may be composed of an area which determines the specificity of the antibody and a hydrophobic area which interacts with the hydrophobic area of the antigen.

It is interesting that very similar conclusions may be drawn for the binding of TMVP peptides with antibodies to TMVP produced in the mouse. Recent experiments showed that intradermal injection of mice (CSW) with 10 μg TMVP in Freund's Complete Adjuvant followed 3 weeks later by an aqueous subcutaneous booster injection with 10 μg TMVP produced antibodies capable of binding with [^{125}I] Tyr-Thr-Thr-Ala-Glu-Thr-Leu-Asp-Ala-Thr-Arg (henceforth referred to as [^{125}I] tyrosyl-decapeptide) (Table 1).

Table 1

The Binding of Non-Immune and TMVP-Immune Mouse Serum with ^{125}I-tyrosyl-decapeptide*

Mice	Serum (ml)	CPM Bound
TMVP-Immune	0.05	44,000
	0.10	84,000
	0.30	100,000
Non-Immune	0.05	300
	0.10	500
	0.30	1,500

*The peptide was used at 0.1 nMoles representing approximately 200,000 cpm.

Experiments on the inhibition of the reaction between ^{125}I tyrosyl-decapeptide and anti-TMVP by various peptides (Table 2) reveal that, as expected, the reaction is inhibited to the extent of 50% by the non-iodinated homologous peptide at an inhibitor to antigen ratio of 1:1. The same degree of inhibition is achieved by the decapeptide and by its C-terminal nonapeptide at inhibitor to antigen ratio of

Table 2

The Inhibition of the Binding Between ^{125}I-tyrosyl-decapeptide and Mouse Anti-TMVP by Various Peptides*

Inhibitor	Moles Inhibitor/Moles Test Antigen Required for 50% Inhibition
Tyr-Thr-Thr-Ala-Glu-Thr-Leu-Asp-Ala-Thr-Arg	1:1
Thr-Thr-Ala-Glu-Thr-Leu-Asp-Ala-Thr-Arg	5:1
Thr-Ala-Glu-Thr-Leu-Asp-Ala-Thr-Arg	100:1
Ala-Glu-Thr-Leu-Asp-Ala-Thr-Arg	>10,000:1
Glu-Thr-Leu-Asp-Ala-Thr-Arg	>10,000:1
Thr-Leu-Asp-Ala-Thr-Arg	>10,000:1
Leu-Asp-Ala-Thr-Arg	>10,000:1
Octanoyl-Ala-Thr-Arg	30% inhibition at 100:1

*Test antigen was used at 0.1 nMoles; anti-TMVP was used at 0.1 ml represeting antibody deficiency.

5:1 and 100:1 respectively. The data indicates that while the N-terminal octapeptide and shorter N-terminal peptides were not inhibitory even at ration of 10,000:1, the octanoyl-tripeptide inhibited 30% of the reation at a ratio of 100:1. Since it was technically impractical to use higher concentrations of octanoyl tripeptide for inhibition it was impossible to ascertain whether or not the entire antigenic specificity of the decapeptide can be attributed to the tripeptide Ala-Thr-Arg. However, the data demonstrate, that, as is in the case with the raction between rabbit anti-TMVP and the TMVP antigenic peptide, mouse anti-TMVP bind with the decapeptide and with its C-terminal nonapeptide. Moreover the data indicate the importance of hydrophobicity for the binding and that Ala-Thr-Arg constitutes part of a specific determinant. Although the hydrophobicity may be essential for the system under study it need not necessarily apply universally to all antigen antibody interactions. It is possible that for some antigen-antibody interactions, especially those involving aromatic hydrophobic haptens, the antigenic specificity and the hydrophobicity are conferred by the same chemical grouping. As indicate by Porter (1972), this would be in agreement with the observations that the binding of polysaccharides with antibodies is generally lower than the binding of antibodies with their homologous aromatic haptens.

The size of the antigenic pentapeptide of TMVP is of the order of the size of many antigenic determinants of proteins and polysaccharides (Kabat, 1968; Porter, 1972). It is tempting to suggest that the complementary antibody site is of a similar size. Indeed many studies on the size of the antibody combining site to a variety of antigenic structures put it in the order of less than 20 amino acids (not necessarily sequentially adjacent in the chain); conclusive proof is forthcoming from X-ray crystallographic studies.

Further insight into antigenic specificity was gained by investigating the binding of rabbit anti-TMVP with the pentapeptide Leu-Asp-Ala-Thr-Arg and with its synthetic analogs (Young et al., 1968). Results of these investigations showed the exquisite specificity of the C-terminal portion of this peptide. Substitution of alanine by leucine or by glycine, substitution of the threonine by leucine or glycine, or omitting the C-terminal arginine resulted in peptides with no demonstrable binding. Substitution of the threonine with serine yielded a peptide with demonstrable binding but lower than that of the native pentapeptide. On the other hand, changes in the

Table 3

The Comparative Binding of Anti-TMVP with the N-[^{14}C]-Acetylated Antigenic Peptide of TMVP and with Acetylated Analogs*

N-[^{14}C]-Acetyl Peptide	Comparative Binding
Leu-Asp-Ala-Thr-Arg	1.00
Ala-Asp-Ala-Thr-Arg*	0.15
Ile-Asp-Ala-Thr-Arg	0.33
Tyr-Asp-Ala-Thr-Arg	0.36
D-Leu-Asp-Ala-Thr-Arg	0.44
Leu-Glu-Ala-Thr-Arg	0.00
Leu-Asn-Ala-Thr-Arg	0.56
Leu-Asp-Leu-Thr-Arg	0.04
Leu-Asp-Gly-Thr-Arg	0.01
Leu-Asp-Ala-Leu-Arg	0.05
Leu-Asp-Ala-Gly-Arg	0.00
Leu-Asp-Ala-Ser-Arg	0.31
Asp-Ala-Thr-Arg	0.00
Leu-Asp-Ala-Thr	0.01
Arg-Thr-Ala-Asp-Leu	0.01
N-^{14}C-Octanoyl-Ala-Thr-Arg	2.84
N-^{14}C-Octanoyl-Thr-Arg	0.17

*After Young et al., 1968.
**Substituted position is underlined.

N-terminal dipeptide portion of the pentapeptide could be made provided the changes maintained hydrophobicity of this portion of the peptide. Thus, substitution of leucine with alanine, isoleucine, tyrosine or D-leucine, resulted in active peptides. In fact, substituting the N-terminal dipeptide with octanoic acid resulted in a peptide with higher binding than that of the native pentapeptide. The results strongly support the conclusions presented earlier that antigenic specificity is governed by the C-terminal tripeptide portion of the pentapeptide while enhanced binding through enhanced hydrophobicity is contributed by portions N-terminally to the tripeptide Ala-Thr-Arg. Moreover, these data as well as others (Benjamini et al., 1969) indicate the high degree of specificity of the area which contributes to antigenic specificity compared to the low degree of specificity exhibited by the hydrophobic area.

RELATIONSHIP BETWEEN ANTIGENIC STRUCTURE AND CELL-MEDIATED IMMUNITY

The relationship between antigenic structure and cell-mediated immunity has been ascertained in guinea pigs. Immunization of guinea pigs with TMVP induces delayed hypersensitivity to the antigen. Thus challenge of sensitized animals with the protein TMVP elicits delayed skin reactions. Moreover, challenge of such TMVP-sensitized guinea pigs with the decapeptide, its C-terminal pentapeptide, and its N-butyryl, hexanoyl and octanoyl-C-terminal tripeptide elicit specific delayed skin reactions in the sensitized animals (Spitler et al., 1970). Also, there was a good correlation between the capacity of a peptide to elicit delayed skin reactions and its ability to elicit M.I.F. production by peritoneal exudate cells from TMVP-immunized guinea pigs. Considering the low molecular weight of the antigenic peptides and the fact that they are non-immunogenic (vide infra), they may be considered haptens. Numerous studies throughout the past 15-20 years have demonstrated that in a classical hapten-carrier situation antibodies are elicited with specificity to the hapten whereas delayed hypersensitivity is directed towards the carrier. In this context, the results which demonstrate the ability of the peptides haptens to elicit delayed skin reactions and M.I.F. do not conform to the classical hapten-carrier situation.

From immunochemical studies performed on many protein antigens including those of known amino acid sequence and/or structure (reviewed by Benjamini et al., 1972), it appears that antigenic areas of proteins may be divided into three major categories (a) those recognized by antibodies and B cells (b) those recognized by T cells and (c) those recognized by antibodies, B cells and T cells. Results of the investigations with the antigenic peptides of TMVP indicate that these peptide determinants fall into the third broad category - they are recognized by circulating antibodies implying B cell recognition, and they are also capable of eliciting delayed type hypersensitivity (DTH) implying T cell recognition as well as T cell activation. With respect to recognition, it is interesting to note that the antibody specificity and the specificity of DTH are similar if not identical. Thus elicitation of DTH and binding with antibodies seem to depend upon the pentapeptide or more precisely upon its C-terminal tripeptide Ala-Thr-Arg. If one accepts that the antigen receptor on the B cell is of the same specificity as the antibody which this B cell ultimately produces and that the DTH is elicited by virtue of activation of T cell with receptor(s) to a given determinant, then the above findings suggest that the B cell and T cell receptors to the peptide(s) are similar if not identical. This conclusion is in agreement with recent findings which indicate identity of idiotypes on the T cells and on the B cells (Black et al., 1975; Binz and Wigzell, 1977; Eichmann, 1977; Krawinkel et al., 1977).

The ability of the peptides to elicit DTH (i.e. activate T cells) in spite of their univalence and their non-immunogenicity (*vide infra*) indicate that perhaps the requirements for activating the T cells which participate in DTH may differ from the requirements for activating other T cells (such as helper cells) or B cells which are essential for immunogenicity. It is still not clear by what mechanisms these peptides, which seem univalent with respect to their reactivity with antibodies or immunogenicity, activate the T cells for DTH.

RELATIONSHIP BETWEEN STRUCTURE AND IMMUNOGENICITY

Whereas it could be easily demonstrated that the eicosapeptide, its C-terminal decapeptide, pentapeptide and octanoyl-tripeptide exhibited binding with anti-TMVP and elicited DTH in guinea pigs immunized with TMVP, we could not demonstrate the immunogenicity of these peptides. The peptides could not elicit, *in vivo* or *in vitro* a primary response (to the peptides or to TMVP) in animals subsequently immunized with TMVP or a secondary response in TMVP-primed animals (Spitler et al., 1970). The capacity of the peptides to elicit DTH and MIF in TMVP-sensitized guinea pigs is sharply contrasted with their non-immunogenicity in guinea pigs. These findings point to a fundamental difference in the capacity of univalent peptides to elicit DTH and to induce either cell mediated immunity or circulating antibodies. It is well accepted that although antibodies are produced by cells belonging to the B cell lineage, T cells participate in several functions such as helper function, DTH, and suppression. Since a given peptide is capable of eliciting T cell functions (DTH) in TMVP-sensitized guinea pigs in spite of their non-immunogenicity, it appears that the requirements for immunogenicity differ from the requirements for activating DTH participating T cells either *in vivo* or *in vitro*. It is well established that there exist several T cell subpopulations which differ in their antigenic markers and functions (Cantor et al., 1975; Fathman et al., 1975). It is possible that there exist two subpopulations of T cells: one which is activated by the univalent peptides and which participates in DTH, and another, which participates in immunogenicity, and which cannot be activated by the peptides. Since no antibodies have ever been detected in animals injected with the peptides it can be concluded that the peptides were unable to activate B cells An alternative explanation for the non-immunogenicity of the peptides despite their ability to elicit DTH is that the same T cell may participate in both, but perhaps the requirements for activation for these two purposes differ. These two possibilities await resolution.

In view of the non-immunogenicity of the peptides, the specificity of antibodies induced by the peptides was studied using peptide conjugated to protein carriers. The various peptides (shown in Table 4) were conjugated to succinylated bovine serum albumin (SuBSA) by use of 1-ethyl-3-(3-dimethylaminopropyl) carbodiimide (Fearney et al.

Table 4

The Specificity of Antibodies from Rabbits Immunized with TMVP and with Peptides Conjugated to Succinylated Bovine Serum Albumin*

	Test Antigen: N-[^{14}C]-Acetyl				
Immunogen: Peptide Conjugated to Succinylated Bovine Serum Albumin	Leu-Asp-Ala-Thr-Arg	Leu-Asp-Gly-Thr-Arg	Leu-Asp-αABu**-Thr-Arg	Leu-Asp-Ala-Gly-Arg	Thr-Thr-Ala-Glu-Thr-Leu-Asp-Ala-Thr-Arg
TMVP	+	-	+	-	+
Leu-Asp-Ala-Thr-Arg	1.00	0.00	4.90	0.00	2.22
Leu-Asp-αABu-Thr-Arg	0.35	0.00	1.00	0.08	1.70
Leu-Asp-Ala-Gly-Arg	0.00	0.00	0.02	1.00	0.04
Thr-Thr-Ala-Glu-Thr-Leu-Asp-Ala-Thr-Arg	0.30	0.00	0.35	0.02	1.00

*Plus or minus signs signify binding or no binding respectively. All numbers are relative to the binding of antibodies to a given conjugate with the homologous peptide valued at 1.00. (Benjamini, 1977).

**αABu signifies α-aminobutyric acid.

1971); the conjugates contained 10-15 groups of peptide per molecule of carrier proteins. Following immunization of rabbits with the various conjugates the serum from each rabbit was tested for binding with the homologous peptide as well as with several closely related analogs. The results (Table 4) are presented relative to the binding of a certain peptide with antibodies produced by the same peptide conjugated to a carrier. Also, depicted in the table (as + or -) is the capacity of each peptide to bind with rabbit anti-TMVP. Although only a single rabbit was immunized with each immunogen and only a small number of analogs were tested, it appears that the specificities of the induced antibodies differ greatly, with the best binding exhibited by the homologous peptide. Moreover, conjugates of peptides which bind with rabbit anti-TMVP elicit antibodies capable of binding with those peptides which exhibit binding with anti-TMVP, but not with peptides which do not bind anti-TMVP. Thus, it appears that the specificity of antibodies produced by immunization with the protein TMVP is broadly similar to the specificity of antibodies produced by conjugates of those peptide determinants which bind with anti-TMVP. It is therefore tempting to suggest that these results confirm the notion that the specificity of the receptor on the cells which participate in antibody production is similar (if not identical) to the specificity of the produced antibodies.

It is intersting that rabbit antibodies produced in response to immunization with a conjugate consisting of the decapeptide and SuBSA were capable of binding not only with the peptides but also with the parent protein TMVP (Fearney et al., 1971). These findings suggest that the conformation of the decapeptide on the carrier is similar to its conformation on the protein TMVP. Moreover, the findings suggest that the decapeptide (which appears to be a random coil) is a sequential rather than conformational determinant. This is supported by the findings that its C-terminal pentapeptide protion, lacking a specific conformation, is capable of completely inhibiting the binding between the decapeptide and anti-TMVP.

To date, attempts to elicit anti-peptide antibodies by immunization of several strains of mice with a conjugate consisting of the decapeptide and SuBSA have failed. We were also unsuccessful in eliciting significant titers of anti-peptide antibodies by immunization of mice with the decapeptide conjugated to bovine gamma globulin (BGG) using carbodiimide or by immunization with a conjugate consisting of BGG to which the N-tyrosyl-decapeptide was attached by diazolization with bis diazotized benzidine (Arquilla, 1970). The conjugates contained 6 and 15 groups peptide per molecule BGG respectively. In view of the above, it was suspected that perhaps the conjugation resulted in a preparation in which the decapeptide's conformation or composition has been changed. To test this possibility, the capacity of the conjugate to inhibit the reaction between mouse anti-TMVP and ^{125}I-tyrosyl-decapeptide was tested. The results presented in Table 5 show that the inhibition of the reaction was achieved without

Table 5

The Capacity of TMVP Peptides and of Peptide-Protein Conjugates to Inhibit the Binding Between ^{125}I-Tyr-Thr-Thr-Ala-Glu-Thr-Leu-Asp-Ala-Thr-Arg and Mouse Anti-TMVP*

Inhibitor	Moles Inhibitor/Moles Test Antigen Required for 50% Inhibition
Tyr-Thr-Thr-Ala-Glu-Thr-Leu-Asp-Ala-Thr-Arg	1:1
Thr-Thr-Ala-Glu-Thr-Leu-Asp-Ala-Thr-Arg	5:1
BGG-Thr-Thr-Ala-Glu-Thr-Leu-Asp-Ala-Thr-Arg (carbodiimide)	2:1**
BGG-Tyr-Thr-Thr-Ala-Glu-Thr-Leu-Asp-Ala-Thr-Arg (diazotization)	2:1**

*Test antigen used at 0.1 nMoles with 0.1 ml antibodies representing antibody deficiency.

**Calculated from moles peptide per protein of 6 and 12 for conjugation by use of carbodiimide and by diazotization respectively.

necessitating significant excess of inhibitor. This indicates that the decapeptide on both conjugates is presented in a way similar to that of the free decapeptide or to that of the decapeptide on TMVP since it is recognized by and binds with anti-TMVP. The reasons for our failure to produce, in mice, anti-peptide antibodies by immunization with conjugates is not clear. Our attempts to achieve this goal are continuing.

GENETIC CONTROL OF THE IMMUNE RESPONSIVENESS TO ANTIGENIC AREAS OF TMVP

Throughout the years of investigations on the ability of anti-TMVP sera to bind with the decapeptide and shorter peptide, it became apparent that all the tested animals (rabbits, mice, guinea pigs and sharks) produced antibodies capable of binding with TMVP or with the decapeptide. However, variations were noted in the capacity of various rabbit antisera to bind with C-terminal shorter peptides (Benjamini et al., 1968a,b). Thus some rabbits produced antibodies capable of binding with the C-terminal pentapeptide, while the hexapeptide or heptapeptide was required for demonstrable binding with anti-TMVP produced by other rabbits. Also, it was shown that anti-TMVP produced by various rabbits exhibited different binding affinities with the decapeptide and shorter peptides. However, in spite of all these variations it was demonstrated that the anti-TMVP antibodies produced by all rabbits exhibited binding with the octanoyl tripeptide (octanoyl Ala-Thr-Arg), and that only few variations existed in the specificity of the antibodies to this test antigen (Benjamini et al., 1969). Since all of the rabbit antisera tested exhibited the capacity to bind with N-octanoyl-Ala-Thr-Arg but not necessarily the capacity to bind with the pentapeptide Leu-Asp-Ala-Thr-Arg, it is postulated that antisera produced by all the rabbits immunized with TMVP contained antibodies which recognize Ala-Thr-Arg; however antibodies produced by some rabbits do not possess sufficient hydrophobic areas in the correct juxtaposition to express measurable binding with Leu-Asp-Ala-Thr-Arg. The hydrophobic interaction with these antibodies is enhanced by reacting with the highly hydrophobic antigen N-octanoyl-Ala-Thr-Arg. It therefore appears that differences exist between individual rabbits with respect to their ability to produce antibodies with high enough affinity to Leu-Asp-Ala-Thr-Arg for the expression of measurable binding. Regarding the specificity of antibodies produced by the different rabbits it appears that, in general, the degree of specificity for Ala-Thr-Arg is remarkably high. This is true for antibodies produced by a given rabbit and also for antibodies produced by different rabbits (Benjamini et al., 1969).

During the course of the investigations on the immune response of mice to TMVP and its antigenic peptides, it became apparent that while antibodies produced by all the tested strains exhibit the capacity to bind with TMVP, dramatic differences were found in the capacity of anti-TMVP produced by various strains to bind with the antigenic decapeptide (summarized by Benjamini, 1977). Of particular interest are two congenic strains, CSW and CWB, both of $H\text{-}2^b$ histocompatibility but with CSW and CWB having Ig^a and Ig^b immunoglobulin allotypes respectively. In response to immunization with TMVP, both strains produce antibodies which exhibit identical binding with TMVP. However, whereas anti-TMVP produced by CSW exhibits a high degree of binding with the antigenic decapeptide, antibodies produced by the CWB mice exhibit only marginal binding (if any) with this peptide. Subsequent experiments showed that the low response could be attributed to the reduced concentration of antipeptide antibodies (approximately one fourth of that present in high responder's sera) and, more importantly, to the fact that the binding affinity of antipeptide CSW antibodies was forty times higher than that of the CWB antibodies (K_o of 1.6×10^7 and 4×10^5 liters per mole for CSW and CWB respectively) (Benjamini, 1977). Preliminary genetic analysis revealed that the segregation of the responsiveness to the antigenic decapeptide was associated, in a general way, with the immunoglobulin allotype, Ig^a being high responders and Ig^b being low responders. However, the correlation between responsiveness and allotype was not absolute (Herzenberg, 1972). Nevertheless, considering the above results several explanations may be proposed for the low responsiveness of the CWB strain. One possibility is that the CWB strain lacks high affinity decapeptide-recognizing cells. Experiments are currently in progress to ascertain this possibility. Another possibility is that the low responsiveness of the CWB strain is due to specific suppression of the response to the decapeptide determinant. The identical H-2 of the two strains affords the unique opportunity to perform adoptive transfer experiments within as well as between the strains. Accordingly the possibility of suppression was recently investigated by measuring the secondary anti-peptide response of CSW mice in the presence of unprimed or of TMVP-primed CWB spleen cells. The experiment was performed as follows: CSW mice were primed with 100 μg TMVP in Freund's complete adjuvant. Eight weeks following the priming, when the anti-decapeptide titer reduced to minimal levels the animals were sacrificed and the spleen cells were harvested. The cells (2×10^8 cells representing cells from two spleens) were mixed with 2×10^8 spleen cells obtained from normal CSW or CWB mice, or with 2×10^8 cells obtained from CWB mice which have been primed 10 days earlier with 100 μg TMVP in Freund's complete adjuvant. The cells (the above number of cells per recipient) were transfered into CSW mice which have been lethally irradiated (800R) and supplemented with normal CSW bone marrow cells. One day after the transfer the recipients received a booster injection consisting of 50 μg of TMVP in phosphate buffered saline. The animals (three recipients per group) were bled one week after transfer and the capacity of their sera to bind with ^{125}I-tyrosyl decapeptide was

Table 6

The Induction of Antibodies, Capable of Binding with ^{125}I-N-tyrosyl-decapeptide, in Irradiated Bone Marrow Reconstituted CSW Mice Following Transfer of TMVP Primed CSW Spleen Cells Supplemented with Normal CSW or CWB Spleen Cells or With TMVP-Primed CWB Spleen Cells*

Spleen Cells Supplement	Serum (ml)	CPM Bound**
Normal CSW	0.10	2483
	0.05	1044
	0.01	427
Normal CWB	0.10	3583
	0.05	1036
	0.01	330
TMVP-Primed CWB	0.10	2681
	0.05	1230
	0.01	736
Control (receiving normal CSW cells only)	0.1	50

*Recipients were irradiated with 800R and received normal CSW bone marrow cells. Recipients were given 50 μg TMVP in saline 1 day following transfer and bled one week following transfer; ^{125}I-N-tyrosyl-decapeptide was used at 0.1 nMoles (approx. 30,000 cpm).
**Numbers represent average of three recipients.

assessed. Results in Table 6 clearly indicate that the ability of the CSW recipients to mount, *in vivo*, a secondary response to the decapeptide was not affected by the unprimed or primed CWB cells, suggesting that the latter are not suppressive for the secondary response. Experiments are in progress to further ascertain the genetic basis of the immune response to the antigenic area peptide of TMVP and to gain insight into the mechanism underlying this phenomenon. Of particular interest is the possibility that the low responsiveness is due to an allotype linked idiotype suppression.

REFERENCES

Anderer, F.A., Uhlig, H., Weber, E., and Schramm, G. (1960). *Nature* *186*, 922.

Arquilla, E.R. (1970) in: *Methods in Immunology and Immunochemistry* (Williams, C.A., and Chase, M.W., eds.) *Vol. 3*, Academic Press, New York.

Benjamini, E. (1977) in: *Immunochemistry of Proteins*, (Atassi, M.Z. ed.) *Vol. 2*, 265, Plenum Press, New York.

Benjamini, E., Young, J.D., Shimizu, M., and Leung, C.Y. (1964) *Biochemistry* *3*, 1115.

Benjamini, E., Young, J.D., Peterson, W.J., Leung, C.Y., and Shimizu, M. (1965) *Biochemistry* *4*, 2081.

Benjamini, E., Scibienski, R.J., and Thompson, K. (1972) *Contemp. Top. Immunochem.* *1*, 1.

Benjamini, E., Shimizu, M., Young, J.D., and Leung, C.Y. (1968a) *Biochemistry* *7*, 1253.

Benjamini, E., Shimizu, M., Young, J.D., and Leung, C.Y. (1968b) *Biochemistry* *7*, 1261.

Benjamini, E., Shimizu, M., Young, J.D., and Leung, C.Y. (1969) *Biochemistry* *8*, 2242.

Binz, H., and Wigzell, H., (1977) *J. Supramolec. Structure Suppl.* *1*, 222.

Black, S.J., Hammerling, G.J., Berek, C., Rajewski, K., and Eichmann, K. (1976) *J. Exp. Med.* *143*, 846.

Cantor, H., Simpson, E., Sato, V.L., Fathman, C.G., and Herzenberg, L.A. (1975) *Cell. Immunol.* *15*, 180.

Eichmann, K. (1977) *J. Supramolec. Structure, Supp.* *1*, 214.

Fathman, C.G., Small, M., Herzenberg, L.A., and Weissman, I.L. (1975) *Cell. Immunol.* *15*, 109.

Fearney, F.J., Leung, C.Y., Young, J.D., and Benjamini, E. (1971) *Biochim. Biophys. Acta*, *243*, 509.

Herzenberg, L.A. (1972) in: *Genetic Control of Immune Responsiveness* (McDevitt, H.O., and Landy, M., eds.) pp. 171, Academic Press, New York.

Kabat, E.A. (1968) *Structural Concepts in Immunology and Immunochemistry*, Holt, New York.

Karush, F. (1962) *Adv. Immunol.* *2*, 1.

Knight, C.A. (1975) Chemistry of Viruses, 2nd ed., Springer-Verlag, Berlin, New York.

Krawinkel, U., Cramer, M., Mage, R., Kelns, A., and Rajewski, K. (1977) J. Exp. Med. 146, 792.

Merrifield, R.B. (1964) Biochemistry 3, 1385.

Metzger, H., Wofsy, L., and Singer, S.J. (1963) Arch. Biochem. Biophys. 103, 206.

Porter, R.R. (1972) in: Contemp. Top. Immunochem. 1, 145.

Singer, S.J. (1965) in: The Proteins, 2nd ed. (Neurath, H., ed.) Vol. 3, pp 269, Academic Press, New York.

Spitler, L., Benjamini, E., Young, J.D., Kaplan, H., and Fudenberg, H.H. (1970) J. Exp. Med. 131, 133.

Steward, J.M., Young, J.D., Benjamini, E., Shimizu, M., and Leung, C.Y. (1966) Biochemistry 5, 3396.

Tsugita, A., Gish, D.T., Young, J., Fraenkel-Conrat, H., Knight, C. A., and Stanley, W.M. (1960) Proc. Natl. Acad. Sci. U.S. 46, 1463.

Young, J.D., Benjamini, E., and Leung, C.Y. (1968) Biochemistry 7, 3113.

Young, J.D., Benjamini, E., Stewart, J.M., and Leung, C.Y. (1967) Biochemistry 6, 1455.

IMMUNOBIOLOGIC PROPERTIES OF THE MAJOR ANTIGENIC DETERMINANTS OF THE FERREDOXIN MOLECULE

Barbara Kelly and Julia G. Levy

Department of Microbiology
University of British Columbia
Vancouver, British Columbia, Canada V6T 1W5

There was considerable interest, about a decade ago, in the precise structure of the antigenic determinants on proteins. Such studies involved the testing, usually of tryptic or other peptides from a given antigen, in terms of their ability to interfere with the reaction of the whole protein with its homologous antibody. A number of peptide antigenic determinants were chemically characterized at that time from proteins or peptides such as tobacco mosaic virus protein (TMVP) (Benjamini *et al.*, 1964, 1965), lysozyme, both native (Arnon and Sela, 1968; Shinka *et al.*, 1967) and carboxymethylated (Thompson and Levy, 1970; Gerwing and Thompson, 1968) and glucagon (Senyk *et al.*, 1971). The peptide sequences elucidated as determinants by these studies did not demonstrate any obvious similarities. However, sequences identified as determinants in a number of proteins frequently constituted terminal sequences or sterically prominent regions of the molecule. In this laboratory, an in-depth study of the major antigenic regions of the ferredoxin molecule from *C. pasteurianum* was undertaken.

The ferredoxin molecule is a small (55 amino acid residues) molecule which probably arose as a result of a gene duplication event, since there are repeating sequences in the amino and carboxy halves of the molecule. The total amino acid sequence is known (Fig. 1). Preliminary studies implied that the regions in which cysteines were located were not involved in the antigenicity of the molecule. This was indicated by the observation that ferredoxin molecules in which the cysteine residues had been modified by carboxymethylation or performic acid oxidation reacted equally as well as native ferredoxin with antiserum prepared against the native molecule (Fig. 2) (Nitz *et al.*, 1969). Because of these observations, further work was carried out using oxidized

Ala-Tyr-Lys-Ile-Ala-Asp-Ser-Cys-Val-Ser-Cys-Gly-Ala-Cys-Ala-Ser-Ala-Cys-Pro-Val-Asn-Ala-Ile-Ser-Gln-Gly

Asp-Ser-Ile-Phe-Val-Ile-Asp-Ala-Asp-Thr-Cys-Ile-Asp-Cys-Gly-Asn-Cys-Ala-Asn-Val-Cys-Pro-Val-Gly-Ala-Pro-Val-Gln-Glu

FIGURE 1. The amino acid sequence of *Clostridium pasteurianum* ferredoxin.

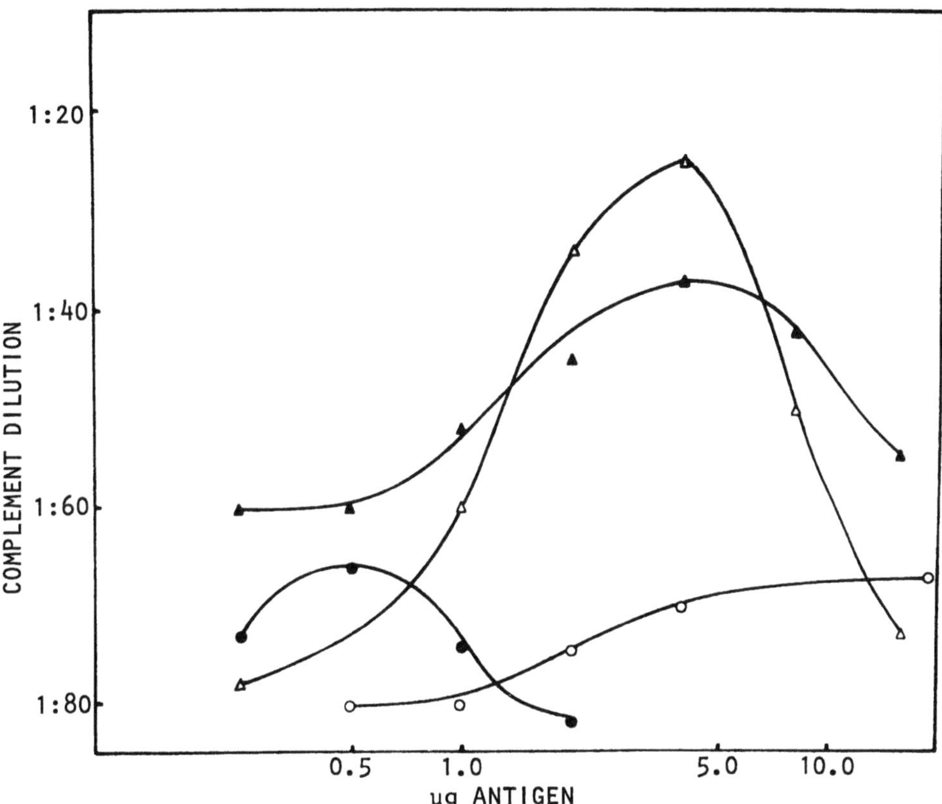

FIGURE 2. Complement fixation reaction of antiserum against native ferredoxin at 1:40 with various antigenic preparations ●——●, native ferredoxin △——△, TCA-precipitated ferredoxin; ▲——▲, alkylated ferredoxin; O——O, O-Fd. Complement dilution represents the actual dilution of guinea pig serum used in the test.

ferredoxin (O-Fd) and its homologous antiserum. The amino acid sequences lying in regions of the molecule not containing cysteinyl residues were synthesized by the solid phase Merrifield method (1964) and tested for their ability to inhibit the reaction of performic acid oxidized ferredoxin (O-Fd) with its homologous antiserum. These studies indicated that the NH_2-terminal heptapeptide and the COOH-terminal pentapeptide of the molecule (subsequently termed the N and C determinants) constituted two major antigenic determinants of O-Fd (Table 1). Further studies using ^{14}C-acetylated peptides in equilibrium dialysis established that these two peptides accounted for essentially all the antibody synthesized in rabbits to O-Fd (Fig. 3) (Kelly and Levy, 1971).

TABLE 1. The amino acid composition of the C and N terminal peptides of O-Fd

N hapten :	H_2N - Ala - Tyr - Lys - Ile - Ala - Asp - Ser - COOH
C hapten :	H_2N - Ala - Pro - Val - Gln - Glu - COOH

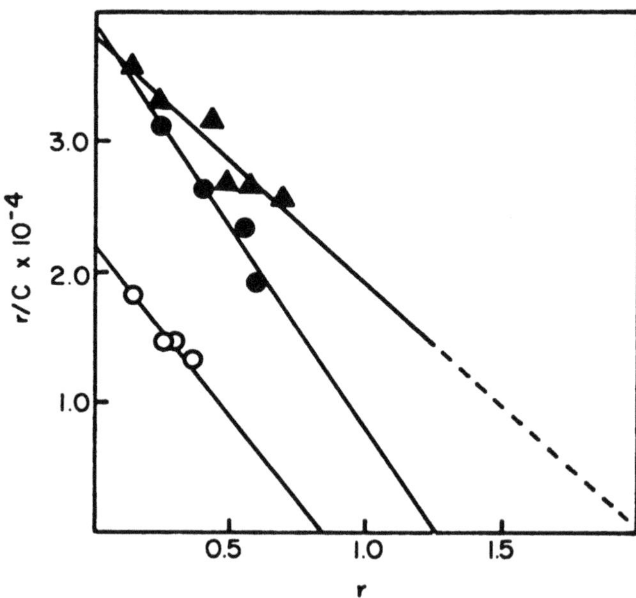

FIGURE 3. The binding of the NH_2-terminal heptapeptide (Ala^1 to Ser^7), the COOH-terminal pentapeptide (Ala^{51} to Glu^{55}), and a combination of both peptides by purified antiserum to O-Fd (O)= NH_2-terminal heptapeptide, (●)= COOH-terminal pentapeptide, and (▲)= combined peptides. r which is the moles of hapten bound per mole of antibody protein, is plotted vs. r/c (M^{-1} x 10^{-4}) in which c is the amount of free hapten present.

Our knowledge of these determinants enabled us to seek a number of answers regarding basic requirements for the immunogenicity of a given molecule. Subsequent work involved the synthesis of a number of peptides containing various combinations of these determinants (Table 2). Briefly, N-5-C contained the N and C determinants bridged by 5 glycine residues, N-10-C contained the two determinants bridged by 10 glycine residues, C-mal-10-C contained two identical and symmetrical C-determinants bridged by 10 glycine residues and a malonic acid, and N-8-N contained two

TABLE 2. The amino acid composition of the various synthetic peptides used in this study.

Peptide	Sequence
N-5-C	H_2N - Ala - Tyr - Lys - Ile - Ala - Asp - Ser - $(Gly)_5$ - Ala - Pro - Val - Gln - Glu - COOH
N-10-C	H_2N - Ala - Tyr - Lys - Ile - Ala - Asp - Ser - $(Gly)_{10}$ - Ala - Pro - Val - Gln - Glu - COOH
N-8-N	H_2N - Ala - Tyr - Lys - Ile - Ala - Asp - Ser - $(Gly)_8$ - Ala - Tyr - Lys - Ile - Ala - Asp - Ser - COOH
C-Mal-10-C	HOOC - Glu - Gln - Val - Pro - Ala - $(CH_2)_2$ - $(Gly)_{10}$ - Ala - Pro - Val - Gln - Glu - COOH.

TABLE 3. A summary of the immunological properties of various synthetic peptides containing the N and C determinants from ferredoxin.

Tests in O-Fd sensitized guinea pigs	N-5-C	N-10-C	C-Mal-10-C	N-8-N	N.determinant	C.determinant
MIF	+	+	+	+	+	+
Arthus	-	+	+	+	-	-
Delayed skin reaction	+	+	+	+	+	+
Lymphocyte stimulation	-	+	-	+	-	-
Immunogenicity						
In guinea pigs	-	+	+	+		
In rabbits (as assessed by circulating antibody)	-	+	-	+		

N-determinants bridged by 8 glycine residues. The immunological behaviour of these peptides are summarized in Table 3, and have been published in detail elsewhere (Levy _et al._, 1972; Kelly _et al._, 1973). It can be seen that the peptide N-5-C appears to be too small to initiate a number of immunological reactions. In fact, the only two reactions in which this peptide was reactive were the MIF test and the induction of a delayed skin reaction in guinea pigs previously sensitized to O-Fd or N-10-C. This is not surprising since these reactions have been shown previously to be elicited by single antigenic determinants (Spitler _et al._, 1970; Waterfield _et al._, 1971). All the other peptides appeared to constitute immunogenic molecules to the extent that they elicited Arthus and delayed skin reactions in immunized guinea pigs. The symmetrical C-determinant-containing peptide (C-mal-10-C) appeared to be a somewhat weaker antigen than did N-8-N, since it was unable to stimulate lymphocyte transformation in N-10-C or O-Fd immunized lymph node cells, and did not stimulate the formation of measurable antibody in rabbits. These data supported cell cooperation models in immune responsiveness and indicated that while both the N and C determinants reacted at both the T and B cell level and were presumably recognized by both cell types, the N determinant appeared to be the stronger of the two in controlling immune responsiveness and possibly had a stronger influence on the generation of help.

Studies using ^{125}I labeled conjugates of the N or C determinants and autoradiographic development of lymphoid cells from Balb/C mice supported this possibility (Table 4). Anti-Thy-1 treatment of unimmunized cells resulted in a relative increase of both N and C binding cells, indicating that most of the cells being detected in these animals were B lymphocytes. However, in N-10-C and N-8-N sensitized animals, this treatment resulted in a relative increase of C determinant binding cells and a slight but not significant decrease in N binding cells. These data support the possibility of an amplification of N-reactive T cells after immunization with N-10-C or N-8-N (Kelly et al., 1974).

The observations made earlier that lymphocyte transformation of sensitized cells could be stimulated by either N-10-C, N-8-N or C-mal-10-C but not by single determinants (N or C) suggested the possibility that T-T cell interaction might be involved in this immunological test. This possibility was tested in the following way: Lymph node cells from O-Fd sensitized guinea pigs were subjected to antigen suicide with ^{125}I-labeled N- or C-determinant conjugates. Depletion of either population resulted in a significant drop in the stimulation indices (Table 5). This effect was specific for the O-Fd system (Pearson _et al._, 1975). This evidence for T-T cell interaction was further substantiated by Feldmann _et al._ (1975), who, using N or C determinants conjugated to bovine serum albumin (BSA), showed synergy between

TABLE 4. Distribution of N hapten and C hapten ABC in spleen cells from N-10-C and N-8-N immunized BALB/c mice.[a)]

		Test antigen							
		^{125}I-N-10-C		^{125}I-PDG-N			^{125}I-PDG-tyr-C		
Immunogen	Treatment of cells	No.of ABC[b)] per 10^4 cells	No. of cells counted	No.of ABC[b)] per 10^4 cells	p[c)]	No.of cells counted	No.of ABC[b)] per 10^4 cells	p[c)]	No.of cells counted
N-10-C	NRS	10.60	280.000	4.46	0.3	66.000	3.91	0.05	65.000
N-10-C	Anti-Thy-1	-	-	4.04		72.000	6.33		60.000
N-8-N	NRS	-	-	4.20	0.3	75.000	-		-
N-8-N	Anti-Thy-1	-	-	3.66		60.000	-		-
Non-immunized	NRS	3.17	120.000	1.02	0.3	40.000	0.50	0.2	40.000
Non-immunized	Anti-Thy-1	-	-	3.20		40.000	1.19		40.000

a) Spleen cells were treated with either NRS or anti-Thy-1 serum prior to incubation with ^{125}I-labeled antigens for autoradiography. In each test group, a minimum of 6 animals was used.

b) The number of ABC is the averaged number of ABC for the number of animals tested in each group.

c) p values are based on the results obtained from Student's t-test, where the number of ABC from NRS treated cells are compared with the number of ABC from anti-Thy-1 treated cells for each immunogen.

TABLE 5. O-Fd stimulation[a] of (^{3}H)dThd incorporation in cultures of O-Fd sensitized guinea pig lymph node cells treated with high specific activity ^{125}I-labeled S-BSA and peptide conjugates.[b]

Cell treatment	S.I.[c] ± S.D.	P[d]	P[e]	P[f]
Control	2.76 ± 1.41			
^{125}I-S-BSA	2.50 ± 0.53	N.S.		
^{125}I-N-S-BSA	1.37 ± 0.79	< 0.005	< 0.005	< 0.025
^{125}I-C-S-BSA	1.70 ± 1.04	< 0.005	< 0.005	N.S.
^{125}I-N-S-BSA / ^{125}I-C-S-BSA mixture	2.02 ± 1.54	< 0.005	< 0.01	

a) (^{3}H)dThd added at 96 h and cultures harvested 16 h later.

b) Specific activities of labeled preparations ranged from 200-1000 μCi/μg. The antigen dose used was 1.0 μg/2 x 10^7 lymphocytes.

c) The stimulation index (S.I.) is the ratio of (^{3}H)dThd incorporation in triplicate cultures containing O-Fd (4.8 μg) to those without O-Fd. The S.I. presented is the average (± standard deviations) from 10 experiments.

d-f) P values are based on results obtained from paired T-analysis where data is compared with untreated control cultures (d), with ^{125}I-labeled S-BSA-treated cultures (e), and where data from the mixed cultures are compared with cultures ^{125}I-N-S-BSA and ^{125}I-C-S-BSA-treated cultures (f). P values of 0.025 are considered nonsignificant (N.S.).

N- and C-sensitized T cells from mice when they were co-cultured to generate helper cells _in vitro_ in generating a DNP-O-Fd response (Table 6, Fig. 4). These data show significant increases in helper function when the _in vivo_ generated N-sensitive and C-sensitive T cells are mixed _in vitro_, which strongly supports the model for T-T cell interaction.

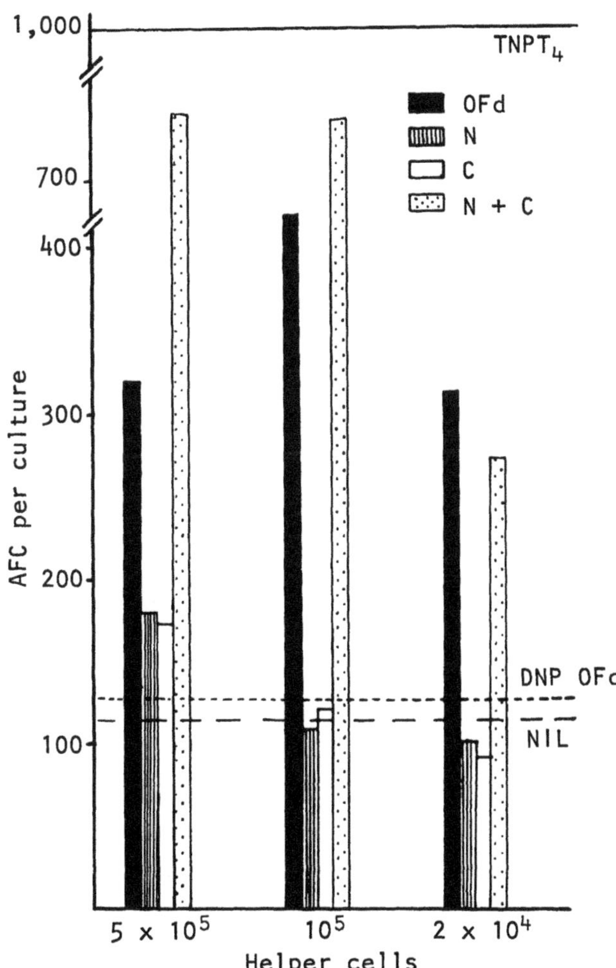

FIGURE 4. Synergy between N and C primed T cells. Spleen cells were treated with a cytotoxic rabbit anti-mouse B cell antiserum, prepared by repeated injection (3 or 4) of anti-θ treated spleen cells which had been depleted of dead cells and red cells. About 10^8 cells were injected a 2-weekly intervals, half intramuscularly emulsified in Freund's, and the rest intravenously. B cell contamination after treatment with the antiserum and complement ranged from 0-3% in replicates. Significant helper cells to OFd were only induced provided OFd primed T cells, or a mixture of N and C-BSA primed spleen cells were used. The dots above the bars indicate the upper limit of standard error.

TABLE 6. Synergy between N- and C-primed T cells in the generation of helper cells to O-Fd.

	Cells cultured	Helper cell induction: Treatment	Helper cell induction: Antigen	Helper cell induction: Helper cells transferred	Cell cooperation: Antigen	Cell cooperation: Anti-DNP response (AFC per culture)
(1)	O-Fd primed spleen	Nil	O-Fd	10^5	DNP O-Fd	173 ± 22
	N-primed spleen	Nil	O-Fd	10^5	DNP O-Fd	13 ± 10
	C-primed spleen	Nil	O-Fd	10^5	DNP O-Fd	0
	N- + C-primed spleen (1:1)	Nil	O-Fd	10^5	DNP O-Fd	217 ± 33
	-	-	-	-	DNP O-Fd	3 ± 43
					DNPPOL	553 ± 160
					Nil	27 ± 33
(2)	O-Fd primed spleen	Nylon wool	O-Fd	5×10^5	DNP O-Fd	320 ± 122
				10^5	DNP O-Fd	417 ± 65
		Nylon wool		2×10^4	DNP O-Fd	313 ± 100
	N-primed spleen	Nylon wool	O-Fd	5×10^5	DNP O-Fd	187 ± 53
				10^5	DNP O-Fd	110 ± 47
	C-primed spleen	Nylon wool	O-Fd	5×10^5	DNP O-Fd	173 ± 30
				10^5	DNP O-Fd	123 ± 62
	N-primed + C-primed (1:1)	Nylon wool	O-Fd	5×10^5	DNP O-Fd	743 ± 105
				10^5		717 ± 82
				2×10^4	DNP O-Fd	267 ± 17
	-	-	-	-	DNP O-Fd	127 ± 25
					TNP T_4	920 ± 110
					Nil	113 ± 54

Another area of research in which chemically-defined antigens may be of importance is in asking the question as to whether T and B cells "see" the same antigenic determinants. There are some interesting observations in the literature pertaining to this. We observed that antibodies to native lysozyme showed virtually no cross-reactivity with S-carboxymethylated lysozyme (Gerwing and Thompson, 1968). However, complete cross-reactivity between these two molecules was observed when assays were carried out for cell-mediated immunity (Thompson et al., 1972). Parish (1971a, b) observed that the affinity of anti-flagellin antibodies for flagellin was lost as the degree of acetoacetylation of the flagellin increased, while even highly substituted flagellin elicited delayed hypersensitivity in animals sensitized to native flagellin. Similar observations, indicating differences in T and B cell recognition have been made by others (Schirrmacher and Wizzell, 1972, 1974; Parish, 1972; Marin et al., 1972). Some experiments were undertaken in this laboratory, using the O-Fd system, to explore this area. O-Fd molecules were subjected to a variety of modifications including alkylation with N-ethyl maleimide (NEM-Fd), dinitrophenylation (DNP-O-Fd), carboxymethylation (CM-Fd) and methylation (meth-O-Fd). These modified molecules were tested for their ability to fix complement with antisera to O-Fd (antibodies were taken as representative of B cell recognition) or to induce lymphocyte proliferation in splenic lymphocytes of O-Fd sensitized mice. The 5 day proliferative study was shown to involve only anti-Thy-1 sensitive cells (Table 7). With respect to the T cell response, only NEM-Fd and unmodified Fd gave significant stimulations indicating that the other modifications to which the molecules had been subjected had modified the molecules sufficiently to prohibit recognition by sensitized T cells. Alternately, most of these modifications did not interfere with the ability of antibodies raised against O-Fd to react with them (Figure 5). Only meth-O-Fd was apparently incapable of reacting in this way. Since this modification affects carboxyl groups, and these are present in both the N and C determinants, this is not surprising (Gregerson et al., 1976 a). Thus, although inconclusive, these results support the possibility that recognition between antigen and B or T cells, may involve slightly different mechanisms.

The specificity of recognition between antibody and T cell surfaces was investigated further, using analogues of the N-determinant and assessing their ability to either induce MIF production in sensitized splenic lymphocyte populations, or to inhibit complement fixation with specific antiserum and O-Fd (Gregerson et al., 1976 b). The modified peptides used are shown in Table 8. The MIF results (Table 9) showed that the smallest peptide to react in this assay was N_4, that modification of the tyrosine and NH_2-terminal with DNP did not prohibit reactivity,

TABLE 7. Responses of O-Fd-sensitized and unsensitized spleen cells from DBA mice to modified ferredoxin antigens at 16 μg/ml.*

Hours†	NEM-Fd	Meth-O-Fd	CM-Fd	TCA-Fd	Native-Fd	DNP-O-Fd	Immune status
24	1.79 ± 0.32††	1.00 ± 0.03	0.84 ± 0.08	1.18 ± 0.17	1.13 ± 0.13	1.05 ± 0.04	Immune
24	1.08 ± 0.23	1.00 ± 0.05	0.83 ± 0.15	1.10 ± 0.08	1.12 ± 0.04	0.93 ± 0.09	Non-immune
	<0.05+						
72	2.19 ± 0.55	0.74 ± 0.09	0.95 ± 0.26	0.99 ± 0.14	1.32 ± 0.47	0.83 ± 0.26	Immune
72	1.01 ± 0.27	0.79 ± 0.12	0.72 ± 0.29	1.01 ± 0.07	0.72 ± 0.08	0.63 ± 0.15	Non-immune
	<0.05				<0.10		
120	2.99 ± 0.68	0.97 ± 0.11	0.90 ± 0.18	1.16 ± 0.13	1.94 ± 0.31	1.04 ± 0.28	Immune
120	0.86 ± 0.17	0.98 ± 0.16	1.03 ± 0.12	1.18 ± 0.18	1.04 ± 0.07	0.73 ± 0.09	Non-Immune
	<0.025				<0.005		

*Represents the pooled results of five experiments and nine determinations per experiment.

†Hours in culture prior to labelling.

††Stimulation index ± s.e.m.

+t-probabilities.

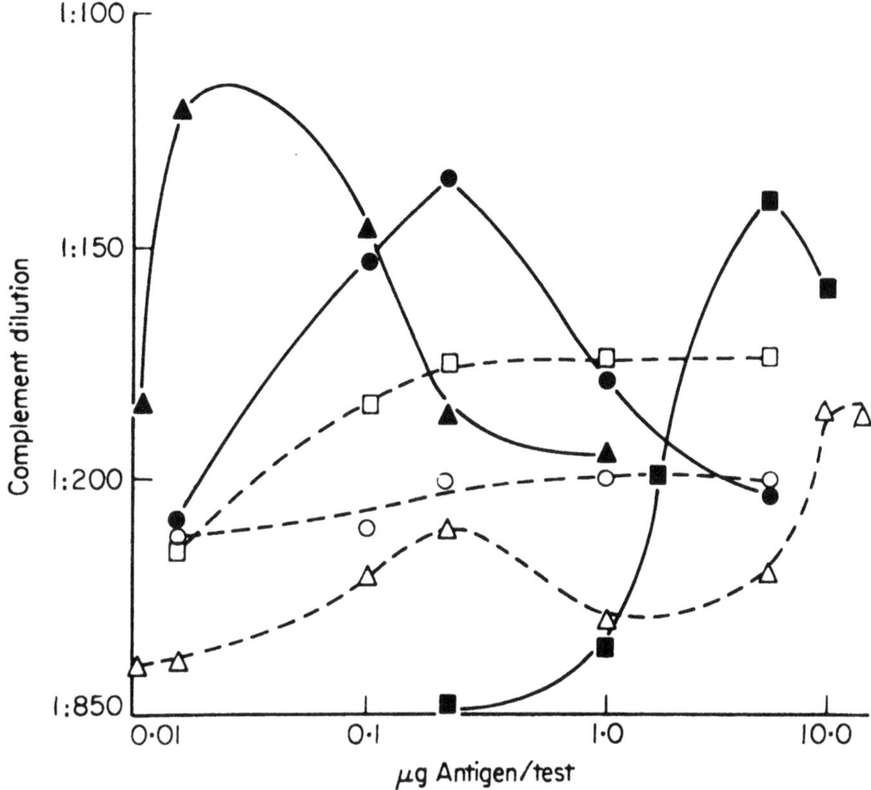

FIGURE 5. Complement fixation reactions of pooled antisera against O-Fd at a 1:40 dilution with several preparations of ferredoxin: ■——■, TCA-Fd; ▲——▲, DNP-O-Fd; △——△, NEM-Fd; ●——●, O-Fd; □——□, CM-Fd; O——O, meth-O-Fd.

but that modifications at the COOH terminal end of the molecule with glycine ethyl ester and benzoylation at the serine residue, destroyed immunological reactivity. The observation that the aspartic residue was not essential for MIF stimulation support the possibility that the serine, alanine and isoleucine residues may be important in recognition but that the free carboxyl of aspartic acid is not. The observations on hapten inhibition studies using these peptides yielded quite different results (Figure 6). Only N_7 and N_6 were active in terms of the different-sized peptides, and with the modified peptides, only N_4-Bzl-Ser and N-M-Asp showed significant inhibition. Although inconclusive, these results again support the possibility that mechanisms for recognition on B and T cells may be different.

TABLE 8. Names and structures of synthetic peptides.

Name	Structure
N_2	asp - ser
N_3	ala - asp - ser
N_4	ile - ala - asp - ser
N_5	lys - ile - ala - asp - ser
N_6	· - lys - ile - ala - asp - ser
N_7	ala - tyr - lys - ile - ala - asp - ser
N-M-Asp	ala - tyr - lys - ile - ala -------- ser
DNP-N_7	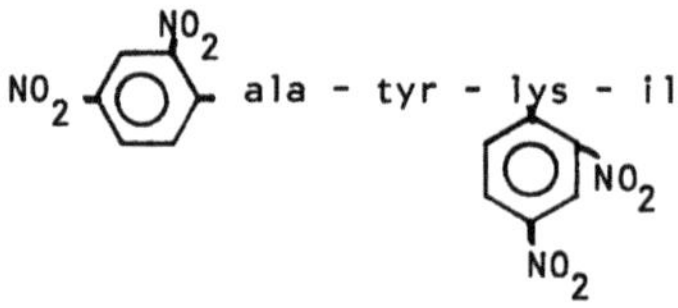 NO_2-(ring)-NO_2 - ala - tyr - lys(ring-NO_2, NO_2) - ile - ala - asp - ser
GEE-N_7	ala - tyr - lys - ile - ala - asp($CONHCH_2COOCH_2CH_3$) - ser - $CONHCH_2COOCH_2CH_3$

An N_7 peptide diaminated with glycine ethyl ester.

Name	Structure
N_4-Bzl-Ser	ile - ala - asp - ser(O-CH_2-ring) 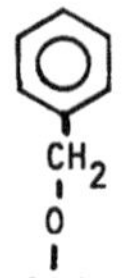

An N_4 peptide with intact O-benzyl protecting group

Name	Structure
NC_7	ser - leu - ala - tyr - asp - lys - ala

Leucine is substituted for isoleucine for identification purposes.

TABLE 9. Inhibition of migration of spleen cells from O-Fd immune and non-immune guinea pigs.

Antigen	O-Fd Immune	Unimmunized	t-test**
N_7*	0.70 ± 0.04†	0.99 ± 0.04	<0.0005
N_6	0.79 ± 0.04	1.02 ± 0.08	<0.01
N_5	0.73 ± 0.05	0.92 ± 0.07	<0.01
N_4	0.71 ± 0.0[illegible]	0.94 ± 0.06	<0.005
N_3	0.90 ± 0.05	0.96 ± 0.08	<0.40
N_2	0.91 ± 0.07	0.97 ± 0.09	<0.40
NC_7	0.93 ± 0.06	1.09 ± 0.08	<0.10
N-M-	0.88 ± 0.06	1.14 ± 0.07	<0.005
GEE-N_7	0.86 ± 0.09	1.06 ± 0.08	<0.10
N_4-Bzl-Ser	0.92 ± 1.10	0.90 ± 1.10	>0.40
N8N 0.025 µmoles/ml	0.67 ± 0.10	0.87 ± 0.14	<0.05
O-Fd 16 µg/ml	0.78 ± 0.03	1.06 ± 0.06	<0.0005
N_7-BSA 10 µg/ml	0.78 ± 0.05	1.01 ± 0.11	<0.01
N_7-PDG 10 µg/ml	0.79 ± 0.05	0.98 ± 0.09	<0.025
N_7-PLL 10 µg/ml	0.73 ± 0.02	0.92 ± 0.09	<0.01
DNP-N_7††	0.69 ± 0.13	0.92 ± 0.31	<0.001

* All peptides used at 0.05 µmoles/ml.

† Mean ± s.e. mean.

** Probability calculated from the student's t-test that the ratio of migration in immune animals is different from that in unimmunized animals.

†† From previously published work using animals immunized to a synthetic analogue of O-Fd (Waterfield _et al._, 1974).

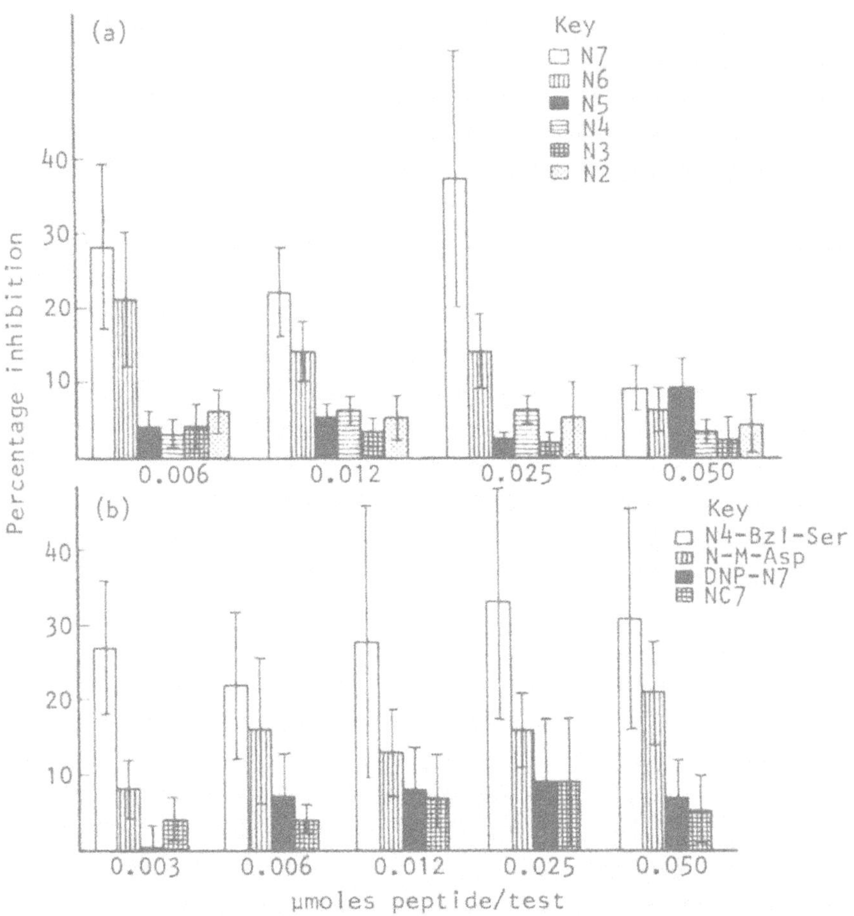

FIGURE 6. (a) and (b). Inhibition of the complement fixation reaction between O-Fd and homologous antisera by peptide analogues of the amino terminal determinant of O-Fd. Bars indicate the standard error of the means.

Because peptide antigenic determinants can be subjected to specific modification, it may be possible to use these as a tool in studying the specificities of Ir genes. One of the problems in the past has been the difficulty in developing sensitive assays for antibody-forming cells in responding mice. With the development of the technique of protein A plaque assays, it is now possible to do these definitive experiments in mice using antigens such as ferredoxin to possibly corroborate and extend data already available in the TG-AL system.

REFERENCES

Arnon, R., and Sela, M. (1969) Proc. Nat. Acad. Sci. 62: 163.

Benjamini, E., Young, J.D., Shimizu, M., and Leung, C.Y. (1964). Biochemistry 3: 1115.

Benjamini, E., Young, J.D., Peterson, W.J., Leung, C.Y., and Shimizu, M. (1965). Biochemistry 4: 2081.

Feldmann, M., Kilburn, D.G., and Leung, J.G. (1975). Nature 256: 741.

Gerwing, J., and Thompson, K.E. (1968). Biochemistry 7: 3888.

Gregerson, D.S., Kelly, B., and Levy, J.G. (1976) (a). Immunology 31: 371.

Gregerson, D.S., Kelly, B., and Levy, J.G. (1976) (b). Immunology 31: 379.

Kelly, B., and Levy, J.G. (1971). Biochemistry 10: 1763.

Kelly, B., Levy, J.G., and Hull, D. (1973). Eur. J. Immunol. 3: 574.

Kelly, B., Kaye, B., Yoshizawa, W., Levy, J.G., and Kilburn, D.G. (1974). Eur. J. Immunol. 4: 356.

Levy, J.G., Hull, D., Kelly, B., Kilburn, D.G., and Teather, R.M. (1972). Cellular Immunol. 5: 87.

Maron, E., Webb, C., Teitelbaum, D., and Arnon, R. (1972). Eur. J. Immunol. 2: 294.

Merrifield, R.B. (1964). Biochemistry 3: 1385.

Nitz, R.M., Mitchell, B., Gerwing, J., and Christensen, J. (1969). J. Immunol. 103: 319.

Parish, C.R. (1971) (a). J. Exptl. Med. 134: 1.

Parish, C.R. (1971) (b). J. Exptl. Med. 134: 21.

Parish, C.R. (1972). Eur. J. Immunol. 2: 143.

Schirrmacher, V., and Wizzell, H. (1972). J. Exptl. Med. 136: 1616.

Schirrmacher, V., and Wizzell, H. (1974). J. Immunol. 113: 1635.

Senyk, G., Williams, E.B., Nitecki, D.E., and Goodman, J.W. (1971). J. Exptl. Med. 133: 1294.

Shinka, S., Imanishi, M., Miyagawa, N., Amano, T., Inouye, M. and Tsugita, A. (1967). Biken J. 10: 89.

Spitler, L., Benjamini, E., Young, J.D., Kaplan, H., and Fudenberg, H.H. (1970). J. Exptl. Med. 131: 133.

Thompson, K.E., and Levy, J.G. (1970). Biochemistry 9: 3463.

Thompson, K., Harris, M., Benjamini, E., Mitchell, G. and Noble, M. (1972). Nature (New Biol.) 238: 20.

Waterfield, D., Levy, J.G., Kilburn, D.G., and Teather, R.M. (1972). Cell. Immunol. 3: 253.

IN VITRO RESPONSES OF MYOGLOBIN-PRIMED LYMPH NODE CELLS TO MYOGLOBIN AND MYOGLOBIN SYNTHETIC ANTIGENIC PEPTIDES

A. B. Stavitsky[a], M. Z. Atassi[b], G. T. Gooch[a], G. L. Manderino[a], W. W. Harold[a], and R. P. Pelley[c]

[a]Department of Microbiology, School of Medicine, Case Western Reserve University, Cleveland, Ohio 44106; [b]Department of Immunology, Mayo Medical School, Rochester, Minnesota 55901; [c]Division of Geographic Medicine, Department of Medicine, School of Medicine, Case Western Reserve University, Cleveland, Ohio 44106

INTRODUCTION

The ultimate objective of the newer immunology is to understand various immune responses and reactions in cellular and molecular terms. The relevant molecules include various antigenic determinants, receptors and antigen-binding molecules on lymphocytic surfaces, molecules produced and secreted by lymphocytes, and lymphocytic surface molecules that recognize and are triggered by helper and/or regulatory molecules produced by other cells (Cold Spring Harbor Symposia, 1976). These cellular and

* Abbreviations: ATG, goat anti-rabbit thymocyte globulin; CFA, complete Freund's adjuvant; G, bovine glucagon; HSA, human serum albumin; Ig, immunoglobulin; KLH, keyhole limpet hemocyanin; LNC, lymph node cells; MIF, macrophage inhibitory factor; Mb, metmyoglobin from the sperm whale; MbX, the major chromatographic component No. 10 obtained from crystalline sperm whale myoglobin (Atassi, 1964); O-Fd, performate-oxidized ferredoxin from _Clostridium pasteurianum_; TCA, trichloroacetic acid; TMV, Tobacco mosaic virus.

molecular mechanisms have been illuminated by studies with hapten-protein and synthetic peptide systems in inbred strains of mice. Beginning in the early 1970's Goodman utilized glucagon, Benjamini Tobacco mosaic virus protein and then Levy ferredoxin to obtain much new information about the relationships between antigenic structure of these proteins and their peptides and the capacity of these molecules to induce various immune reactions. We assumed that many questions about such relationships could be approached incisively with peptides derived from proteins of known molecular and antigenic structure. It was also hoped that the complexity of immune responses would be reduced by studying the results of adding single peptides to lymphocytes; this was based on the assumption that some of this complexity was due to the response of different clones of T and/or B lymphocytes to the different antigenic determinants on a protein. We proposed to utilize small peptides approximating in size one antigenic determinant, i.e., a tetrapeptide (Schechter et al., 1966) because such peptides would not effect the cross-linkage of receptors considered necessary for lymphocytic activation (Fanger et al., 1970).

We chose sperm whale myoglobin (Mb)* because its three-dimensional structure (Kendrew et al., 1961) and amino acid sequqnce (Edmundson, 1965) were known and there was a great deal of information about its antigenically active regions (Table 1). Small Mb peptides inhibited precipitation of Mb by early course rabbit and goat antisera to Mb (see Atassi, 1975 for review of this information). Mb contains five antigenically active regions in the following locations: (1) sequence 16-21, +1 or 0 residue on one side only, depending on the antiserum (Koketsu and Atassi, 1974a); (2) sequence 56-62 (Koketsu and Atassi, 1974b); (3) sequence 94-99 (Pai and Atassi, 1975); (4) sequence 113-119 (Atassi and Pai, 1975); (5) sequence 146-151, + lysine 145 with some antisera. Each peptide used here, therefore, comprises an intact antigenic region with some peptides (e.g. 54-62; 146-153; 112-120) carrying in addition one or two extraneous amino acids on one end or the other (or both) of the reactive region. Peptide 1-6 does not react with early course antisera to Mb (Pai and Atassi, 1975) and presumably is not part of a reactive region.

The <u>first aim</u> of our studies was to induce antibody formation with single Mb peptides, which has not been accomplished previously. The injection of small peptides of TMV (Spitler et al., 1970), of G (Senyk et al., 1971) and of 0-Fd (Waterfield et al., 1973) into guinea pigs did not induce antibody production. We had induced antibody production *in vitro* by adding keyhole limpet hemocyanin (KLH) to rabbit lymph node cells (LNC) previously primed *in vivo* with this protein (Stavitsky and Cook, 1974). Therefore, we added Mb or Mb peptide(s) to rabbit LNC previously primed with Mb. The *second aim* was to induce the production of macrophage inhibitory factor (MIF) upon addition of single peptides to LNC. The addition of peptides from TMV protein (Spitler et al., 1970), from G (Senyk et al., 1971) and from 0-Fd (Waterfield et al., 1972) induced MIF production by guinea pig lymphoid cells immunized with the homologous protein. The *final aim* was to induce IgG, protein, DNA and RNA syntheses by adding Mb peptides to Mb primed LNC. DNA synthesis was not enhanced by the addition of TMV peptides to TMV protein primed guinea pig LNC (Levy et al., 1972; Waterfield et al., 1972; Kelly et al., 1973). However, enhanced DNA synthesis was observed when G peptides were added to guinea pig LNC primed with G (Senyk et al., 1971). The induction by peptides of IgG, protein or RNA syntheses by protein-primed lymphoid cells has not been reported previously.

This paper recapitulates our previously published observations (Stavitsky et al., 1975) of enhanced antibody or MIF production when single Mb peptides were added to cultures of Mb-primed rabbit LNC. Then newer findings are described, including the induction of IgG, protein, DNA and RNA syntheses upon addition of these peptides to these cells; on the inhibition of antibody and protein syntheses when peptides are added to cultures of LNC primed for only a week or two; on the molar ratios of peptide/Mb required for these responses; on the thymus dependency of some of these responses.

MATERIALS AND METHODS

Myoglobin in these experiments was the major component No. 10 (MbX) obtained by CM-cellulose chromatography of twice crystallized Mb (Atassi, 1964). All MbX preparations were homogeneous by starch gel, acrylamide gel and disc electrophoresis.

The amino acid sequence, molecular weight and molar excess (to cause maximum inhibition of precipitation) of each Mb peptide are listed in Table 1. The methods of synthesis and purification of these peptides were as follows: 1-6, 94-100 (Pai and Atassi, 1975); 16-23 (Koketsu and Atassi, 1974a); 54-62, 56-62, 56-63, 57-63 (Koketsu and Atassi, 1974b); 112-120, 113-119 (Atassi and

Table 1. Amino Acid Sequence, Molecular Weight and Antigen Activity of Myoglogin Peptides

Peptide	Amino acid sequence	M.W.	Molar excess to cause max. inhibition of precipitation[a]	Reference[b]
1-6	Val-Leu-Ser-Glu-Gly-Glu	614.7	No inhibition with 600-700 molar excess	1
16-23	Lys-Val-Glu-Ala-Asp-Val-Ala-Gly	788.0	Dependent on antiserum, usually between 250-300 for max. inhib.	2
15-22	Ala-Lys-Val-Glu-Ala-Asp-Val-Ala	802.0	Dependent on antiserum, usually between 250-300 for max. inhib.	3
56-63	Lys-Ala-Ser-Glu-Asp-Leu-Lys-Lys	919.0	Usually between 150-200	4
57-63	Ala-Ser-Glu-Asp-Leu-Lys-Lys	789.9	Usually between 150-200	4
54-62	Glu-Met-Lys-Ala-Ser-Glu-Asp-Leu-Lys	1050.2	Usually between 150-200	4
56-62	Lys-Ala-Ser-Glu-Asp-Leu-Lys	789.9	Usually between 150-200	4
94-100	Ala-Thr-Lys-His-Lys-Ile-Pro	794.1	Between 250-300	1
112-120	Ile-His-Val-Leu-His-Ser-Arg-His-Pro	1095.4	Between 250-300	5
113-119	His-Val-Leu-His-Ser-Arg-His	885.1	Between 250-300	5
146-153	Tyr-Lys-Glu-Leu-Gly-Tyr-Glu-Gly	957.2	Between 250-300	6
146-151	Tyr-Lys-Glu-Leu-Gly-Tyr	771.9	Between 250-300	6

[a]The reaction of each peptide was performed with several antisera. The molar excess (relative to MbX) necessary for 50% of maximum inhibition depends on the antiserum (see the references indicated). Also, the minimum molar excess to achieve maximum inhibition (which is not as well defined) depended on the antiserum.

[b]1. Pai and Atassi (1975); 2. Koketsu and Atassi (1974a); 3. Atassi (1975); 4. Koketsu and Atassi (1974b); 5. Atassi and Pai (1975); 6. Koketsu and Atassi (1973).

Pai, 1975); 146-151, 146-153 (Koketsu and Atassi, 1973). Following exhaustive purification, each peptide used possessed purity of 99% or better as determined by elution and 570 nm absorption of the ninhydrin-positive spots from heavily loaded peptide maps. Complete characterization of the peptides is given in the aforementioned references.

Rabbits were injected with 5 mg Mb in complete Freund's adjuvant (CFA) into each hind foot pad. At different intervals cultures were prepared from the popliteal LNC (Stavitsky and Cook, 1974). The cultures were incubated with Mb or Mb peptide for 0-24 hr. The LNC were then washed twice with Hank's balanced salt solution and placed in fresh medium. The medium removed at the end of 24 hr was utilized for the assay of MIF (David and David, 1971) employing rabbit peritoneal exudate macrophages whose migration was much more susceptible to inhibition by rabbit MIF than guinea pig peritoneal macrophages (Pelley, R. P. and Stavitsky, A. B., umpublished observations). ^{14}C-uridine 0.5 μCi (50 mCi/mM) or 5.0 μCi ^{3}H-thymidine (54 Ci/mM) was added to cultures during 24-48 hr of incubation, the period of maximal incorporation. ^{14}C-L-leucine - - 0.5 μCi (312 mCi/mM) was added during 72-120 hr of culture to radioactively label antibody, IgG and TCA-precipitable protein. Newly synthesized radioactive antibody was assayed by a highly sensitive method (Self et al., 1974) employing the immunosorbent bromoacetyl cellulose-Mb. The assays of DNA, RNA and protein syntheses were described previously (Stavitsky and Cook, 1974). IgG synthesis was assayed as previously described (Bernier and Fanger, 1972) utilizing goat anti-rabbit IgG to precipitate the radioactive IgG. At least three cultures were prepared from each incubation mixture and the average value in antibody CPM/10^7 cells is reported. The antibody CPM for replicate cultures varied by 10% or less. The standard error usually was about 7%. The data were subjected to analysis according to "Student's" *t* test and the confidence limits of the data are reported.

RESULTS

Antibody, Protein and IgG Syntheses. Preliminary experiments indicated that when Mb or Mb peptides were incubated either with unprimed LNC or LNC primed *in vivo* 1 or 2 weeks earlier antibody synthesis was not enhanced. However, when either Mb or one of its peptides was added to LNC primed *in vivo* at least 21 days earlier antibody synthesis was induced (Stavitsky et al., 1975). Table 2 summarizes data from two experiments in which antibody synthesis was induced over the background (no added antigen) level upon addition of Mb or one of the peptides from each antigenic region - - as well as 1-6 - - to LNC primed for 30 days or 175 days. Additional data from many experiments were presented in our original paper (Stavitsky et al., 1975). Antibody synthesis was consistently induced when Mb or one of its peptides was added to LNC primed for 30-60 days and less commonly when added to cells primed for shorter or longer periods. In one of two experiments that employed LNC from rabbits primed 6 months earlier (7491) the addition of peptides induced antibody synthesis; in the

Table 2. *In Vitro* Induction of Antibody Synthesis upon Addition of Mb or Mb Peptides to Mb-Primed Rabbit Lymph Node Cells [a]

	Antibody Synthesis (CPM x $10^{-3}/10^{7}$ cells)[c] induced by									
	Myoglobin - nmoles			Peptides - 200 nmoles added						
Days[b]	0	.0057	.057	1-6	15-22	16-23	56-62	94-100	113-119	146-151
30	0.6		2.9[e]	2.0	2.0			2.1	1.5	2.7
175	0.5	2.1	3.2	1.5		2.2	1.8			2.0

[a] These data were published previously (Stavitsky, et. al., 1975).

[b] Interval between *in vivo* priming with 5 mg Mb in complete Freund's adjuvant in each hind foot pad and the removal of the popliteal lymph nodes for culture and antigenic challenge.

[c] CPM of ^{14}C-leucine incorporated into antibody by cells cultured for 120 hr, with the radiosotopic amino acid present during 96-120 hr of culture.

[d] Mb and peptides were added to 10^{7} cells for 24 hr, then washed out.

[e] The difference between the underlined CPM and the control was significant (*t*-test: $p < 0.025$).

other (data not shown) the peptide did not elicit antibody formation.

Antibody synthesis was induced in 14 of 19 experiments in which the 54-62 or 146-151 peptides were incubated with LNC primed for 30 days with 5 mg Mb in CFA. Antibody formation was induced less frequently when LNC primed in this manner were challenged with the other peptides. Antibody production occurred much less frequently when LNC primed with lesser amounts of Mb in CFA or with alum-precipitated Mb were challenged with any of the peptides.

LNC induced by peptide(s) to produce antibody were derived from rabbits obtained from a single local dealer. In preliminary experiments LNC obtained from another dealer were not induced to produce antibody upon addition of Mb peptides or indeed Mb *per se*.

Table 3 presents the typical results when Mb or peptide was added to LNC primed for only 6 or 14 days. Peptides 56-62 or 145-151 consistently *reduced* antibody synthesis below the background level. Peptides from other regions have not been added to LNC primed for these short periods. In 5 of 16 experiments

Table 3. In Vitro Inhibition of Antibody Synthesis upon Addition of Mb or Mb Peptides to Mb-Primed Rabbit Lymph Node Cells [a]

Antibody Synthesis (CPM x $10^3/10^7$ cells) induced by							
Rabbit number	Days	Myoglobin - nmoles				Peptides 100 nmoles added	
		0	0.057	.057	5.7	56-62	145-151
8208	6	2.2	1.4	2.2	0.7[b]	0.5	1.5
8209	14	0.5	0.3	0.19	1.1[c]	0.68	0.04

[a] See legend for Table 2.

[b] Underlined data indicate significant inhibition compared to control; (t-test: $p < 0.025$).

[c] Underlined data indicate significant enhancement compared to control; (t-test: $p < 0.025$).

the addition of Mb or one of its peptides from all six regions, i.e., including 1-6, to LNC primed for 90 or more days inhibited antibody synthesis.

Table 4 shows two experiments in which the addition of Mb or peptide induced protein synthesis. Induction of protein synthesis was observed in only 15% of experiments. Occasionally (7491 in Tables 2 and 4) the induction of antibody and protein syntheses were correlated, but this was always so. The addition of Mb or Mb peptide to unprimed LNC did not result in enhanced protein synthesis.

Another new finding was that protein synthesis was inhibited when Mb or peptide(s) was added to LNC primed for 6 or 14 days (Table 5). In one experiment (8209, Tables 3 and 5) the reduction in antibody synthesis was part of a generalized reduction in protein synthesis.

The introduction of Mb or peptide(s) into cultures of Mb-primed LNC can induce IgG synthesis (Table 6). Tables 2, 4 and 6 present data on the induction of antibody, protein and IgG syntheses when Mb or peptide was added to aliquots of LNC from rabbit 7491. Antigen induced IgG synthesis comprised about 50% of total induced protein synthesis. Induced antibody synthesis was about 7% of total protein synthesis and 14% of total IgG synthesis. The incubation of Mb or peptide with LNC from unprimed animals did not cause an increase in IgG or protein syntheses.

Table 4. *In Vitro* Induction of Protein Synthesis upon Addition of Mb or Mb Peptides to Mb-Primed Rabbit Lymph Node Cells[a]

Protein Synthesis (CPM x $10^{-3}/10^{7}$ cells)[b]									
Rabbit number	Days	Myoglobin nmoles		Peptides - 200 nmoles added					
		0	0.057	1-6	16-23	56-62	57-63	146-151	146-153
7423	50	30.0	58.0			71.2			73.0
7491	175	8.2	38.0	28.3	31.0	26.0	31.0	28.4	

[a] See legend for Table 2.

[b] CPM of ^{14}C-leucine incorporated into TCA-precipitable protein when this isotope was present in medium during 96-120 hr of culture.

[c] Underlined data significant by *t*-test: at least at p 0.025 level.

Table 5. *In Vitro* Inhibition of Protein Synthesis upon Addition of Mb or Mb Peptides to Mb-Primed Rabbit Lymph Node Cells[a]

Protein Synthesis (CPM x $10^{-3}/10^{7}$ cells)							
Rabbit number	Day	Myoglobin - nmoles				Peptides 100 nmoles added	
		0	.057	.57	5.7	56-62	145-151
8209	14	35.1	27.0	31.2	16.0	12.5	6.1

[a] See legends for Tables 2, 3 and 4.

Table 6. *In Vitro* Induction of IgG Synthesis upon Addition of Mb or Mb-Primed Rabbit Lymph Node Cells[a]

IgG Synthesis (CPM x $10^{-3}/10^{7}$ cells) induced by									
Rabbit number	Day	Myoglobin - nmoles			Peptides - 200 nmoles added				
		0	.0057	.057	1-6	16-23	56-62	94-100	146-151
7491	175	1.8	15.2	18.0	12.4	15.3	13.7	18.4	14.0

[a] CPM of ^{14}C-leucine incorporated into IgG co-precipitated with IgG-anti-rabbit IgG from culture medium when isotope present during 96-120 hr of culture.

DNA and RNA Syntheses. In 3 of 10 experiments the addition of peptide to Mb primed LNC increased the level of incorporation of thymidine into DNA (Table 7) and uridine into RNA (data not shown). The correlations between the enhanced incorporation of thymidine into DNA or of uridine into RNA with the enhancement of antibody, protein and IgG syntheses generally were poor. The addition of Mb or peptide to LNC cultures from unprimed rabbits did not induce any of these syntheses.

The introduction of peptides of all six regions into cultures of LNC primed for 6 months inhibited both thymidine and uridine incorporation into DNA and RNA of these cells (two experiments).

Molar Ratios of Peptide to Mb Required for Induction of Protein and DNA Syntheses. Table 7 also presents typical data on the molar ratios of peptide to Mb required for the induction of protein and DNA syntheses by Mb-primed LNC. In this and other experiments from 200 to 4000 molar excess of peptide was needed for the induction of comparable levels of ^{14}C-leucine incorporation into protein or ^{3}H-thymidine incorporation into DNA. Not enough experiments were done with LNC primed for varying lengths of time to determine the relationship, if any, of the length of time between *in vivo* priming and *in vitro* antigenic challenge to the molar ratio of peptide/MB required for induction of these syntheses. In a few preliminary experiments it appears that a ratio of peptide/ Mb of at least 1000 is also required for the induction of antibody synthesis.

MIF Production and Correlation between Induction of Antibody and MIF Production. We previously reported (Stavitsky et al., 1975) that the addition of Mb peptides from all five regions, but not 1-6, into Mb-primed LNC cultures consistently induced MIF production. LNC obtained 30-180 days after priming were utilized in these experiments. Table 8 summarizes typical data. MIF was most consistently induced upon addition of sequences from the 54-63 and 146-151 regions. In control experiments utilizing unprimed LNC there was neither background MIF production (minus antigen) nor MIF production upon addition of Mb or any of its peptides.

Table 9 indicates two experiments in which the addition of a single peptide induced MIF (7500) or antibody (7491) production. Indeed, in the seven experiments in which this question was examined (Stavitsky et al., 1975) there were only 3 instances in which a single peptide induced both MIF and antibody production as opposed to 17

Table 7. Relative Concentrations of Mb and of Mb Peptides Required for Induction of Thymidine Incorporation and of Protein Synthesis by Mb-Primed Lymph Node Cells

Rabbit number	Day	Additions: nmoles	Additions: Antigen	CPM (x 10^{-3})[a] Tdr incorp.	CPM (x 10^{-3})[b] Protein Synthesis
7423	56	0	none	1.3	30.6
		.005	Mb	1.8	28.2
		.05	Mb	15.3	38.2
		.5	Mb	2.8	58.8
		50	56-62	2.6	27.5
		100	56-62	2.5	26.5
		200	56-62	12.2	71.8
		50	146-153	6.1	43.5
		100	146-153	4.7	64.0
		200	146-153	11.4	73.4

[a] Antigen was present 0-24 hr of culture, then washed out. ^{3}H-Thymidine (0.5 μC) was present 24-48 hr of culture, the time of maximal incorporation.

[b] CPM in TCA precipitable protein in culture medium after 120 hr of culture, with ^{14}C-leucine present during 96-120 hr.

Table 8. *In Vitro* Induction of MIF Activity upon Addition of Mb or Mb Peptides to Mb-Primed Rabbit Lymph Node Cells[a]

	MIF activity[b] induced by									
	Myoglobin - nmoles			Peptides - 100 nmoles added						
Days	.057	.57	5.7	1-6	15-22	56-62	57-63	94-100	113-119	146-151
30	60±11	77±5			26±5[c]		80±4			46±5
35		32 7	60±3	0					26±5	
78	42±10	57±17	90 4	0		43±11				36±8
86			34±1	14±5		27±11[d]		31±11[d]		34±9
180	88±3									87±5

[a] These data were published previously (Stavitsky, et.al., 1975).

[b] $$\%MIF = \frac{\text{Area control migration} - \text{Area experimental migration} \times 100}{\text{Area control migration}}$$

Rabbit macrophages were employed in this assay. At least 8 capillaries/culture fluid were utilized with a standard error of 10% or less. Culture fluid was harvested after 24 hr of incubation of Mb-primed LNC with the antigen preparation.

[c] The underlined data were significant (*t*-test: $p < .01$).

[d] These data were significant (*t*-test: $.025 < p < 0.05$).

Table 9. Correlation between Induction of MIF and Antibody Synthesis upon Addition of Mb or Mb Peptides to Mb-Primed Rabbit Lymph Node Cells[a]

Rabbit number	Days	Additions	MIF[b]	AB[b]
7500	86	Mb	↑	↑
		1-6	--	--
		16-23	↑	--
		56-62	↑	--
		94-100	↑	--
		146-151	↑	--
7491	175	Mb	↑	↑
		1-6	--	↑
		16-23	--	↑
		56-62	--	↑
		94-100	--	↑
		146-151	--	↑

[a] Some of these data were published previously (Stavitsky, et. al., 1975).

[b] ↑ increase; -- no change.

instances in which either MIF or antibody was produced. The incorporation of peptide 1-6 in the LNC cultures frequently induced antibody formation, but in none of 10 experiments did it induce MIF production (7500 and 7491, for example).

The MIF assay employed culture media which always contained Mb or Mb peptide. Therefore, it was imperative to show that neither the Mb nor its peptides *per se* inhibit the migration of the rabbit peritoneal macrophages employed in the assay. It was, therefore, significant that none of the cultures containing Mb or Mb peptides plus unprimed LNC ever inhibited the migration of these macrophages.

Thymus Dependency of Mb or Mb Peptide Induced Responses. We utilized a highly specific goat anti-rabbit thymocyte globulin (ATG) to demonstrate that the *in vitro* anamnestic antibody, protein, DNA and RNA synthetic responses of antigen-primed rabbit LNC to keyhole limpet hemocyanin (KLH) (Stavitsky and Cook, 1974) and to human serum albumin (HSA) (Stavitsky et al., 1974) were thymus dependent. Table 10 presents the results of one of a number of experiments in which the thymus dependency of Mb and Mb peptide induced *in vitro* responses was examined. The induction of protein, DNA and RNA syntheses was inhibited when 400 μg ATG was added to the LNC culture at the same time as the Mb or one of its peptides, e.g., 56-62. Inhibition ranged from 40-50%. However, antibody synthesis induced by Mb or Mb peptide was inhibited in only 20% of experiments. The 40-50% inhibition of Mb or Mb peptide induced syntheses is in striking contrast to the 90-95% inhibition of KLH (Stavitsky and Cook, 1974) or HSA (Stavitsky et al., 1974) induced syntheses.

Table 10. Thymus Dependency of Mb and Mb-Induced Protein Synthesis and Thymidine and Uridine Incorporation by Mb-Primed Lymph Node Cells

Additions			CPM ($x 10^{-3}/10^7$ cells in		
Mb (nmoles)	56-62 (100 nmoles)	ATG[a] (400 μg)	Protein[b]	DNA[c]	RNA[d]
0		0	34.4	2.9	24.7
0		+	29.7		
.0057		0	45.0	6.3	31.0
.0057		+	31.5		
.057		0	52.1[e]	8.1	31.0
.057		+	30.0		
.57		0	61.0	14.3	49.0
.57		+	35.2		
	+	0	67.0	13.19	44.0
	+	+	41.0	7.6	24.0

[a] Goat anti-rabbit thymus globulin--added together with antigen for 0-24 of culture, then washed out.

[b] TCA-precipitable protein collected after 120 hr of culture; ^{14}C-leucine in medium 96-120 hr of culture.

[c] ^{3}H-thymidine incorporation into DNA during 24-48 hr of culture.

[d] ^{3}H-uridine incorporation into RNA during 24-48 hr of culture.

[e] Significant enhancement over control (0 antigen) or inhibition by ATG compared to control (minus ATG): (*t*-test: p at least < 0.05).

DISCUSSION

Antibody, IgG and protein syntheses were assayed by the incorporation of ^{14}C-leucine. Antibody production usually is demonstrated by the hemolytic plaque assay. Our approach permits the determination whether Mb or a peptide induces or inhibits antibody synthesis exclusively or whether this synthesis merely reflects increases or decreases in total protein synthesis. Studies of antibody responses exclusively by the plaque assay do not permit determinations of the relationship of antibody to other syntheses. We showed that Mb or Mb peptide induced antibody synthesis usually was part of a general elevation of protein and IgG synthesis. There is some, but much less, evidence that the inhibition of antibody synthesis observed upon addition of Mb or peptide to LNC primed for 6 or 14 days was part of a general inhibition of protein synthesis. It would be ideal to have information both about the number of cells producing antibody and the actual extent of antibody and other syntheses so that the level of these syntheses per antibody producing cell could be determined.

The level of Mb or peptide induced syntheses is compared to the background of "spontaneous" responses by primed LNC that occur in the absence of added antigen. These "spontaneous" antibody responses to KLH (Stavitsky et al., 1974) and HSA (Tew et al., 1973) were found to be due to residual antigen - - on dendritic type cells (Tew and Stavitsky, 1974) - reacting with T and B memory cells in lymph nodes (Stavitsky et al., 1974). The "spontaneous" antibody, and presumably other, responses by primed LNC to Mb or peptide presumably also require the interaction of residual Mb determinants with T and B memory cells, but there is no hard evidence for the role of T cells in antibody formation. The most persuasive evidence for the role of memory cells is the consistent finding that the addition of Mb or peptide to unprimed LNC does not induce any of these responses. Presumably, the increases or decreases in *in vitro* responses caused by added Mb determinants involve the added determinant, T and B memory cells and residual determinants in the node.

Local immunization with Mb would be expected to induce the development in the draining lymph node of T and/or B memory cells reactive with and activatable by one or more of the antigenic regions of this protein. However, there was no precedent for predicting whether any of these small peptides *per se* would activate LNC cultures for antibody production. Indeed, since the cross-linking of lymphocytic surface immunoglobulin (Ig) by anti-globulin was required for in vitro blast transformation (Fanger, et al., 1970) it might have been expected that small peptide would not activate B cells. Nevertheless, the addition of single small Mb peptides from each of the five antigenic regions defined by Atassi (1975) as well as from the putatively non-antigenic 1-6 sequence induced suitably primed LNC cultures to synthesize antibody to Mb. The most direct interpretation of these findings is that peptides of 6-9 residues can initiate cellular events that culminate in antibody synthesis. The physical state of these peptides in culture is not known; they may be effectively multivalent through non-specific binding to macrophages, dendritic type cells or lymphocytes or to proteins in the medium. A tetrapeptide is the minimum sized determinant for binding to antibody (Schechter et al., 1966) and presumably for binding to surface Ig receptors. Therefore, the non-specifically bound peptides would have to expose at least a tetrapeptide segment for activation of lymphocytes, which seems unlikely. Moreover, it appears that the activation of lymphocytes for at least protein and DNA syntheses requires a large molar ratio of peptide/Mb (Table 7). This finding indicates that these small molecules are much less efficient than Mb per se in lymphocyte activation, presumably because the peptides exist mainly in the free, uncomplexed state in the cultures. The lower limit - - ratio of peptide/Mb concentration of 400 - - approximates the ratio of peptide to Mb required for inhibition of precipitation (Table 1). However, a higher ratio might be expected to be required for activation of lymphocytes than for inhibition of precipitation and the ratio usually is closer to 1000 for the former reaction.

At least three types of peptide-lymphocyte interactions resulting in antibody synthesis can be postulated on the assumption -- which has been only partially supported by evidence (Table 10) -- that the antibody response to Mb is thymus-dependent. The first assumes that peptide can activate both T and B cells for antibody formation. The second postulates that the peptide can activate only T cells; the B cells are stimulated by Mb persisting from the original priming injection. The occurrence of a "spontaneous" antibody response of from 500 to 2,200 CPM to Mb in the absence of added antigen (Tables 2 and 3) indicates that Mb immunogen is present in LNC cultures prepared from 6-175 days after priming. The third mechanism assumes that T cells are stimulated by the residual Mb immunogen and the B cells by the Mb peptide. All of these mechanisms assume that two signals are required to activate B cells for antibody synthesis, one provided by antigen and the other by some other agent(s) -- such as specific or non-specific soluble factors produced by antigen stimulated T cells (Katz and Benacerraf, 1972).

The specificity of the antibodies synthesized upon addition of Mb or peptide(s) has not been determined because Mb *per se* was employed in the radioimmunoassay for these antibodies. A given peptide conceivably can induce antibodies of more than one specificity, perhaps not even including antibody to the added peptide *per se*; this may especially be true of peptide 1-6 which from previous studies is not antigenic (Pai and Atassi, 1975). The induction by 1-6 of antibody to another non-cross reacting Mb peptide would then be analogous to the demonstration (Stavitsky and Self, 1972) that the addition of KLH to LNC primed with both KLH and the non-cross reacting HSA will induce the synthesis of antibodies to both KLH and HSA. By 21-30 days after immunization with Mb LNC reactive with peptide 1-6 presumably have appeared in the local lymph node. Mechanism 2 may account for the observed results: peptide 1-6 triggers peptide-specific T cells to produce soluble factor that promotes the antibody response of B cells to residual Mb determinants. Thus the 1-6 determinant is utilized only for recognition by and activation of T cells. It is imperative that the specificity of the antibodies produced in response to this determinant be identified.

Of special interest was the observation that the addition of Mb or one of its peptides to LNC primed for 6 and 14 days - - or occasionally for 90+ days - - leads to inhibition of antibody and protein syntheses relative to the spontaneous responses (Tables 3 and 5). No information is available on the thymus-dependency of this inhibition so no conclusions can be drawn about the possible role of T suppressor cells. It may be noteworthy that frequently the inhibition of antibody synthesis reflected the inhibition of protein synthesis (8209, Tables 3 and 5), both antigen induced events.

Striking differences were observed in the *in vitro* antibody response of LNC from different dealers to Mb and its peptides; LNC from one dealer was unresponsive, i.e., did not produce antibody or any other macromolecules. These results prompted us to investigate the genetic control of the antibody response to Mb and its peptides in different inbred strains of mice. These results will be reported elsewhere.

The 56-62 and 146-151 regions of Mb are immunodominant, i.e. antibody, MIF and protein production occur earlier and much more frequently to these peptides than to the other three sequences. Derivatives of the 56-62 and 146-151 peptides are being employed to attempt to gain information about the relationship between the structure of these peptides and their immunogenicity.

It was hoped that the complexity of the cellular immune responses would be reduced by adding single peptides to the LNC. However, a wide variety of permutations of responses was still observed when a single peptide was added to LNC from a single Mb-primed rabbit, including, for instance, the induction of antibody, IgG and protein syntheses (e.g. 7491, Tables 2, 4 and 6), but not DNA or RNA syntheses (data not shown). In other instances, the addition of a single peptide induced the synthesis of antibody, IgG, protein, DNA and RNA. Some of this complexity might be reduced if a single peptide were added to purified T or B cells and especially if added to functionally more homogeneous populations, e.g., T helper cells. However, together with other findings (e.g. IgM and IgG antibody to DNP (Plotkin et al., 1968), it is evident that a single antigenic determinant *per se* can evoke a very complex immune response, comprising antibody, immunoglobulin, protein, DNA and RNA syntheses. The most reasonable interpretation is that even a single peptide reacts with numerous T and/or B cell populations.

All of the peptides, except 1-6, induced MIF production by Mb-primed LNC (Table 8). In previous studies small peptides (with as few as five amino acids) from TMV protein (Spitler et al., 1971), G (Senyk et al., 1971) and 0-Fd (Waterfield et al., 1972) elicited MIF production in *in vitro* immune systems. There is strong evidence that T cells are implicated in lymphokine production - - perhaps by producing a soluble factor which with antigen induces B cells to produce these agents (Wahl and Rosenstreich, 1976). Thus the collective data strongly suggest that small peptides can activate peptide-specific T and/or B cells for lymphokine production.

A single peptide rarely induced both MIF and antibody production by Mb primed LNC from a single rabbit (Table 9, and Stavitsky et al., 1975). One explanation is that different peptide-specific T cell populations function as helper cells for antibody synthesis and for lymphokine production. However, experiments with mouse T cells indicate that T helper cells and T cells involved in delayed hypersensitivity both possess the same Ly phenotype (Huber et al.,

1976). Peptide 1-6 induced only antibody synthesis, never MIF production which can be explained by assuming that there are 1-6 reactive T cells for antibody production but not for MIF production. However, alternative interpretations of the cellular basis of these observations can be offered.

Thus far we have not been able to inhibit any of the Mb - or Mb peptide-induced responses by more than 50% by adding ATG together with antigen to Mb-primed LNC (Table 10). Antibody synthesis has been inhibited only infrequently. These results constrast sharply with the 90-95% inhibition by this ATG of KLH (Stavitsky and Cook, 1974) and HSA (Stavitsky et al., 1974) induced antibody and other syntheses. It is unlikely that the Mb-induced responses are thymus-independent. It is more likely that both T helper and T suppressor cells reactive with Mb exist and that the net effect depends on the ratio of these populations. If there is a close balance between T help and T suppression, the addition of ATG to the LNC would not be expected greatly to affect the antigen induced responses. The resolution of this question will require the separation of the T helper and T suppressor cells and their separate and collective stimulation by antigen in the presence of B cells.

The antigenic structure of Mb has been analyzed by extensive chemical and synthetic approaches (Atassi, 1974, 1975). Insofar as the present study utilized more than one peptide in the 16-21, 56-62 and 146-151 regions there are no discrepancies between the sequences that react with humoral antibody and those that react with and activate Mb primed LNC, presumably through specific cell receptors. There has been only limited analysis of the efficiency of peptides of varying length in inducing various cellular synthetic responses. Moreover, in contrast to the _in vitro_ studies (Atassi, 1975) which employed early course goat and rabbit antisera to Mb, our experiments utilized antigen-reactive cells from rabbits immunized 21-180 days earlier. It is, therefore, conceivable that LNC from rabbits immunized for more than 30 days can react with peptides from regions other than the six thus far indicated in the studies from this laboratory and that of Atassi.

These experiments have raised many questions about the molecular and cellular mechanisms whereby small peptides can induce suitably-primed LNC to produce antibody, protein, IgG, DNA, RNA and lymphokines. The system described here should permit the study of many of these questions, including the nature of the receptors on T cells; the structural features of peptides that are involved in immunodominance and lymphocyte activation; and the interrelations of the cell populations and mechanisms involved in various cellular and humoral immune responses (Bretscher, 1974).

SUMMARY

Rabbits were injected in the hind foot pads with 5 mg Mb in CFA. At various days thereafter the draining popliteal LNC were removed for the preparations of cultures. These cultures (1×10^7 LNC) were challenged for the first 24 hr with different amounts of either Mb or synthetic Mb peptides which were then washed out. The medium collected after 24 hr of culture was employed for the assay of MIF. ^{14}C-leucine was added to LNC during 72-120 hr of culture to radioactively label newly synthesized antibody to Mb as well as IgG and TCA-precipitable protein. The medium collected at 120 hr was then utilized for the assay of radioactive antibody to Mb, and of radioactive IgG and protein. Radioactive antibody to Mb was assayed by binding of the antibody to an immunosorbent (bromacetyl cellulose-Mb). ^{3}H-thymidine or ^{3}H-uridine was added to some cultures during 24-48 hr - - the time of maximal incorporation into DNA and RNA, respectively. Mb and synthetic peptides corresponding to 6 regions of Mb, i.e., sequences 1-6, 15-22 (or 15-23 or 16-22), 54-62 (or 56-62 or 57-63), 94-100, 113-119 and 146-151 induced LNC primed at least 21 days earlier to synthesize antibody to Mb. Peptides 56-62 and 146-151 most consistently induced antibody synthesis. LNC collected as long as 175 days after priming sometimes produced antibody upon challenge with 16-23, 56-62 and 146-151. In contrast, antibody and protein synthesis by LNC primed for only 6 or 14 days was reduced upon addition of peptides from these 6 regions. LNC from unprimed rabbits did not produce antibody upon challenge with any of these peptides or indeed Mb itself. Peptides from all of these regions -- except 1-6 -- induced cultures of LNC primed for at least 30 days to produce MIF. The addition of a single peptide to a culture usually induced either antibody or MIF, not both. The addition of Mb or any peptide to unprimed rabbit LNC did not induce MIF production.

The addition of Mb or peptides from the 6 regions to LNC primed for 30-175 days also induced the production of IgG, protein, DNA and RNA, but much less consistently then the synthesis of antibody. The addition of Mb or Mb peptides from these 6 regions to LNC primed only for 6 or 14 days also led to decreased synthesis of protein compared to control cultures. In a series of cultures from a single lymph node, there were poor or only fair correlations in the induction of different responses upon the addition of Mb or a single peptide to the Mb-primed cells. For instance, antibody synthesis might be induced by 56-62, but not DNA or RNA synthesis. Generally, there were better correlations between the induced synthesis of antibody and of IgG and protein, although the amount of antibody synthesis usually was only a fraction of total IgG synthesis and antibody plus IgG synthesis only a fraction of total protein synthesis.

The molar ratios of peptide/Mb required for protein and DNA synthesis generally were from 200-4000, suggesting that the peptides are much less efficient than Mb itself in activating lymphocytes for the antibody response.

The induction by Mb or Mb peptides of protein synthesis, thymidine and uridine incorporation was thymus-dependent; these reactions were inhibited when an anti-rabbit thymus globulin was incorporated in the medium together with the antigen.

At least three types of peptide-lymphocyte interactions were postulated, assuming that the antibody response to Mb is thymus-dependent: first that the peptide can activate both T and B cells for antibody formation; second that the peptide activates only T cells; the B cells are stimulated by Mb persisting from the original priming injection; third that T cells are stimulated by the residual Mb immunogen and the B cells by the Mb peptide. The second type of interaction presumably explains the capacity of 1-6 - - a putative non-antigen, i.e., non reactive with antibody to Mb - - to induce antibody formation to Mb. All three types of interaction may be dependent upon the peptide(s) being effectively multivalent through non-specific binding to lymphocytes, macrophages and/or dendritic types cells and/or to proteins in the medium.

ACKNOWLEDGEMENTS

The authors appreciate the valuable assistance of Dr. J. Koketsu, Mr. R. C. Pai and Mr. Roger Karp. This work was supported by grants from the National Institutes of Health, U. S. Public Health Service to ABS (AI-11420) and to MZA (AM-13389).

REFERENCES

1. Atassi, M. Z. (1964) Nature, Lond. 202, 496.
2. Atassi, M. Z. (1975) Immunochemistry 12, 423.
3. Atassi, M. Z. and Pai, R. C. (1975) Immunochemistry 12, 735.
4. Bretscher, P. A. (1974) Cell. Immun. 13, 171.
5. Bullock, W. W. and Rittenberg, M. B. (1970) J. Exp. Med. 132, 926.
6. Cold Spring Harbor Symposia on Quantitative Biology, XLI, Parts 1 and 2, 1976.
7. David, J. R. and David, R. (1971) in In Vitro Methods in Cell Mediated Immunity (Edited by Bloom, B. R. and Glade, P. R.) p. 249. Academic Press, New York.
8. Edmundson, A. B. (1965) Nature, Lond. 205, 883.
9. Fanger, M. W. and Bernier, G. M. (1973) J. Immunol. 111, 609.
10. Fanger, M. W., Hart, D. A., Wells, J. V. and Nisonoff, A. (1970) J. Immun. 105, 1484.
11. Feldmann, M. and Nossal, G. J. V. (1972) Transplantation (Rev.) 13, 3.
12. Gorczynski, R. M. (1974) J. Immun. 112, 1815.
13. Huber, B., Devinsky, O., Gershon, R. K. and Cantor, H. J. (1976) J. Exp. Med. 143, 1534.
14. Katz, D. H. and Benacerraf, B. (1972) Adv. Immunol. 15, 1.
15. Kelly, B., Levy, J. G. and Hull, D. (1973) Eur. J. Immunol. 3, 574.
16. Kendrew, J. C., Watson, H. C., Strandberg, B. E., Dickerson, R. E., Phillips, D. C. and Shore, V. C. (1961) Nature, Lond. 190, 666.
17. Koketsu, J. and Atassi, M. Z. (1973) Biochim. Biophys. Acta 328, 289.
18. Koketsu, J. and Atassi, M. Z. (1974a) Immunochemistry 11, 1.
19. Koketsu, J. and Atassi, M. Z. (1974b) Biochim. Biophys. Acta 342, 21.
20. Levy, J. G., Hull, D., Kelly, B., Kilburn, D. G. and Teather, R. M. (1972) Cell. Immunol. 5, 87.
21. McDonough, R. J. and Inman, F. T. Analyt. Biochem. 36, 495.
22. Pai, R. C. and Atassi, M. Z. (1975) Immunochemistry 12, 285.

23. Plotkin, D. H., Kontiainen, S., Stavitsky, A. B. and Makela, O. (1968) Immunol. 15, 799.
24. Robbins, J. B., Haimovich, J. and Sela, M. (1967) Immunochemistry 4, 11.
25. Schechter, I., Schechter, B. and Sela, M. (1966) Biochim. Biophys. Acta 127, 438.
26. Self, C. H., Tew, J. G., Cook, R. G. and Stavitsky, A. B. (1974) Immunochemistry 11, 227.
27. Senyk, G., Williams, E. B., Nitecki, D. E. and Goodman, J. W. (1971) J. Exp. Med. 134, 1294.
28. Spitler, L., Benjamini, E., Young, J. D., Kaplan, H. and Fudenberg, H. H. (1970) J. Exp. Med. 131, 133.
29. Stavitsky, A. B. and Cook, R. G. (1974) J. Immun. 112, 583.
30. Stavitsky, A. B. and Self, C. H. (1972) Immun. Commun. 1, 491.
31. Stavitsky, A. B., Tew, J. G. and Harold, W. W. (1974) Immun. 113, 2045.
32. Stavitsky, A. B., Atassi, M. Z., Gooch, G. T., Pelley, R. P. and Harold, W. W. (1975) Immunochemistry 12, 959.
33. Tew, J. G., Self, C. H., Harold, W. W. and Stavitsky, A. B. (1973) J. Immun. 111, 416.
34. Tew, J. G. and Stavitsky, A. B. (1974) Cellul. Immunol. 14, 1.
35. Wahl, S. M. and Rosenstreich, D. L. (1976) J. Exp. Med. 144, 1175.
36. Waterfield, D., Levy, J. G., Kilburn, D. G. and Teather, R. M. (1972) Cell. Immun. 3, 253.
37. Yoshida, T., Sonosaki, H. and Cohen, S. (1973) J. Exp. Med. 138, 784.

DISCUSSION

Sidney Leskowitz

Department of Pathology, Tufts Medical School
Boston, Massachusetts 02111

After a short and not very intense internal discussion I decided to forego the usual prerogative of a discussant which is to ignore everything that was said previously and present my own data. I decided to do this for two reasons. One, of course, is that so much good stuff has already been presented and the second is that I don't have any slides anyway. So what I would like to do is to try to take all the information that we've had so far and that we are bound to get more of and before drowning, try to come up with some generalizations that will at least help me understand where we're going and what the field is like. The first thing that I would like to say is that it strikes me, from what I've heard about the nature of an antigenic determinant as far as the B cell is concerned, is that while it's extremely complex operationally, it is totally intelligible on structural grounds. Now the work we heard last night, especially the beautiful work by Dr. Atassi, our host, went very far, in fact, in laying out the strategy of how to go at this, and before fatigue set in, it seemed to me last night that I was able to grasp the principles of how to determine what the specific antigenic determinant that any B cell recognizes would be, so it seems to me that this is a kind of problem where the technology now exists to allow us to approach just about any molecule and with enough effort and patience get out the antigenic determinants. This has been amply borne out, I think, by a lot of work that was presented both last night and today as well by Benjamini and others. The interesting question remaining at least to me in my own prejudiced state is what is the nature of antigenic determinants that T cells see, or that is specific for T cells, and here it seems to me we're still confronted with conceptual difficulties which are making the task difficult for us. I would like now to make some generalizations, really wide ranging generalizations with no data, to give my impression of what the problem is. In the first place, it seems that there is already ample evidence which suggests that T cells and B cells probably see antigens a little differently and that T cells have a slightly more limited repertory of what they see. Now, what do I mean by that? Well, we've heard evidence already that for any given antigen, T and B cells may recognize different antigenic determinants and a key case in point is the evidence that Dr. Goodman presented with the beautifully simple glucagon molecule, one determinant is seen by the T cells and one by the B cells. There is also a vast literature that goes back more years than most of you here can probably remember having to do with denaturation of antigens and unfolding of proteins and so on, and a lot of it is coming back up again, it's current. It seems to suggest that when you denature a protein, when you remove conformation, you destroy antigenic determinants that B cells see but frequently you do nothing as far as a T cell is concerned. A T cell is amply capable of recognizing these drastically altered proteins. The second bit of information is again buried in ancient literature and that is that there are almost no examples that I know of anyway, in which polysaccharides are active as antigens in a T cell phenomenon while they are well studied and characterized for B cells specificity. And the third one, about which I have some personal knowledge, and Dr. Goodman has also done some work, is that virtually any hapten will suffice for B cell triggering and activation on the appropriate carrier, but the number of haptens to which T cells will show reactivity is limited in a very peculiar and as yet not completely understood way, all of which suggests that T cells cannot see everything. So, what kind of a unified field theory can we come up with to encompass this mass of information? I would suggest, along with a lot of other people, that what is involved here is something which almost has not been uttered in the conference so far, namely, the macrophage. It is amply clear, I think, that regardless of what is needed for triggering the B cell, by virtue of the fact that its receptors are immunoglobulin molecules, an antigenic determinant whether it be hapten, polysaccharide or protein is seen directly as is on almost any carrier. The T cell, we are beginning to learn now, sees antigens only on macrophage, and in particular, only with some kind of association with the Ia molecules of the macrophage and that to me suggests the nature of the whole problem. In order to understand the peculiar antigenic specificity required for T cell triggering it seems to me that first and foremost we must learn how macrophages process antigens, what they do to various kinds of antigenic determinants, and, in particular, how they take these antigenic determinants and either associate them with Ia antigens, or, as my own personal prejudice goes, at least as far as this present meeting is concerned, how they couple them directly to Ia antigen and present that as the determinant which is finally recognized by the T cells. So I would suggest, and as I indicated it is only my prejudice, that the kind of thing that I am going to be looking forward to in the rest of this meeting and the kind of message I wish to take home is how to get some handle on this problem of antigenic determinants as far as T cells are concerned, to try and get some sense of how we can at least approach the problem of what macrophages do to antigenic determinants in order to present them to T cells. Now I have listed some specific questions that I have for speakers but we are so far over time that I think I will take the second prerogative of being a discussant and stop right now and leave the floor open for anybody else that has anything to say.

GENETIC CONTROL OF THE ANTIBODY RESPONSE TO SPERM WHALE MYOGLOBIN IN MICE

Jay A. Berzofsky

Metabolism Branch, National Cancer Institute

National Institutes of Health, Bethesda, Maryland 20014

ABSTRACT

The antibody response to the main chromatographic component IV of sperm whale myoglobin in mice has been shown to be under the control of both H-2-linked and non-H-2-linked genes, using an assay which measures antibody concentration independent of affinity. The effect of non-H-2 background genes was such that for a given H-2 haplotype, mice of the A background were higher responders than those of the B10 background. Among congenic mice of all the same background, mice of haplotypes $H\text{-}2^{d,s}$ were high responders, while those of haplotypes $H\text{-}2^{k,b,q}$ were low responders. Use of intra-H-2 recombinant strains B10.A, B10.A(5R), A.TL, and D2.GD allowed mapping of at least two H-2-linked Ir genes, both within the I region, one tentatively mapping in I-A, designated Ir-Mb-1, and one mapping to the right of I-E and left of H-2D, designated Ir-Mb-2. Strains bearing both genes or only Ir-Mb-1 were high responders, while those bearing Ir-Mb-2 were intermediate responders.

When the concentration of antimyoglobin antibodies which bound to [^{14}C]-fragment (132-153) of myoglobin was measured in the same sera described above, levels in the B10.A sera were low like those of the B10.BR rather than intermediate between the levels of the B10.BR and the high-responding B10.D2, as for myoglobin, whereas levels in the D2.GD sera were still high. It is therefore suggested that the 2 or more genetically defined H-2-linked Ir genes each control the response to a different chemically defined determinant or group of determinants on myoglobin. Further studies with other fragments are in progress to test this hypothesis.

INTRODUCTION

The immune responses to only a few natural protein antigens have been found thus far to be under major histocompatibility complex-linked Ir-gene control. One such is staphylococcal nuclease, discussed elsewhere in this symposium (Berzofsky et al. 1977a). The ability to compare native and non-native conformations, and the presence of several determinants which each occur only once per molecule, have led to some results not readily obtained with synthetic antigens. Myoglobin, similar in size and complexity to nuclease, has several potential additional advantages as a model antigen for Ir-gene studies. The five major antigenic determinants have been very precisely defined in the elegant immunochemical studies of Atassi and coworkers (Atassi, 1975). Also, myoglobins from closely related species that differ in only a few amino acid residues can be compared to localize relevant determinants under control. In addition, the heme prosthetic group allows the use of physical (optical, magnetic) probes.

The only previous search for genetic control of the antibody response to myoglobin in mice (Young and Ebringer, 1976) revealed no straightforward genetic effects. The current study demonstrates the existence of both H-2-linked and non-H-2-linked genetic controls, indicates more than one I-region gene involved, and approaches the question of whether the responses to different determinants are under the control of different genes.

MATERIALS AND METHODS

Sperm whale myoglobin (Biozyme, England) was fractionated on CM-Sephadex C-50 by the method of Hapner et al. (1968) to obtain the major chromatographic component IV in the notation of Garner et al. (1974) (corresponding to MbX in the notation of Atassi (1964)). Only this homogeneous component was used throughout the study.

Mice, obtained from Jackson Laboratories, or Drs. D.H. Sachs or R.H. Schwartz, were immunized intraperitoneally with 200 μg of myoglobin emulsified 1:1 in complete Freund's adjuvant, bled at 3 weeks, and then boosted with 100 μg myoglobin in saline and bled and boosted at 10-day intervals.

To measure the concentration of antimyoglobin antibodies, a radiobinding assay was used, similar to that we described for nuclease (Berzofsky, et al. 1977b,c). Myoglobin was labeled selectively at the amino-terminal α-amino group by carbamoylation with $K^{14}CNO$ as previously described.[1] Increasing concentrations of labeled myoglobin were mixed with a constant 1:5 dilution of antiserum and the immunoglobulin and bound antigen separated from free antigen with polyethylene glycol (MW 6,000; final concentration 10% W:W). When the concentration of bound antigen reached a plateau, at large antigen excess, the antibodies were considered to be saturated and the level of the plateau was taken as the molar concentration of antibody binding sites, independent of affinity.[1] Binding by preimmune sera from the same animals (usually less than 5% of total cpm added) was subtracted from each value. The same data were plotted according to the Scatchard format to assess affinity.

The C-terminal fragment of myoglobin extending from residues 132 to 153, denoted Mb(132-153), was prepared by cyanogen bromide cleavage and purified by the method of Marshall et al. (1974). Its purity was confirmed by amino acid analysis to be > 99.5%. The fragment was carbamoylated preferentially at the N-terminal α-amino group with $K^{14}CNO$ by the same method as for myoglobin, to obtain a final specific activity of 69 Ci/mole. Binding of the fragment by antibodies in antimyoglobin sera was assessed by the same type of binding assay used for whole myoglobin.

RESULTS AND DISCUSSION

In order to assess *H-2* linkage of any genetic control found, congenic resistant series of inbred strains were used which had different *H-2* haplotypes bred onto a common "background" genome of non-*H-2* genes (Klein, 1975). Thus, all mice on a given background were genetically identical except for genes closely linked to *H-2*. Three different backgrounds were used, the B10 (short form of C57BL/10), A (from A/WySn), and DBA/2. The parental and recombinant *H-2* haplotypes of strains of mice used are shown in Table I, with the haplotype of origin of each subregion of *H-2* indicated.

Congenic Strains on the B10 Background

Binding curves for antisera from three congenic strains of mice on the B10 background, after three immunizations with myoglobin, indicated clear *H-2*- linked genetic differences (Fig. 1). The B10.BR mice ($H\text{-}2^k$) gave a barely measurable response; the B10.D2 mice ($H\text{-}2^d$) gave a high response; and the B10.A mice ($H\text{-}2^a$) gave an intermediate response. However, since the $H\text{-}2^a$ haplotype

---

[1]Berzofsky, J.A., manuscript submitted for publication.

Table I

Strain	K	I-A	I-B	I-J	I-E	I-C	S	G	D
				H-2 Type in Subregion					
B10.D2, DBA/2	d	d	d	d	d	d	d	d	d
B10.S, A.SW	s	s	s	s	s	s	s	s	s
B10, A.BY	b	b	b	b	b	b	b	b	b
B10.BR	k	k	k	k	k	k	k	k	k
A.TL	s	k	k	k	k	k	k	k	d
B10.A, A/J	k	k	k	k	k	d	d	d	d
B10.A(5R)	b	b	b	k	k	d	d	d	d
B10.A(4R)	k	k	b	b	b	b	b	b	b
D2·GD	d	d	b	b	b	b	b	b	b
B10.DA	q	q	q	q	q	q	q	q	s

Assignments based on Shreffler and David (1975), Shreffler et al. (1976), Sachs (1977) and Murphy et al. (1976).

of the B10.A mice is a recombinant between $H\text{-}2^d$ and $H\text{-}2^k$ (Table 1), the intermediate response of this strain suggests that at least 2 H-2-linked Ir genes are operative in the B10.D2 strain, that the B10.BR strain has neither of these, and that the recombinant B10.A strain has one but not the other.

Both of these results were borne out when more strains were studied. In order to show the time course of the response with repeated immunizations for many different strains, each binding curve is represented by a single point corresponding to the plateau level of binding multiplied by the dilution factor (1:5 in every case), with error bars indicating the uncertainty of measurement of the plateau (Fig. 2). All the differences described were found to be true for all 3 bleeds, by which time the response in most cases appeared to be leveling off. Among the 4 prototype or parental H-2 haplotypes tested (Fig. 2A), $H\text{-}2^d$ (B10.D2) and $H\text{-}2^s$ (B10.S) conferred high responsiveness and $H\text{-}2^k$ (B10.BR) and $H\text{-}2^b$ (B10) produced low responses. Since the (B10 x B10.D2) F_1 hybrid mice gave a high response, the high responsiveness of the $H\text{-}2^d$ was dominant (Fig. 2B).

The intermediate responsiveness of the B10.A mice was confirmed by other bleeds of the same mice (Fig. 2B), by a second group of B10.A mice (data not shown), and by a statistical

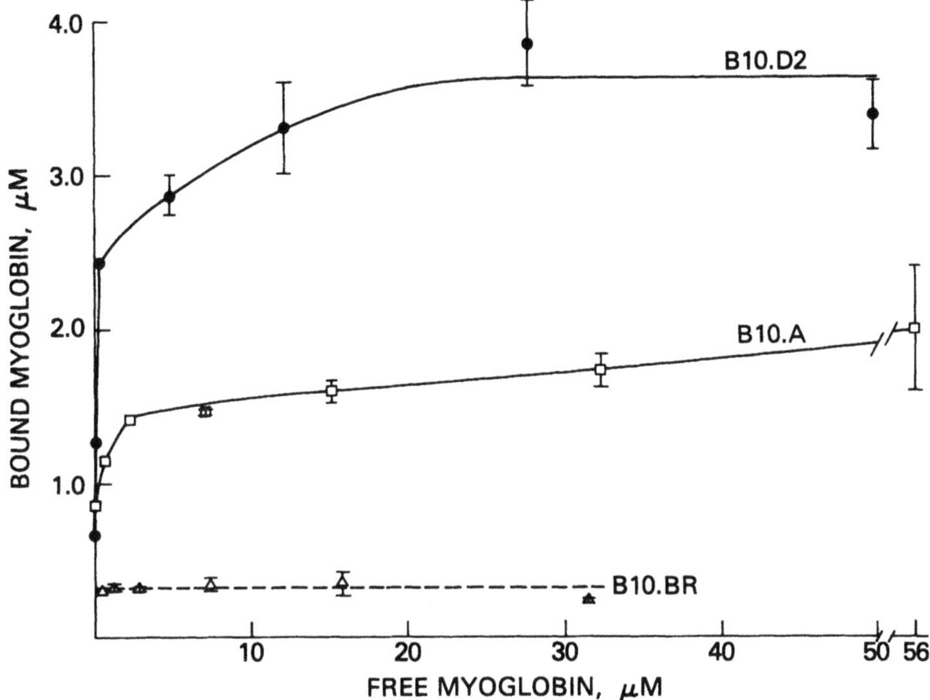

Fig 1. Binding of ^{14}C-myoglobin by antimyoglobin antisera from B10.D2, B10.A, and B10.BR mice after three immunizations with myoglobin. All sera were tested at a constant 1:5 dilution with increasing concentrations of labeled myoglobin. Sera were pools of equal aliquots from 7, 6, and 5 mice, respectively. Error bars represent range of duplicates (shown only for points on or near a plateau). Binding by preimmune sera from each group (< 5% of myoglobin added) has been subtracted.

analysis of the binding by sera from individual mice of the several strains.[1] In addition, the same conclusion was confirmed by the intermediate response of the B10.A(5R) strain (Fig. 2B). This strain bears the same $\underline{H-2^d}$ alleles at the right side of $\underline{H-2}$ as the B10.A, but the left side derived from a recombination with the $\underline{H-2^b}$ haplotype of B10, a low responder (Table I). Thus, whether the left side of $\underline{H-2}$ comes from $\underline{H-2^k}$ or $\underline{H-2^b}$, the response of these recombinant strains is lower than that of the $\underline{H-2^d}$ strain (B10.D2), but higher than those of the pure $\underline{H-2^k}$ or $\underline{H-2^b}$ strains. In contrast, the B10.A(4R) recombinant between two low responder strains is a low responder.

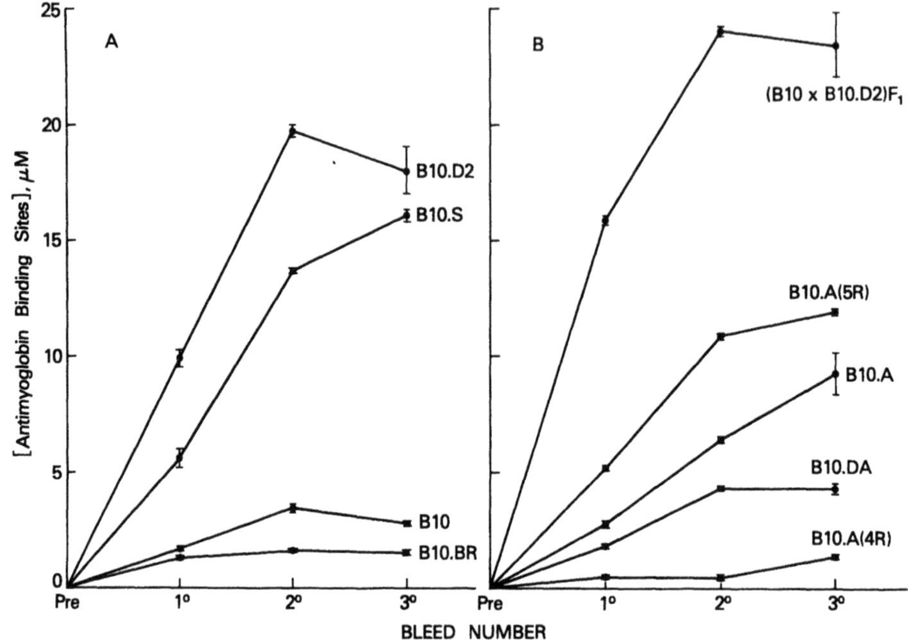

Fig 2. Antimyoglobin antibody binding site concentration as a function of successive immunization over time for nine congenic strains of mice on the B10 background. Each point represents the plateau value of bound myoglobin obtained from a complete binding curve as in Fig. 1. The mean of determinations for points on the plateau is shown, with S.E.M. of these points as an estimate of experimental uncertainty. All sera were pooled from equal aliquots of sera from 5 to 9 mice. Binding by preimmune sera (< 5% of total myoglobin added) was subtracted. Panel A. Strains of parental H-2 haplotypes. Panel B. Strains of F_1 hybrid or recombinant H-2 haplotypes.

This fairly strong evidence for the existence of at least two H-2-linked Ir genes for myoglobin is unusual in that most two-gene Ir systems involve complementation between two low responders, in an F_1 hybrid or recombinant strain (e.g. Benacerraf and Dorf, 1976). In the myoglobin system, there is no evidence that the two genes complement one another. If, in fact, they function independently, then one explanation may be that each gene controls the response to a different determinant or group of determinants on the antigen molecule. This hypothesis can be tested by analyzing the specificity of the populations of antibodies made by different strains, using fragments of the antigen (see below). Until further subdivisions become possible, I shall designate Ir-Mb-1 as the gene (or genes) for high responsiveness to myoglobin which maps to the left of the recombination event in the B10.A strain and Ir-Mb-2 as the gene (or genes) to the right of the recombination event.

Finally, the low responsiveness of the B10.DA strain (Fig. 2B) suggests that $H\text{-}2^q$ is also a low-responder haplotype.

Congenic Strains on the A Background

When several strains on the A background were examined in a fashion similar to that of Fig. 2, the first striking observation was that all the responses were about 5-fold higher than those of the H-2-identical strains on the B10 background (Fig. 3). Thus, a non-H-2 linked gene (or genes) must also be involved in the regulation of the antibody response to myoglobin. The direction of this difference between B10 and A backgrounds is the same as in the case of staphylococcal nuclease (Berzofsky et al. 1977 a,b), and the magnitude is similar. However, whereas the non-H-2-linked control completely masked the H-2-linked effects in the overall magnitude of the response after three immunizations with nuclease (Berzofsky, et al., 1977 a,b)[2], in the case of myoglobin, the H-2-linked differences remained just as apparent after 3 immunizations as after one, despite the non-H-2-linked effect.

Comparing strains on the same background, the A.SW strain ($H\text{-}2^s$) gave a high response, while the A.BY strain ($H\text{-}2^b$) gave a low response (Fig. 3) similar to the findings for the B10.S and B10 mice. Thus, the H-2 linkage of these differences is confirmed. The alternative explanation of genetic drift between the supposedly identical background genomes of B10.S and B10 is excluded, since identical drift in two different backgrounds is exceedingly unlikely.

The low response of the A.TL strain (Fig. 3) leads to several conclusions. This strain has a recombinant H-2 haplotype in which the K and D ends come from the $H\text{-}2^s$ and $H\text{-}2^d$ haplotypes (both high-responder haplotypes) respectively, but all of the subregions in between, including the whole I region, derive from the $H\text{-}2^k$ (low-responder) haplotype (Table I). Since the A.TL strain is a low responder, like the $H\text{-}2^k$ strain on the B10 background, rather than high like the $H\text{-}2^s$ or $H\text{-}2^d$ strains, the Ir genes for myoglobin in these strains can be mapped to the right of H-2 K and left of H-2D, i.e. within the I, S, or G regions. Of these, the I region is the most likely, since most Ir genes have been mapped there, while the

[2] Pisetsky, Berzofsky, and Sachs, manuscript in preparation.

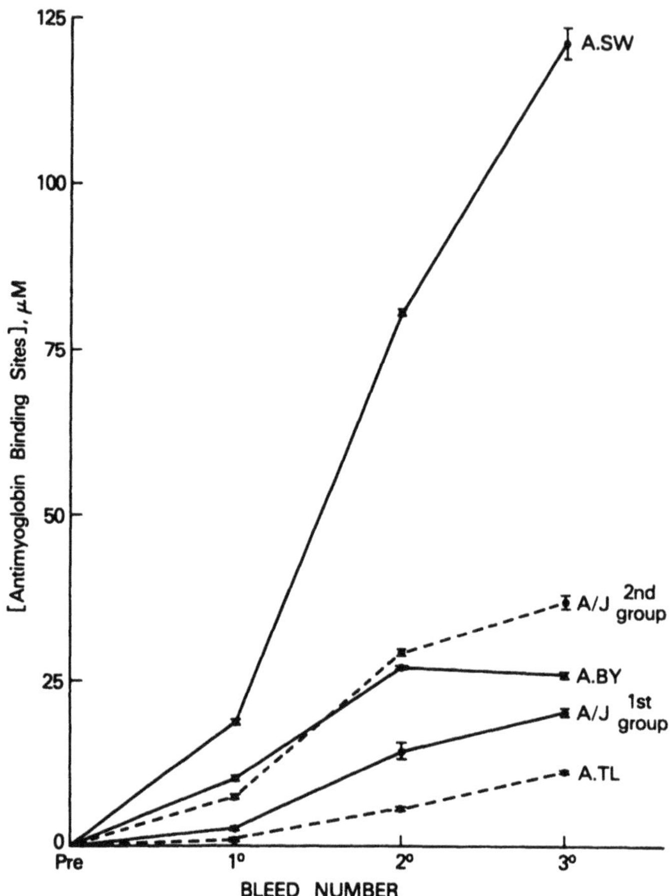

Fig. 3. Antimyoglobin antibody binding site concentration as a function of successive immunization for four congenic strains of mice on the A background. Each point represents the plateau of a complete binding curve on pools of equal aliquots from 5 to 8 mice as detailed in the legend of Fig. 2. The 2nd group of A/J mice was immunized simultaneously with the A.TL mice (both dashed).

S region codes for a component of complement and the G region for an erythrocyte antigen; but the strains are not available to formally prove this supposition. In addition, the low response of the A.TL strain confirms on a second background the low responsiveness associated with the I^k haplotype on the B10 background.

Finally, two different groups of A/J mice gave responses higher than did the A.TL mice but lower than did the A.SW mice (Fig. 3). Since no pure $H\text{-}2^k$ or $H\text{-}2^d$ strains exist on the A background, these are the best standards of comparison available. This intermediate status of A/J mice (H-2^a) confirms the observation made on the B10.A (H-2^a) strain on the B10 background. Again, the differences noted were found to be statistically significant when individual mice were studied.[1] The fact that the response of the A/J mice was not greater than that of the A.BY mice (H-2^b) is not formally contradictory to this conclusion, since the H-2^a recombinant haplotype should be compared with its parental haplotypes H-2^k and H-2^d, rather than a different low responder type. Differences between strains bearing the left side of the H-2^b and H-2^k low-responder haplotypes were consistently noted in the same direction, although usually not in a statistically significant fashion. Thus, if one compares the pairs A.BY and A.TL, B10 and B10.BR, B10 and B10.A(4R), and B10.A(5R) and B10.A, the first of each pair always gave the higher response to myoglobin. The meaning of this difference between low responder alleles is not known.

Congenic Strains on the DBA/2 Background

The DBA/2 mice, bearing the same H-2^d as the B10.D2 mice (Table I) but on a different background, produced comparable levels of antibodies to the B10.D2 strain (Fig. 4). Thus, responsiveness of this haplotype was confirmed on a different background, although no low-responder haplotype was available on the DBA/2 background to compare.

The D2.GD strain (Lilly and Klein, 1973) is congenic to the DBA/2 strain but arose from a recombination between the H-2^d haplotype of this and the H-2^b haplotype of the C57BL/6 strain. Only the _H-2K_ and _I-A_ subregions derived from H-2^d, the rest from H-2^b (Table I). Nevertheless, two groups of D2.GD mice produced just as much antimyoglobin as the congenic H-2^d DBA/2 strain (Fig. 4). Therefore, the _Ir-Mb-1_ gene of the H-2^d high-responder haplotype, mapped above to the right of _H-2K_ and left of _I-C_, appears to map in the _I-A_ subregion. However, in contrast to _Ir-Mb-2_ in the B10.A, A/J, and B10.A(5R) strains, this gene(s) appears to confer essentially full responsiveness, rather than intermediate. Results on the B10.HTT strain (recombinant haplotype _s s s s k k k k d_ in the notation of Table I) tend to support this observation for the H-2^s haplotype "allele" of _Ir-Mb-1_.[1]

One possible explanation may be that _Ir-Mb-1_ is a gene or group of genes controlling the response to determinants which represent the large majority of the antibodies made to myoglobin, whereas _Ir-Mb-2_ is a gene (or genes) which controls the response to determinants represented by a minority of antibodies made. Therefore, _Ir-Mb-1_ alone would be hard to distinguish from both genes together, whereas strains bearing _Ir-Mb-2_ alone would be significantly lower responders than strains bearing both. Alternatively,

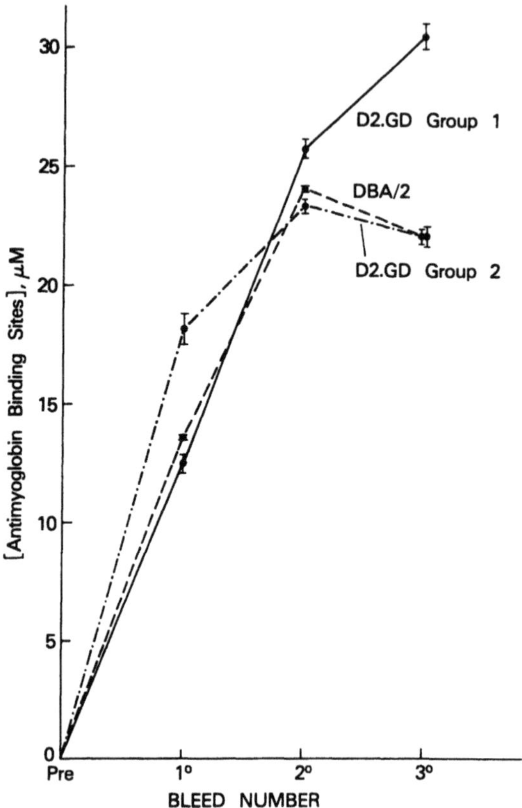

Fig. 4. Antimyoglobin antibody binding site concentration as a function of successive immunization for two congenic strains of mice on the DBA/2 background. Each point represents the plateau of a complete binding curve on pools of equal aliquots as detailed in the legend of Fig. 2. A total of 8 DBA/2 and 13 D2.GD mice were studied.

if the different genes all act on the whole response rather than the response to different determinants as postulated above, one could invoke a rather complex scheme of coupled complementation (Benacerraf and Dorf, 1976), in which only certain combinations of Ir-Mb-1 and Ir-Mb-2 complement. For example, Ir-Mb-2 of $H\text{-}2^b$ would complement with Ir-Mb-1 of $H\text{-}2^d$ but not with that of $H\text{-}2^b$, while in the opposite direction Ir-Mb-2 of $H\text{-}2^d$ would only partially complement with Ir-Mb-1 of $H\text{-}2^b$ (as in the B10.A(5R) strain).

Table II summarizes the assignments made for at least two H-2-linked Ir genes for the strains tested thus far.

Table II
Summary of Response Patterns Attributable to H-2-Linked Ir Genes

Strain	H-2	Ir-Mb-1	Ir-Mb-2	Response
B10.D2,DBA/2	d	+	+	High
B10.S, A.SW	s	+	?	High
D2.GD	g2	+	-	High
B10.A(5R)	i5	-	+	Intermed.
B10.A, A/J	a	-	+	Intermed.
B10.BR	k	-	-	Low
A.TL	tl	-	-	Low
B10,A.BY	b	-*	-	Low*
B10.A(4R)	h4	-	-	Low
B10.DA	qp1	-	-	Low
$(B10xB10.D2)F_1$	b/d	-/+	-/+	High

*Reproducibly not as low as $H\text{-}2^k$, although the differences are not statistically significant for these numbers of mice.

Antibodies Specific for Fragment (132-153)

In order to evaluate the hypothesis elaborated above that the genetically separable H-2-linked Ir genes for myoglobin control the response to chemically distinguishable determinants on the antigen, the prediction is being tested that the recombinant strains bearing only one of the genes should respond like high responders to some determinants and like low responders to other determinants. So far, only one fragment has been adequately tested, that corresponding to residues 132-153, denoted Mb(132-153). This fragment should bear only one major antigenic determinant as defined by Atassi and coworkers (Atassi, 1975).

When the same antimyoglobin antisera studied above were assayed for antibodies binding to $[^{14}C]$-Mb(132-153), the plateau binding for the B10.D2 high responder (third bleed) sera was about 9% of that for whole myoglobin (Fig. 5). In contrast, neither the B10.A nor the B10.BR sera demonstrated much binding at all (Fig. 5). The fact that the B10.A antimyoglobin antisera contained no more antibodies specific for this fragment than did the B10.BR low responder sera even though the identical pool of serum contained much more antibody to whole myoglobin (Fig. 1) suggests that the Ir-Mb-2 gene(s) borne by the B10.A does not confer responsiveness to the determinant on this region of myoglobin. This observation was reproduced with sera from a second group of B10.D2, B10.A, and B10.BR mice (data not shown). In addition, preliminary results comparing the other intermediate responder B10.A(5R) strain with the corresponding low responder B10 strain ($H\text{-}2^b$) showed that the

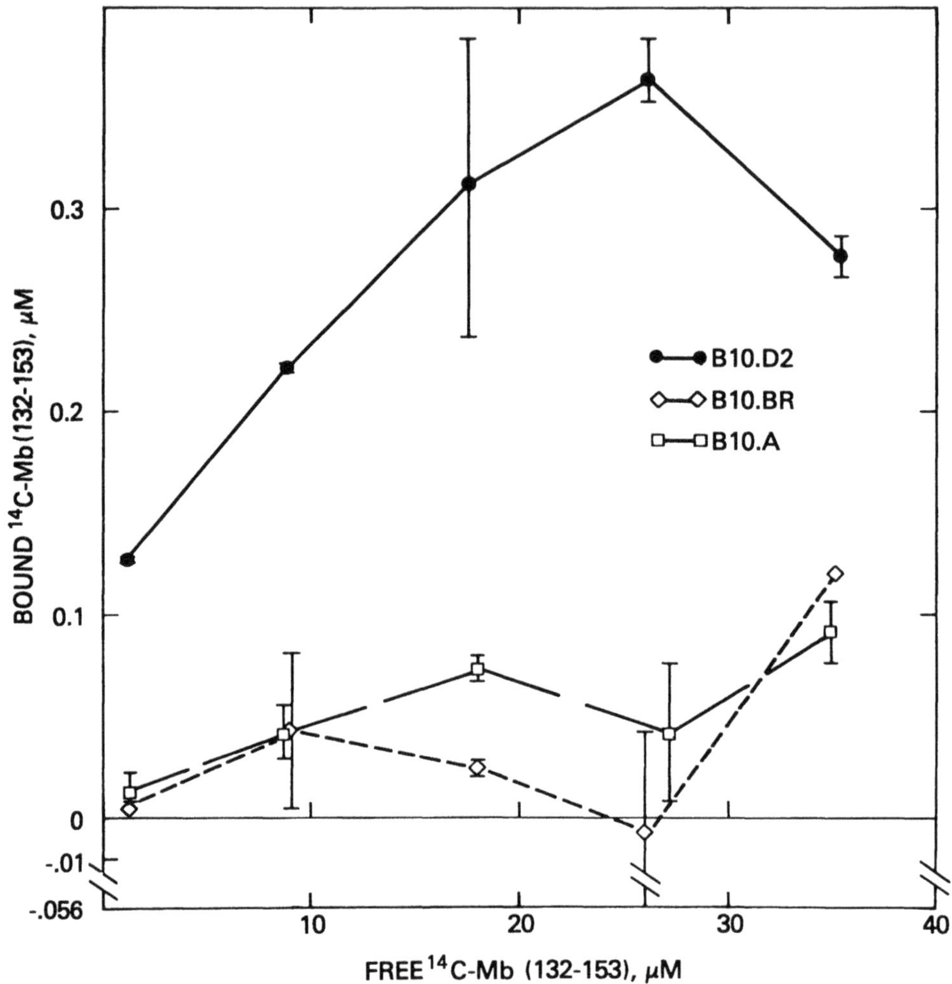

Fig. 5. Binding of ^{14}C-Mb(132-153) fragment by antimyoglobin antisera of B10.D2, B10.A, and B10.BR mice after three immunizations with native myoglobin. The sera were the same as those studied in Fig. 1, and were used at a constant 1:5 dilution. Binding by preimmune sera from the same mice (< 2% of total fragment added) is subtracted.

antimyoglobin sera of the former did not bind significantly more Mb(132-153) than did the sera of the latter. Also, both bound only slightly more than the B10.A and B10.BR sera, consistent with the $\underline{H-2}^b$ vs $\underline{H-2}^k$ difference noted above.

In contrast, the D2.GD antimyoglobin sera contained just as much antibody binding to Mb(132-153) as did the congenic high responder DBA/2 (H-2^d) sera (Fig. 6). Since the D2.GD strain bears only Ir-Mb-1 from the H-2^d parent (Table I and II), one can conclude that Ir-Mb-1 does allow response to the determinant(s) on fragment Mb(132-153).

In summary, the predictions of the hypothesis have proven true so far, for the one fragment tested. The intermediate responder strains B10.A and B10.A(5R), bearing Ir-Mb-2 but not Ir-Mb-1, behaved as low responders for the determinant in this region of myo-

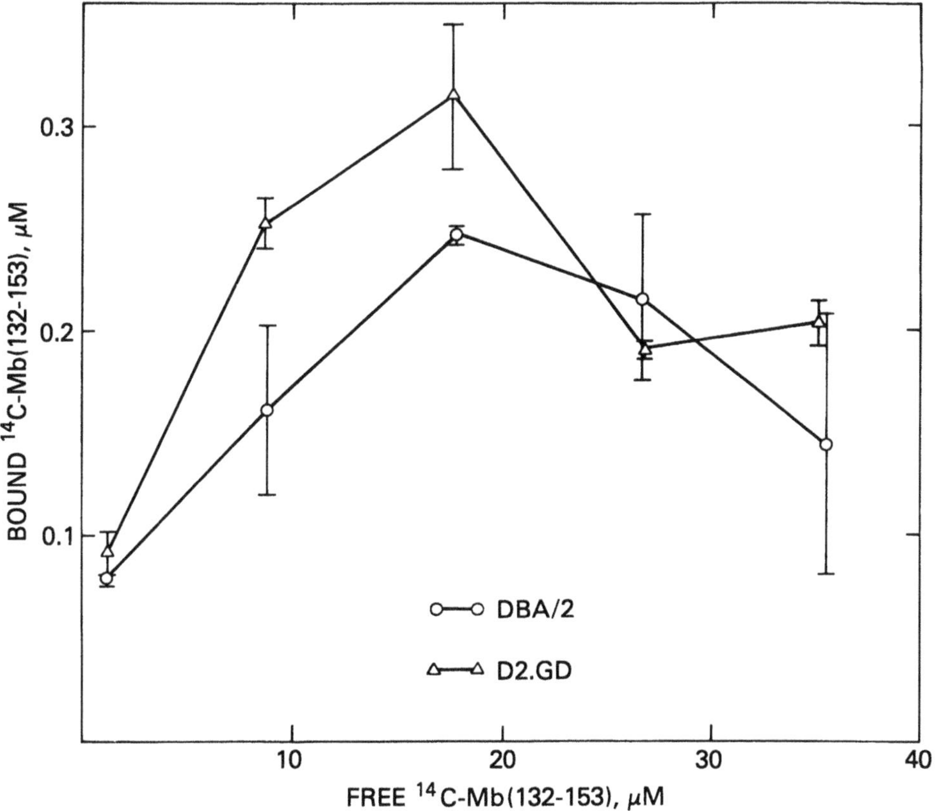

Fig. 6. Binding of ^{14}C-Mb(132-153) fragment by DBA/2 and D2.GD antimyoglobin antisera after three immunizations with native myoglobin. The sera were the same as those studied in Fig. 4 (group 1 of D2.GD), and were used at a constant 1:5 dilution. Binding by preimmune sera from the same mice is subtracted.

globin. The D2.GD strain, bearing only Ir-Mb-1, behaved as a high responder to the determinant(s) on this fragment. The hypothesis is also consistent with our observations on staphylococcal nuclease, for which H-2-linked control regulates the relative proportion of antibodies to different regions of the molecule (Berzofsky, et al., 1977a,b,c). However, we have not demonstrated more than one H-2-linked Ir gene for the antibody response to nuclease. Therefore, the simplest explanation is that the hypothesis is true, i.e. that each of the genetically separable H-2-linked Ir genes for myoglobin controls the response to a different chemically-defined determinant(s), and more specifically, that Ir-Mb-1, not Ir-Mb-2, controls the response to the determinant between residues 132 and 153. This would be the first demonstration of 2 genetically distinct H-2-linked Ir genes which control the response to different determinants on the same antigen molecule. However, these conclusions must remain tentative until the results of binding to other determinants are known. Such studies are in progress.

Acknowledgments. I would like to thank Drs. Thomas A. Waldmann, David H. Sachs, Alan N. Schechter, and Ronald H. Schwartz for helpful discussion and encouragement in the course of this work. I am grateful also to Douglas Killion for excellent technical assistance in the later part of this study, and to Mrs. Teri Cecil for expert preparation of the manuscript.

REFERENCES

Atassi, M.Z. (1964) Nature (Lond.) 202, 496.

Atassi, M.Z. (1975) Immunochemistry 12, 423.

Benacerraf, B., and Dorf, M.E. (1976) Cold Spring Harbor Symp. Quant. Biol. 41, 465.

Berzofsky, J.A., Pisetsky, D.S., Schwartz, R.H., Schechter, A.N., and Sachs, D.H. (1977a) This symposium.

Berzofsky, J.A., Schechter, A.N., Shearer, G.M., and Sachs, D.H. (1977b) J. Exp. Med. 145, 111.

Berzofsky, J.A., Schechter, A.N., Shearer, G.M., and Sachs, D.H. (1977c) J. Exp. Med. 145, 123.

Garner, M.H., Garner, W.H., and Gurd, F.R.N. (1974) J. Biol. Chem. 249, 1513.

Hapner, K.D., Bradshaw, R.A., Hartzell, C.R., and Gurd, F.R.N. (1968) J. Biol. Chem. 243, 683.

Klein, J. (1975) Biology of the Mouse Histocompatibility-2 Complex, Springer-Verlag, New York.

Lilly, F., and Klein, J. (1973) Transplantation 16, 530.

Marshall, R.C., Jones, W.C., Jr., Vigna, R.A., and Gurd, F.R.N. (1974) Zeitschr. Naturforschung 29c, 90.

Murphy, D.B., Herzenberg, L.A., Okumura, K., Herzenberg, L.A., and McDevitt, H.O. (1976) J. Exp. Med. 144, 699.

Sachs, D.H. (1977) in Proceedings of the Third Ir Gene Workshop, H.O. McDevitt, editor, in press.

Shreffler, D.C., and David, C.S. (1975) Adv. Immunol. 20, 125.

Shreffler, D.C., David, C.S., Cullen, S.E., Frelinger, J.A., and Niederhuber, J.E. (1976) Cold Spring Harbor Symp. Quant. Biol. 41, 477.

Young, C., and Ebringer, A. (1976) Immunogenetics 3, 299.

GENETIC CONTROL OF THE IMMUNE RESPONSE TO STAPHYLOCOCCAL NUCLEASE IN MICE

Jay A. Berzofsky, David S. Pisetsky, Ronald H. Schwartz, Alan N. Schechter, and David H. Sachs

National Institutes of Health, Bethesda, Maryland 20014

ABSTRACT

Genetic control of the immune response to staphylococcal nuclease in mice is detectable at several levels. At least one H-2-linked Ir gene controls 1) the relative proportions of antibodies to different determinants on nuclease when whole nuclease is the immunogen; 2) the immunogenicity of isolated fragments of nuclease, corresponding to the same regions or determinants; and 3) the T-lymphocyte proliferative response to nuclease and to its fragments. It is concluded that a model in which Ir-gene control is determined by the recognition by T lymphocytes of a single "carrier" determinant for the whole molecule does not adequately explain this system. Evidence is presented for the existence of more than one such H-2-linked Ir gene in the T-cell proliferative response. In addition, a non-H-2-linked gene(s) is described which controls the overall level of antibodies to nuclease, i.e., the aggregate of all the antibodies of different subspecificities which have in common that they bind to some part of the nuclease molecule. Evidence is also presented that T lymphocytes, as well as the receptors involved in Ir-gene function (whether or not these are T-lymphocyte receptors), are less sensitive to conformational differences between native nuclease and its isolated fragments than are the antibodies ultimately made. This insensitivity to conformation may reflect the recognition of determinants which are shorter or more flexible in the native state than those recognized by antibodies.

Genetic control of the immune response, especially that by Ir genes linked to the Major Histocompatibility Complex in guinea pigs and mice, was discovered with relatively simple synthetic polypeptide antigens such as poly-L-lysine (McDevitt and Benacerraf, 1969). Most of the subsequent studies were done with simple linear or branched copolymers of a few amino acids. To date, only a handful of natural globular protein antigens have been studied for genetic control, primarily those represented in this symposium. Yet, these differ from the synthetic copolymers in that each determinant is unique, occurring only once per molecule. In addition, these have well-defined native three-dimensional conformations. Thus, the constraints on the immune response to these globular proteins may differ from those on the response to synthetic polymers.

The antibody response to one such protein, staphylococcal nuclease, was shown to be under H-2-linked genetic control in mice by Lozner et al. (1974). The extracellular nuclease of *Staphylococcus aureus* is a single polypeptide chain of molecular weight 16,800 (Anfinsen et al., 1971), with a well-defined three-dimensional structure (Cotton and Hazen, 1971). Antibodies specific for nuclease can be detected by their ability to inhibit its enzymatic activity (Lozner et al., 1974; Berzofsky et al., 1977a). Three weeks after a single intraperitoneal immunization with 100 μg of nuclease in complete Freund's adjuvant, mice of H-2 haplotypes a, k, d, and s were high responders, while those of haplotypes b and q were low responders. Linkage to H-2 was demonstrated both by a formal genetic analysis of the F_2 generation of a cross between a high and a low responder strain, and also by use of congenic resistant strains of mice, which differ only in H-2 and closely linked genes. In addition, by use of intra-H-2 recombinant strains, the control of this response was mapped to the I-B subregion of the H-2 complex.

When we studied the effect of repeated immunizations with nuclease, a more complex picture appeared (Fig. 1). While the high responder B10.A strain made more antinuclease initially than did the low responder congenic strain B10, after three immunizations the B10 mice made just as much antibody as their B10.A counterparts (Berzofsky et al., 1977a). The levels of antinuclease in the two strains remained the same through two more successive immunizations. This observation led to two major findings which we shall discuss: 1) After hyperimmunization, the H-2-linked Ir-gene control regulated the relative response to different determinants on the nuclease molecule, not the total level of response, and 2) the overall or aggregate response to all the determinants of nuclease was regulated by a different gene(s) linked neither to H-2 nor to heavy-chain immunoglobulin structural genes.

Non-H-2-linked genetic control. First, let us consider some new data on the non-H-2-linked control, before we discuss fragments of nuclease. In the initial sera a reproducible difference was

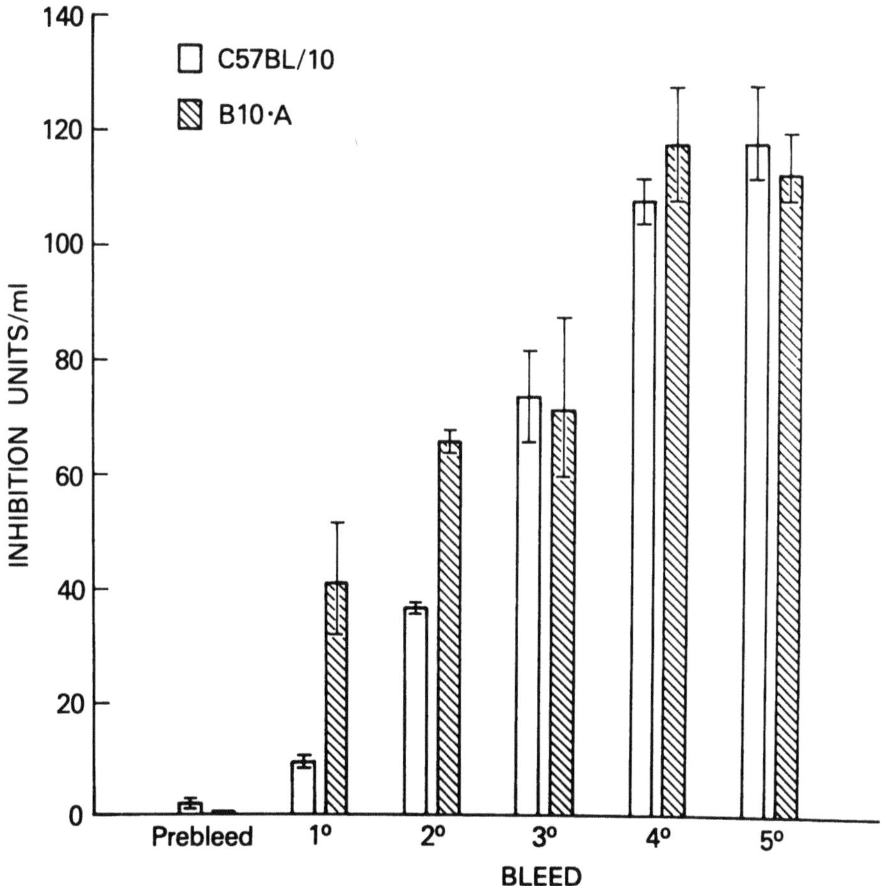

Fig. 1. Effect of repeated immunization with nuclease on the level of antinuclease antibodies expressed as inhibition units/ml, i.e., the number of nuclease activity units which can be inhibited by a ml of serum. Abscissa indicates number of immunizations (100 μg nuclease in complete Freund's adjuvant for 1°, 10 μg nuclease in saline for subsequent boosts). Error bars represent ranges of replicates. Adapted from Berzofsky et al. (1977a).

TABLE I

Antinuclease Levels in Mice Differing Only in H-2 or Only in Non-H-2-Linked Genes

Strain	H-2	C_H Allotype	Antinuclease, Inhibition Units/ml 1st Bleed	5th Bleed
B10.A	a	Ig-1^b	27.3	113
B10	b	Ig-1^b	3.9	120
A/J	a	Ig-1^e	175	920
A.BY	b	Ig-1^e	4.6	1200

seen between the H-2^a-identical B10.A and A/J mice, which must thus be attributed to non-H-2-linked genes (Table I). In contrast, the two H-2^b strains both showed negligible initial response, regardless of background. However, after five immunizations, the two H-2^b strains reached the same total antinuclease level as their respective congenic H-2^a counterparts, and the only significant difference was a 10-fold greater antibody level in the A background strains than in the B10 background strains.

Possible linkage of this non-H-2-linked effect to allotype, a marker of immunoglobulin heavy chain structural genes, was tested in a backcross of (B10.A x A/J)F_1 mice to B10.A parental mice, so that all mice were homozygous for H-2^a (Fig. 2). Although the distribution of high responders was broader than that of low responders, two patterns were clearly discernible. The high response of F_1 mice indicated that high responsiveness was dominant. Among the backcross progeny, both the Ig-1^b/1^b homozygotes and the Ig-1^b/1^e heterozygotes were nearly equally distributed between high and low response types. Thus, the non-H-2-linked control of response was not linked to heavy chain allotype. Although the high responder distribution is too broad to demonstrate an unequivocal 1:1 segregation between high and low responders, the results are not inconsistent with the action of a single genetic locus.

Genetic control of the subspecificities of antinuclease antibodies. In order to see whether the low responder B10 mice, when they finally responded, made antibodies to the same determinants

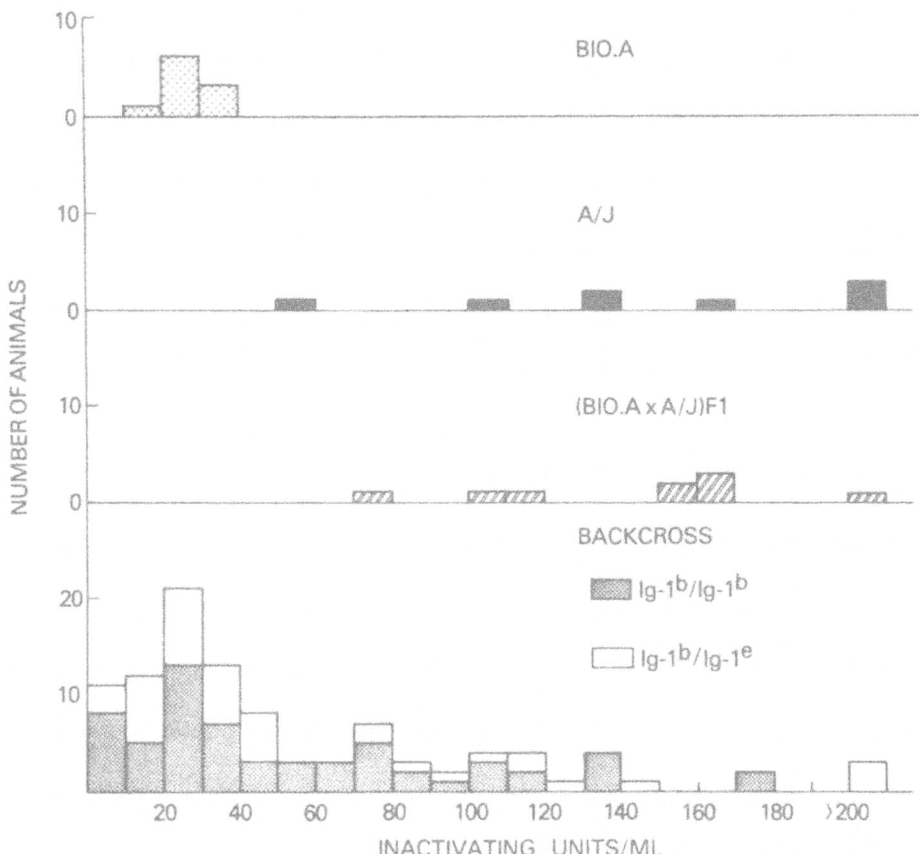

Fig. 2. Distribution of antinuclease antibody levels in parental, F_1, and backcross (B10.A x A/J) x B10.A mice. Units are as in Fig. 1. Of the 101 backcross progeny, 65 were homozygous for the $Ig\text{-}1^b$ allotype of the B10.A parent and 36 were heterozygous $Ig\text{-}1^b/Ig\text{-}1^e$.

of nuclease as the high responder B10.A mice, we examined the ability of the antinuclease antisera to bind to labeled fragments of nuclease.

An artist's representation of the three-dimensional structure of nuclease is shown in Fig. 3. The cyanogen-bromide or proteolytic fragments used were 1) fragment (99-149), the C-terminal third of the molecule containing two of three α-helices in the native structure, 2) fragment (1-126) consisting of most of the molecule except the C-terminal half of the previous fragment, 3) fragment

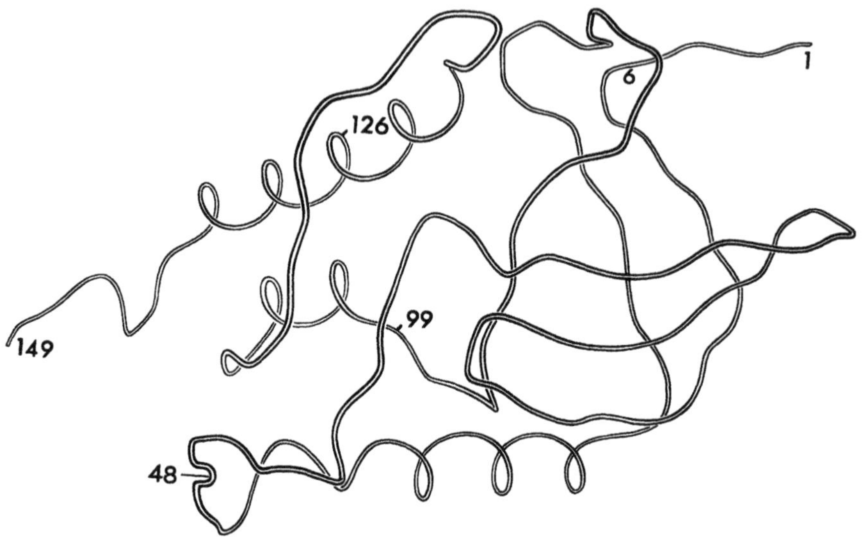

Fig. 3. Artist's representation of the three-dimensional structure of staphylococcal nuclease, with residue numbers indicated where cleavages were made. Reproduced from Berzofsky et al. (1977a).

(49-149), which includes all of the first fragment and overlaps the second, 4) fragment (6-48), roughly the N-terminal third, and 5) the small fragment (127-149).

Fragments were labeled by carbamoylation at the N-terminal α-amino group with $K^{14}CNO$ at neutral pH. The concentration of antibodies which could bind to a particular fragment was determined by incubating a constant dilution of antiserum with increasing concentrations of labeled fragment, precipitating the immunoglobulin with polyethylene glycol, and plotting bound vs free antigen until a plateau was reached, indicating saturation of the antibodies. The concentration of antigen bound at the plateau was then a measure of the concentration of antibodies able to bind that fragment, independent of affinity (Berzofsky et al., 1977 a,b). It had been shown previously that goat antibodies to native nuclease could bind random conformation fragments, but with an apparent affinity about three orders of magnitude lower than that for the native conformation - a difference attributed to the conformational equilibrium constant of the fragment, between non-native and native-like conformation (Sachs et al., 1972).

The first fragment to be examined was fragment (99-149). Three weeks after a single immunization with nuclease in complete Freund's adjuvant, there were no detectable antibodies to this fragment in sera from the B10 mice, in contrast to clear binding by the B10.A sera (Berzofsky et al., 1977a). The same was true of sera from different B10 and B10.A mice after three immunizations, at a time when the total level of antinuclease was the same in both sera (Fig. 4). After five immunizations, the B10 mice did make some antibodies capable of binding to fragment (99-149), but only a third as much as made by the B10.A mice, again in sera for which the total level of antinuclease was comparable in the two strains (Fig. 5).

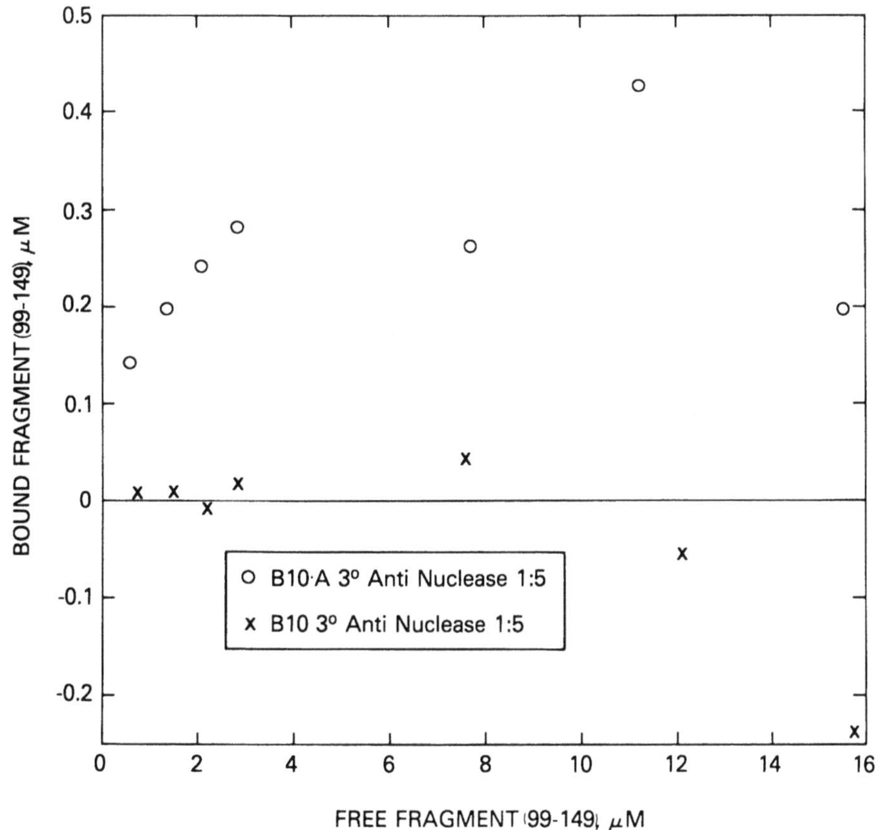

Fig. 4. Binding of [^{14}C]-fragment (99-149) by anti-native nuclease antisera after three immunizations of groups of 5 to 9 B10 and B10.A mice. Increasing concentrations of fragment were added to a constant 1:5 dilution of antiserum. Reproduced from Berzofsky et al. (1977b).

In contrast, B10 and B10.A sera bound the same amount of fragment (1-126) both after one immunization and after five immunizations (Berzofsky et al., 1977b). Thus, if we compare the ratios of antibodies specific for each of these two fragments in sera raised to whole nuclease, a striking H-2-linked effect persists even when no H-2-linked differences exist in the total antinuclease concentration (Table II). The differences must be due to H-2-linked genes since these congenic strains differ only at H-2 and closely linked genes. Moreover, the observation of the same difference between congenic strains on the A background (Table II) mitigates against the possible alternative explanation of genetic drift in the supposedly identical backgrounds of the B10 and B10.A strains. Thus, we conclude that H-2-linked Ir genes can control the relative proportions of antibodies to different determinants on the same antigen molecule.

This result was perhaps surprising, since the hypothesis that H-2-linked Ir genes function at the level of T-cell help for B-cell stimulation, requiring recognition by helper T cells of a "carrier" for the antigen, would have predicted the opposite. Thus, by this hypothesis, if B10 mice can make antibodies to the region (1-126)

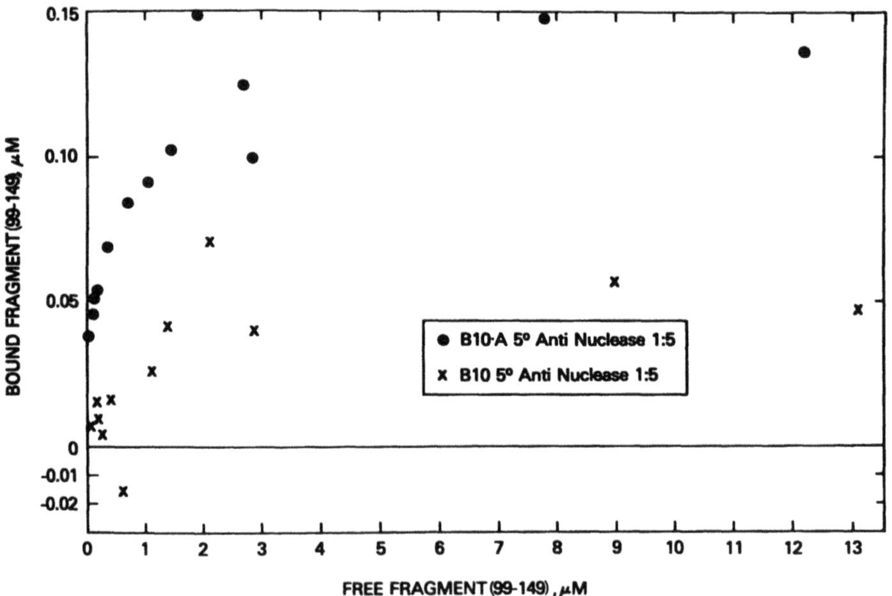

Fig. 5. Binding of [^{14}C]-fragment (99-149) by anti-native nuclease antisera from groups of 7 to 9 B10 and B10.A mice after five immunizations with nuclease. Serum was used at a constant 1:5 dilution. The mice were different groups from those shown in Fig. 4.

TABLE II
Concentrations of Antibodies to Subregions of Nuclease in Antisera to Native Nuclease[a]

Bleed	Strain	Antibody Binding Sites μM Anti-(99-149)	Anti-(1-126)	Ratio Anti-(99-149)/Anti-(1-126)
1°	B10	0.00 ± 0.01	0.61 ± 0.08	0.00
	B10.A	0.34 ± 0.08	0.81 ± 0.11	0.42
	A.BY[b]	≤0.1	1.10 ± 0.19	<0.09
	A/J grp 1[c]	0.58	4.95 ± 0.35	0.12
	grp 2	2.21 ± 0.21	5.44 ± 0.24	0.41
3°	B10	0.01 ± 0.07		
	B10.A	1.47 ± 0.24		
5°	B10	0.26 ± 0.03	1.2 ± 0.15	0.22
	B10.A	0.71 ± 0.03	0.80 ± 0.12	0.89
	A.BY	2.55 ± 0.09	17.2 ± 0.36	0.15
	A/J	5.75 ± 0.3	12.7 ± 0.55	0.45

[a]Data are from Berzofsky et al. (1977b) and Pisetsky, Berzofsky, and Sachs, manuscript submitted for publication.

[b]The 1st bleed sera from A.BY mice came from animals primed with a preparation containing mostly "Nuclease B" and less nuclease. Nuclease B differs from nuclease by the addition of an extra 19 residues at the amino terminus (Davis et al., 1977). This was used in this one case to determine ratios of specificities since A.BY mice produced virtually no antibody to a single immunization with nuclease, and in the case of hyperimmune sera where the response to nuclease and Nuclease B could be compared, there was no difference in the ratio of specificities (Berzofsky, Pisetsky, and Sachs, unpublished observations).

[c]Group 2 of A/J mice were immunized and assayed in parallel with the A.BY mice, and pools were of equal aliquots. Group 1 had been studied much earlier and pools were not of equal aliquots of serum.

of nuclease as well as can the B10.A mice, then they must have T cells capable of recognizing some "carrier" determinant on nuclease (analogous to hapten-carrier complexes) to allow for T-cell help. Therefore, since they have the same B-cell immunoglobulin structural gene repertoire as the B10.A mice, which make antibodies to the region (99-149), they should also be able to make antibodies equally well to this region. The empirical fact that they do not necessitates that some aspect of this model does not apply. One possibility is that no single carrier determinant serves to allow T-cell help for B-cell stimulation by all determinants on the molecule, but rather different determinants serve as carriers for different parts of the molecule. In fact, some evidence we shall discuss below suggests that the determinants recognized by T cells are the same as or closely associated with the determinants recognized by B cells. Thus, the concept of distinct carrier and hapten may break down in this system. An alternative possibility is that H-2-linked *Ir* genes are expressed in B cells in clonal distribution parallel to the immunoglobulin specificity of that B cell.

H-2-linked control of the immunogenicity of nuclease fragments. When mice of five inbred strains were immunized with fragment (99-149), fragment (1-126), or fragment (6-48), instead of whole nuclease and the sera tested by the radiobinding assay, the antibody response to fragment (99-149) paralleled that to whole nuclease, whereas that to the others did not (Berzofsky et al., 1977a). Fragment (6-48) was a very poor immunogen in general, even though it is about the same size as fragment (99-149). A comparison of B10.A and B10 strain responses for fragments (99-149) and (1-126) revealed that both strains could respond to fragment (1-126), whereas the B10 mice failed to produce a statistically significant response to fragment (99-149) even after three immunizations (Table III). In contrast, B10 mice did respond to whole nuclease after three immunizations, as shown above. Thus the response to fragment (99-149) and that to whole nuclease appeared to be under similar control, except that the defect in B10 mice to respond to fragment (99-149) was complete, rather than partial. This result is consistent with the observation above that when the B10 mice did respond to nuclease after hyperimmunization, the response was directed at determinants outside the region of residues 99 to 149.

The finding that the same apparent genetic control is manifested whether the random conformation fragment (99-149) is used as immunogen, or whether the same region 99-149 is presented in the native conformation on whole nuclease, is particularly interesting in view of the fact that the antibodies ultimately made show a striking ability to distinguish these conformational forms (Sachs et al., 1972; Furie et al., 1975). Thus, the recognition structure in *Ir*-gene control appears to be less sensitive to conformational differences than the antibodies made under its control. This result may be a reflection of the possibility that the polypeptide region recognized in the *Ir*-gene control mechanism may be shorter or more flexible and therefore less different in native and random conformations than the regions recognized by antibodies.

H-2-linked control of the T-lymphocyte proliferative response to nuclease and its fragments. To see whether similar genetic constraints would apply to a T-cell response which did not involve B cells, a thymidine-incorporation T-cell proliferative assay using peritoneal exudate T-lymphocyte enriched cells (PETLES) (Schwartz et al., 1975) was employed. Thioglycollate-induced peritoneal exudate cells from mice immunized with nuclease in complete Freund's adjuvant three weeks earlier were passed over nylon wool and the nonadherent population, containing less than 2% B cells, were stimulated with nuclease or fragments *in vitro*. The proliferative response to nuclease was T-lymphocyte dependent in that it was eliminated by treatment of the cells with anti-Thy 1 antiserum and complement.

In a large number of strains tested, mice of haplotypes $H\text{-}2^{a,d,k,s,f}$ were high responders, while PETLES from several strains bearing $H\text{-}2^{b}$ showed a low proliferative response when challenged

TABLE III

Immune Response to Nuclease Fragments[a]

Strain	Fragment	Concentration of Antibody Binding Sites µM ± S.E.M.[b] 1°	2°	3°
B10.A	99-149	0.7 ± 0.6	1.3 ± 0.5	2.0 ± 0.5
	1-126	2.2 ± 0.3	1.9 ± 0.2	1.9 ± 0.4
B10	99-149	0.7 ± 0.7	-0.8 ± 0.4	+0.2 ± 0.5
	1-126	1.4 ± 0.2	0.8 ± 0.4	0.6 ± 0.4

[a]Animals immunized with molar equivalent amounts of each fragment in complete Freund's adjuvant and boosted twice with the same fragment in saline. The 3 successive bleeds are denoted as 1°, 2°, 3°.

[b]Means for 5 to 10 individual animals determined by radioimmunoassay with the corresponding ^{14}C-labeled fragment.

in vitro with whole nuclease as described.[1] Thus, for these haplotypes the *H-2*-linked control of the T-cell proliferative response paralleled that of the antibody response. For the *H-2*^{q} haplotype, both DBA/1 and SWR strains showed wide variability between groups of animals, so the results are uninterpretable at present.

PETLES from mice primed with whole nuclease were then challenged *in vitro* with different fragments of nuclease. The B10.A PETLES (Fig. 6, upper) responded best to fragments (49-149) and (99-149), whereas the response to fragment (1-126) was lower and required a higher molar concentration of antigen to achieve half-maximal stimulation. In contrast, the B10 PETLES (Fig. 6, lower) gave the best response to fragment (1-126) always better than or equal to that to fragment (49-149). The response to fragment (99-149) in this strain was lower and also required more antigen to produce half-maximal stimulation. Thus, the relative response to the fragments was the same as that seen for the antibody responses.

This result suggests that the *H-2*-linked control at the level of individual regions of the molecule, rather than the molecule as a whole, applies to a T-cell response as well as an antibody response. Thus, T-cell-B-cell collaboration is not necessary in order to see these restrictions. Again, a single "carrier" determinant by which T cells recognize the whole molecule does not adequately explain this system.

In addition, the comments made above about the lack of conformational sensitivity of receptors involved in *Ir*-gene control apply to T cell proliferation as well. In contrast to the enormous difference in affinity of antibodies for the native vs random conformations, the T cells respond at least as well to fragments as to native nuclease. The response to native nuclease is reduced by a nonspecific toxicity thought to relate to its enzymatic activity.[1] However, the concentration giving half-maximal response is not less than that for the stimulatory fragments. We conclude that in this nuclease system, both the receptors involved in *Ir*-gene control and those on T cells, whether or not these be the same, recognize determinants which are smaller or more flexible in the native conformation than those recognized by antibodies, and which are therefore less different in the isolated fragments.

When PETLES from nuclease-primed mice of strains bearing recombinant *H-2* haplotypes between *H-2*^{a} and *H-2*^{b} were challenged with fragments *in vitro*, they showed patterns of response different from either parental type. For instance, the B10.A (4R) strain (Fig. 7)

[1] Schwartz, Berzofsky, Horton, Schechter, and Sachs, manuscript in preparation.

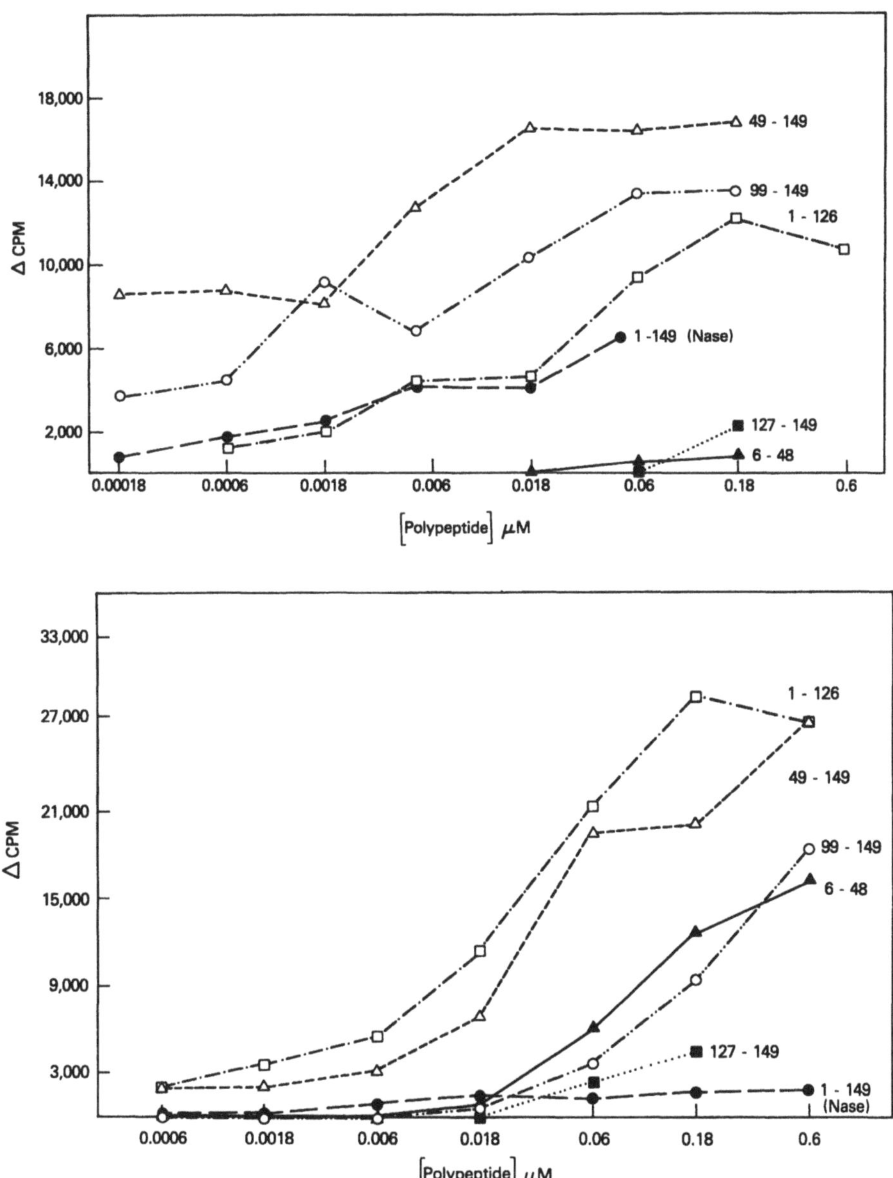

Fig. 6. Dose-response curves of PETLES from nuclease-primed mice to isolated fragments of nuclease and to whole nuclease. The ordinate is the difference in cpm of ^{3}H-thymidine incorporated between triplicate cultures stimulated with fragments and controls stimulated with medium alone. Upper, B10.A; lower, B10.

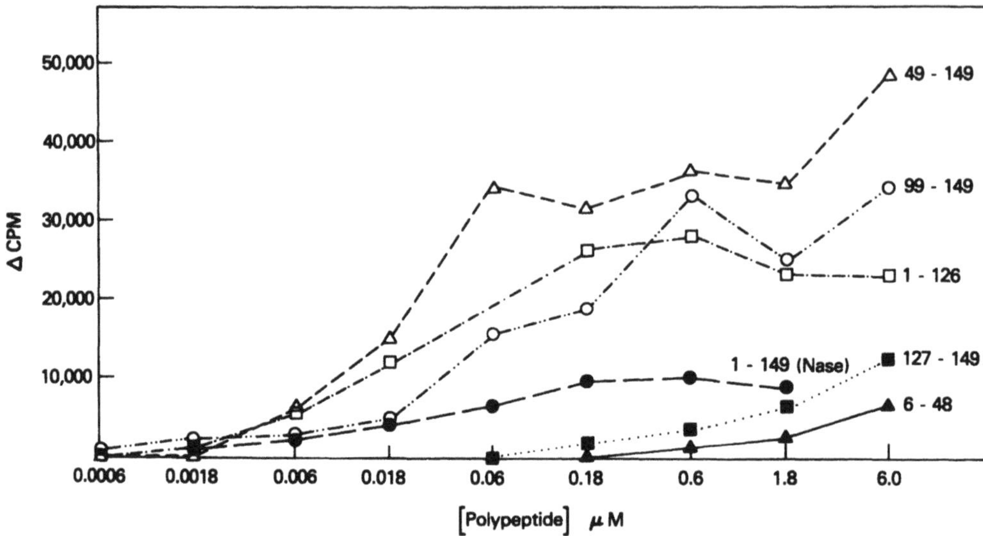

Fig. 7. Dose-response curves of PETLES from nuclease-primed B10.A (4R) recombinant mice to nuclease and its fragments. Ordinate as in Fig. 6.

showed a response to fragment (1-126) which was initially greater than that to fragment (99-149). However, the relative responses were reversed at higher antigen concentration. Also, the response to fragment (49-149) was greater than that to fragment (1-126) and the response to fragment (6-48) was low, as in the B10.A strain. Similar results were found for the B10.A (5R) and B10.A (3R) recombinants, as summarized in Fig. 8, which shows the ratio of responses to the two fragments (99-149) and (1-126). While the ratio was greater than unity for the B10.A PETLES and much less than unity for the B10 PETLES, the ratio for all three recombinants was intermediate, and never very different from unity. All of the ratios converged toward one at very high antigen concentrations.

If the response to nuclease and its fragments were controlled by a single Ir gene (as originally mapped to the I-B subregion for the antibody response), then each recombinant haplotype should behave like one or the other of its parental types, depending on where the crossover took place. The fact that the recombinants showed a pattern which has some features from each parent but which mimicked neither parent exactly can be explained only if more than one H-2-linked Ir gene was operative. The existence of two or more H-2-linked Ir genes for nuclease has not yet been shown for the antibody response, or by complementation of two low responders. However, these results on the T-cell proliferative response of recom-

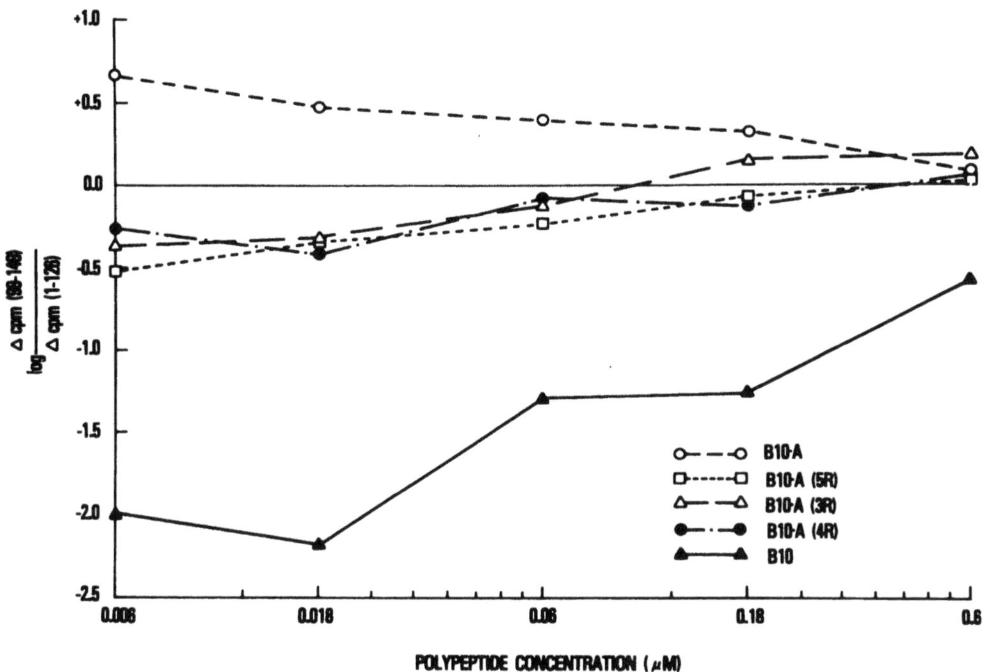

Fig. 8. Ratio of response to fragment (99-149) to that to fragment (1-126), expressed as log of the ratio of Δcpm incorporated, in experiments analogous to those of Figs. 6 and 7, for PETLES from nuclease primed mice of B10, B10.A, and recombinant strains indicated.

binant strains are presumptive evidence for the existence of more than one gene. This observation, in conjunction with the control of the antibody response at the level of a region of the molecule rather than the whole antigen molecule, suggests that different Ir genes may control the response to different antigenic determinants on the antigen. This suggestion can be made even more strongly from the data on the antibody response to myoglobin described elsewhere in this symposium (Berzofsky, 1977), where two H-2-linked Ir genes controlling the antibody response are defined.

In conclusion, we have identified at least one H-2-linked Ir gene that controls the relative proportions of antibodies to different determinants on nuclease, the immunogenicity of the corresponding nuclease fragments, and the T-cell proliferative response to nuclease and its fragments. In addition, a non-H-2-linked gene(s) controls the aggregate level of antibodies to all the determinants of nuclease. Such control implies the existence of a mechanism for sensing the sum of antibodies which have in common only that they bind to the same molecule, even though their specificities and idiotypes (Fathman et al., 1977) are different. This mechanism may, therefore, involve feedback control through the binding of antigen molecules by the antibodies. Consistent with this idea is the reciprocal relationship between affinity and concentration: Antinuclease antibodies of the lower responding B10 background strains have 7- to 10-fold higher affinity for the fragment (1-126) than those of the higher responding A background strains.[2]

In addition to the two genetic control systems described here (i.e., H-2-linked and non-H-2-linked), a system of control of idiotypes of antinuclease antibodies, genetically linked to heavy chain allotype and presumably markers for variable region genes, has been identified (Fathman and Sachs, 1976; Fathman et al., 1977). Antibodies raised against these idiotypes may serve as probes of the cell surface antigen-receptors involved in one or more of the several levels of genetic control elaborated in this paper.

ACKNOWLEDGMENTS

We would like to thank Drs. Thomas A. Waldmann, Gene M. Shearer, and William E. Paul for helpful discussions.

REFERENCES

Anfinsen, C.B., Cuatrecasas, P., and Taniuchi, H. (1971) in The Enzymes, P.D. Boyer, editor, Academic Press, Inc., New York. 4, 177.

Berzofsky, J.A. (1977) This symposium.

Berzofsky, J.A., Schechter, A.N., Shearer, G.M., and Sachs, D.H. (1977a) J. Exp. Med. 145, 111.

Berzofsky, J.A., Schechter, A.N., Shearer, G.M., and Sachs, D.H. (1977b) J. Exp. Med. 145, 123.

Cotton, F.A., and Hazen, E.E., Jr. (1971) in The Enzymes, P.D. Boyer, editor, Academic Press, Inc., New York. 4, 153.

Davis, A., Moore, I.B., Parker, D.S., and Taniuchi, H. (1977) J. Biol. Chem. 252, 6544.

[2]Pisetsky, Berzofsky, and Sachs, manuscript in preparation.

Fathman, C.G., and Sachs, D.H. (1976) J. Immunol. 116, 959.

Fathman, C.G., Pisetsky, D.S., and Sachs, D.H. (1977) J. Exp. Med. 145, 569.

Furie, B., Schechter, A.N., Sachs, D.H., and Anfinsen, C.B. (1975) J. Mol. Biol. 92, 497.

Lozner, E.C., Sachs, D.H., and Shearer, G.M. (1974) J. Exp. Med. 139, 1204.

McDevitt, H.O., and Benacerraf, B. (1969) Adv. Immunol. 11, 31.

Sachs, D.H., Schechter, A.N., Eastlake, A., and Anfinsen, C.B. (1972) Proc. Natl. Acad. Sci. U.S.A. 69, 3790.

Schwartz, R.H., Jackson, L., and Paul, W.E. (1975) J. Immunol. 115, 1330.

PEPTIDES AND AUTOIMMUNE DISEASE

E. H. Eylar

Playfair Neuroscience Unit and
Department of Biochemistry
University of Toronto
Toronto, Canada

ABSTRACT

The use of derived and synthetic peptides has contributed greatly to our understanding of encephalitogenic determinants in the basic protein molecule. Peptides derived from BP by use of trypsin, pepsin, cathepsin D (brain and liver) and BNPS-skatole have proven most useful. Synthetic peptides have served to define the disease-inducing determinants with precision.

A remarkable feature of these studies is that different antigenic determinants serve as encephalitogenic sites in different species. The encephalitogenic sites comprise short peptide domains of the BP polypeptide chain, only 8 residues (rat), 9 residues (guinea pig), and 10 residues (rabbit) in length. In view of the requirement for both haptenic and carrier specificity of an immunogenic molecule, it is impressive that these peptides themselves elicit the autoimmune disease, EAE. While less active than BP on a molar basis, they are nonetheless potent encephalitogens, producing clinical signs in rats and guinea pigs at less than 1 μg dose. The data indicate that for most animal species (guinea pig, rat, monkey) there appears to be only one major encephalitogenic determinant, an unusual finding in view of the number of antigenic determinants for cell-mediated immunity existing in the BP molecule. Possibly a combination of genetic and anatomical factors may account for this phenomenon. A relationship may exist between multiple sclerosis and EAE as shown by peptide studies; lymphocytes are found in MS patients during exacerbation sensitized to the same region of BP active in the monkey. The major encephalitogenic sites are:

Guinea Pig	(9)	Phe-Ser-Trp-Gly-Ala-Glu-Gly-Gln-Lys(Arg)
Rabbit	(10)	Thr-Thr-His-Tyr-Gly-Ser-Leu-Pro-Gln-Lys
Rat	(8)	Ser-Gln-Arg-Ser-Gln-Asp-Glu-Asn
Monkey	(14)	Phe-Lys-Leu-Gly-Gly-Arg-Asp-Ser-Arg-Ser-Gly-Ser-Pro-Hser

---

Autoimmune disease present a class of some of the most serious medical problems. Certain of these diseases such as multiple sclerosis, arthritis, lupus, etc. are chronic diseases and as such pose a special hardship both on the afflicted person and society. One approach to the study of human autoimmune disease has been through animal models where the analogous disease is induced immunologically by injection of the appropriate tissue. Classically, autoimmunity in the animal is elicited by injection of a specific tissue with Freund's complete adjuvant (FCA) which leads to the subsequent immune response to an antigen(s) in the tissue, and ultimately to the development of pathology localized in the same type of tissue that was originally injected. Presumably the immunopathologic response, whether mediated by T lymphocytes or antibody, is directed toward an antigen which is exclusive to the organ or tissue used.

Many of the autoimmune diseases induced in animals mimic to varying degrees certain human diseases. Perhaps the best examples are the Guillian-Barre syndrome, a demyelinating disease of the peripheral nervous system which appears to be cell-mediated (Arneson et al, 1968), perhaps by lymphocytes sensitized to the P2 protein (Sheremata et al, 1975). A disease referred to as experimental allergic neuritis (EAN)*, similar in nearly all respects (clinical, site of attack, histology, duration, etc.) to the Guillian-Barre syndrome, can be induced in monkeys and rabbits by injection of PNS myelin in FCA (Brostoff et al, 1972;Wisniewski et al, 1974). There are also several animal models for rheumatoid

*Abbreviations used are: CNS-central nervous system; PNS-peripheral nervous system; EAE-experimental allergic encephalomyelitis; EAN-experimental allergic neuritis; FCA-Freund's complete adjuvant; BP-myelin basic protein.

arthritis and other autoimmune diseases, but one of the questions which always arise is the relevence of the model to the human disease, i.e., are the pathogenic mechanisms similar. Clearly the human and animal autoimmune diseases must differ in mode of induction. Whereas in the animal disease the immune response to self tissue is induced by injection with FCA, in the human diseases, viruses or other insults may play this role.

Although abundant attention has been directed toward the study of autoimmune diseases, in most cases the responsible antigen is yet unknown. Two cases, however, have been extensively studied and have served as valuable models in which to discern immunologic and biochemical parameters and which relate to particular human disease: experimental autoimmune myesthenia gravis (EAMG) and experimental allergic encephalomyelitis (EAE). Administration of the nicotinic acetylcholine reception, purified from the electric organ of the electric eel or torpedo, into rabbits, mice or rats elicits an immune response leading to clinical and histologic lesions characteristic of human myesthenia gravis such as impaired neuromuscular transmission, and muscular weakness (Patrick and Lindstrom, 1973). The animal disease appears to be mediated by antibody to the receptor since it can be transfered to normal animals by antibody (Toyka et al, 1975); antibody to receptor is also found in most MG patients (Appel et al, 1975). Although the evidence supports the acetylcholine receptor as the responsible antigen, very little is known about the antigenic properties of the receptor, a complex protein from the postsynaptic membrane.

The other example, experimental allergic encephalomyelitis (EAE), is probably the most widely studied autoimmune disease and historically is highly significant since it was one of the first autoimmune diseases studied. In 1933 (Rivers et al), EAE was induced in monkeys by repeated injection of whole brain tissue thus providing evidence for an autoimmune reaction, contrary to the Ehrlich hypothesis. Since 1947, when Kabat et al first demonstrated that induction of EAE was remarkably facilitated by using FCA along with CNS tissue, it has received wide attention as a model to study immunologic and pathologic events associated with autoimmunity. EAE has many properties in common with multiple sclerosis and in some instances may be an appropriate model for this human disease, particularly when studied in monkeys (Eylar, 1972).

Little is known about tissue antigens which are the target for immune attack in autoimmune phenomena. In experimental autoimmune myesthenia gravis the antigen is the acetylcholine receptor; in experimental allergic orchitis, the AP protein (Jackson et al, 1975) and the GPI glycoprotein (Hagopian et al, 1975); in experimental allergic thyroiditis, thyroglobulin (Rose et al, 1968); and in experimental allergic neuritis, probably the P2 protein (Brostoff et al, 1972). These antigens injected with FCA induce the specific autoimmune diseases in appropriate animals. Reaction to other antigens may occur in autoimmune diseases as a consequence of the disease process; to DNA and blood cell membranes in lupus, and to immunoglobulin in rheumatoid arthritis for example. These antigens do not elicit the disease in experimental animals, however.

One of the attractions of EAE, is that the responsible antigen, the myelin basic protein (previously referred to as A1 protein or encephalitogenic protein) has been isolated (Eylar et al, 1969), sequenced (Eylar, 1971a) and well characterized physicochemically in numerous studies (Eylar and Thompson, 1969 and Epand et al, 1974). It is now well founded that EAE is mediated by T lymphocytes sensitized to basic protein (BP). Not only does BP induce EAE, but it also will block disease development if given without FCA in the sensitizing injection (Alvord et al, 1965), or will suppress disease development in monkeys (Eylar et al, 1972) and guínea pigs (Driscoll et al, 1975) if given after clinical signs first appear. Whether the BP could be used to supress human demyelinating diseases such as multiple sclerosis is currently under consideration.

A. ANTIGENIC DETERMINANTS. Antigenic determinants are those portions of a macromolecule which react with antibody or sensitized lymphocytes; they may or may not be immunogenic. Based on studies with synthetic polypeptides, the size of an antigenic determinant reacting *in vitro* with humoral antibody, is approximately 4-6 monomeric units. Considerable information on natural antigenic determinants in humoral immunity has been obtained from the study of proteins such as ribonuclease, myoglobin, lysozyme, ferredoxin, cytochrome C, and others.

Studies on the nature and properties of antigenic determinants for cell mediated immunity are less extensive. It was shown by skin tests in guinea pigs that peptide 17-24 of ACTH (39 residues) defines a major antigenic determinant (Salvin and Liauw, 1967). This peptide is also immunogenic. Tobacco mosaic virus protein has one major antigenic site for cell-mediated immunity localized in residues 108-112 in the protein (Spitler et al, 1970). This peptide region, while not immunogenic, reacts in skin tests and in the macrophage migration inhibition (MI) assay. Glucagon, bovine insulin, and ferredoxin all were found to have a small number of determinants as shown by isolated peptides capable of reacting in skin tests and MI assay. It should be kept in mind that antigenic sites, responsive in cell-mediated immunity, may not be functional for humoral immunity. For example, Ben-Efraim et al (1963) showed that a complex synthetic polypeptide composed of glutamine acid, tyrosine, alanine and lysine induced a prolonged state of delayed hypersensitivity but no detectable antibody in guinea pigs. In rabbits, however, it induced good antibody titers. Thus the nature of the antigenic site may greatly influence the type and degree of the immune response in a given animal species.

Once the BP had been isolated and shown to be homogeneous (Eylar et al, 1969), the rare opportunity existed to search for antigenic sites within the molecule which were responsible for disease induction or were targets for the immunopathologic response.

Fortunately, the BP molecule lacks appreciable secondary structure (Oshiro and Eylar, 1970) and appears to exist in a highly open, double chain conformation (Brostoff and Eylar, 1971) which is very asymmetric (axial ratio 1:10) (Eylar and Thompson, 1969). While not a random coil, the BP apparently contains little internal structure and thus is remarkably stable to denaturation, but liable to proteolytic enzymes (Hashim and Eylar, 1969). It appears likely therefore that disease-inducing determinants might exist in peptide domains of the polypeptide chain rather than in conformational sites composed of distal regions of the polypeptide chain. Encouraging early observations had shown that encephalitogenic material of 3,000-5,000 molecular weight could be derived from degraded CNS tissue (Lumsden et al, 1966). A likely explanation was that this low molecular weight material was derived from proteolysis of the BP yielding peptides which retained activity. Thus the problem was approached by isolation of tryptic and peptic peptides derived from BP, all of which were tested for encephalitogenic activity.

B. PEPTIDES AND EAE. It is indeed fortuitous that the BP molecule exists in an open conformation since many of its properties such as the induction of EAE or receptor function for the enzyme N-acetylgalactosaminyl-transferase can be reproduced by peptide fragments (Hagopian et al, 1971). The use of peptides, both derived and synthetic, has been mainly responsible for elucidation of the disease-inducing and other antigenic sites of the BP molecule. The reason why this strategy, now widespread in EAE work, has been so effective is that the peptide apparently retains nearly the same conformation it possessed as part of the BP molecule. Some of the most useful peptides have been derived using trypsin (Eylar et al, 1971a) pepsin (Hashim and Eylar, 1969a; Eylar et al, 1971), and cathepsin D from brain (Einstein et al 1968) and liver (Brostoff et al, 1974). The most reliable chemical method has been BNPS-skatole (Burnett and Eylar, 1971) which cleaves the COOH-tryptophanyl bond yielding two peptides which are easily purified. This reagent is preferable to N-bromosuccinimide because of fewer side reactions. It should be emphasized that the peptides containing the appropriate antigenic site are themselves immunogenic as well as encephalitogenic since they elicit a cell-mediated response (Eylar, 1972; Spitler et al, 1972). The smaller peptides do not elicit a humoral antibody response, however, which adds further support to the role of cell-mediated immunity as the crucial factor in EAE.

In the study of EAE, particularly with peptides, one of the most important factors is the animal species. The guinea pig particularly exhibits a strong cell mediated response and is probably the most sensitive animal to the BP or peptides. The monkey is of interest because of its similarity to man. The rabbit and the rat have also been used, the latter often for genetic reasons. The mouse is quite resistant to EAE but some strains appear to be susceptible when pertussis organisms are included in the adjuvant.

Several disease-inducing peptides have now been derived from BP

TABLE I
EAE Inducing Peptides Derived From Myelin Basic Protein

Peptide	Sequence*	Derivation	Active in	Reference
113-121(9)	Phe-Ser-Trp-Gly-Ala-Glu-Gly-Gln-Lys	Trypsin	Guinea Pig	Eylar et al (1970)
111-124(14)	Ser-Arg-Phe-Ser-Trp-Gly-Ala-Glu-Gly Gln-Lys-Pro-Gly-Phe	Pepsin	Guinea Pig	Eylar & Hashim (1968)
43-88 (46)	Phe-Gly-Ser-Asp---------Val-His-Phe	Brain tissue	Rabbit	Kibler et al (1969)
43-88 (46)	Phe-Gly-Ser-Asp---------Val-His-Phe	Pepsin	Rabbit	Eylar et al (1971)
116-169(54)	Gly-Ala-Glu-Gly---------Ala-Arg-Arg	BNPS-skatole	Monkey	Eylar et al (1972)
133-169(37)	Tyr-Lys-Ser-Ala---------Ala-Arg-Arg	Pepsin	Monkey	Eylar et al (1972)
153-166(14)	Phe-Lys-Leu-Gly---------Ser-Pro-Hser	Pepsin, CNBr	Monkey	Karkhanis et al (1974)
43-88 (46)	Phe-Gly-Ser-Asp---------Val-His-Phe	Brain tissue (Guinea Pig)	Rat	McFarlin et al (1973)
68-88 (21)	Gly-Ser-Leu-Pro---------Val-His-Phe	Chymotrypsin on Guinea Pig BP	Rat	Chow et al (1977)

*All the sequences shown are from the bovine BP; each peptide is numbered according to its position in bovine BP starting with N-terminal acetylated alanine. The number of residues in each peptide is shown in parenthesis.

(Table I). Some of the peptides or their analogues have also been synthesized by the Merrifield procedure and are equally encephalitogenic. One of the most significant findings is that a species variation exists in response to the BP molecule, i.e., different peptide domains serve as the disease-inducing determinant in different species. Not only are the disease-inducing antigens confined to small peptide regions, there are very few, only one or two, major encephalitogenic sites for a given species.

C. THE GUINEA PIG. The guinea pig is often favoured in the study of EAE because it is very sensitive to the BP; 0.1 - 0.5 ug BP in FCA produces histologic lesions characterized by infiltration of mononuclear cells into the whiite matter, and 5-10 ug elicits clinical signs in most animals as shown by ataxia, hind-leg weakness and paralysis, incontinence, weight loss, etc. (Eylar et al, 1969). The study of EAE in the guinea pig consistently suggests that only one major encephalitogenic determinant exists in BP, and was first isolated in 1968 by Eylar and Hashim as part of a 14 residue peptic peptide (Table I). This peptide, which contains the single tryptophan residue in BP, offered the first indication that the disease-inducing site was confined to a small linear domain of the polypeptide chain. It is important to note that this peptide was highly active; 50-100% as active as BP on a molar basis (Eylar and Hashim, 1968; Lennon et al, 1970). Numerous other peptic and tryptic peptides were tested but none were active except the tryptic nonapeptide also derived from the tryptophan region (Eylar et al, 1970). These results emphasized the tryptophan region as the major, if not the only, encephalitogenic site active in the guinea pig. Later Carnegie (1969) reported that the NH_2-terminal peptide (21 residues), derived from CNBr cleavage of human BP, was weakly active in guinea pigs but this report has not been substantiated.

Our peptide data revealed that the tryptic nonapeptide and 14-residue peptic peptide (Table I) containing the tryptophan region, but none of the other peptides, were disease inducing. The peptides presumably induce a response leading to sensitized T lymphocytes, which, upon migrating to CNS myelin, encounter the same region of the BP molecule and liberate mediators leading to macrophage activation, demyelination and other pathologic events. In guinea pigs sensitized to the nonapeptide, lymphocytes are found which respond to both the peptide and BP as shown by the MI assay and blastogenic response (Eylar, 1972; Spitler et al, 1972). These data suggest that the primary structure of the BP molecular accounts for its EAE activity since it would be most unlikely that the nonapeptide would have the same conformation as that region in the intact BP if folding occured. What are the essential components of the antigenic region? To answer this question we first synthesized the 11 residue peptide (#1) shown in Table II and found that it was approximately as active as the derived peptic or the tryptic nonapeptide. Subsequently, a series of peptides were synthesized by the Merrifield solid state technique, each differing by one residue. In Table II some of the synthetic

TABLE II
Synthetic Peptides Studied in Guinea Pigs

	Peptide	Encephalitogenic Activity
1	Ser-Arg-Phe-Ser-Trp-Gly-Ala-Glu-Gly-Gln-Lys	+
2	Ser-Arg-Phe-Ser-Trp-Gly-Ala-Glu-Gly-Gln	-
3	Ser-Arg-Phe-Ser-Trp-Gly-Ala-Glu-Gly-Gln-ARG	+
4	Ser-Arg-Phe-Ser-Trp-Gly-Ala-Glu-Gly-Gln-ILE	-
5	Ser-Arg-Phe-Ser-Trp-Gly-Ala-Glu-Gly-ILE-Lys	-
6	Ser-Arg-Phe-Ser-Trp-Gly-Ala-ILE-Gly-Gln-Lys	+
7	Ser-Arg-Phe-Ser-PHE-Gly-Ala-Glu-Gly-Gln-Lys	-
8	Ser-Arg-Phe-Ser-VAL-Gly-Ala-Glu-Gly-Gln-Lys	-
9	Ser-Arg-Phe-ALA-Trp-Gly-Ala-Glu-Gly-Gln-Lys	+
10	Ser-Arg-VAL-Ser-Trp-Gly-Ala-Glu-Gly-Gln-Lys	+
11	Phe-Ser-Trp-Gly-Ala-Glu-Gly-Gln-Lys	+
12	Phe-Ser-Trp-Gly-Ala-Glu-Gly-GLU-Lys	±
13	GLY-GLY-Trp-Gly-Ala-Glu-Gly-Gln-Lys-Gly	-
14	ALA-Ser-Trp-Gly-GLY-GLY-Gly-Gln-Lys-Gly	-
15	Phe-Ser-TYR-Gly-Ala-Glu-Gly-Gln-Lys-Gly	-

Peptides 1-12, Ref. Westall et al, 1970; Peptides 13-15, Ref. Hashim and Sharpe, 1975.

peptides are shown which were used to delineate the residues essential for activity. At least three residues were crucial, and could not be replaced without loss of activity: tryptophan, glutamine, and lysine. Arginine (#3), but not isoleucine (#4) could replace lysine, a substitution which occurs naturally in human BP. Numerous peptides were also synthesized in which the terminal lysine was omitted; all of these were inactive (Eylar et al, 1970). Interestingly, the phenylalanine, glutamic acid, and serine residues are replaceable. It should be stressed that in the case of every active peptide, both clinical and histologic signs of EAE were elicited. We concluded (Westall et al, 1970) that at least the three residues are essential components of the antigenic site; the specific immunologic recognition of this site must depend on the simultaneous binding of all three residues. Even deamidation of the glutamine residue (#12) greatly reduces activity; no clinical signs are observed but histologic lesions occur at 3 ug doses. It was gratifying to find as well that the synthetic nonapeptide(#11) was equally as encephalitogenic as the derived tryptic peptide 113-121.

1. Length Limit. What is the length limit of the encephalitogenic region? Based on the synthetic peptide studies, it is clear that the nonapeptide is the smallest active peptide fragment. At the COOH-terminal end, lysine (or arginine) is required and cannot be replaced or omitted. At the NH_2-terminal end, removal but not replacement of the phenylalanine or serine residues inactivates the

peptide (Eylar and Hashim, 1968). These results suggest that the proximity of the terminal amino group to the essential tryptophan residue is inhibitory if separated by less than two residues. Thus the nine residues segment contains the minimum sequence compatible with significant encephalitogenic activity. The dimensions of the tryptophan-containing encephalitogenic determinant are compatible with the length of antigenic determinants found in other cases. Gill and Doty (1962), in a study of several immunologic synthetic polypeptides concluded that the antigenic sites probably consist of short amino acid sequences in the disorded, nonhelical regions of the polypeptide chain. It was concluded that the size of the combining site on the anti-poly-L-alanine antibody would accomodate a maximum of 5 alanyl residues; for poly-L-lysine, the combining site was estimated to be 5-6 residues (Sage et al, 1964; Arnon et al (1965). We can conclude that the essential elements of the disease inducing site in guinea pigs covers seven residues (Trp to Lys), a span in basic agreement with the synthetic polypeptide results. Moreover, since EAE is cell mediated, the tryptophan region must represent a major determinant for cell-mediated immunity; this is indeed the case as shown by MI and other assays (Eylar, 1972; Spitler et al, 1972; Bergstrand, 1972), using lymphocytes sensitized to the peptides. It might be suspected that the BP, because of its highly disorded conformation, may have many antigenic sites if nonhelical regions actually are preferred for cell-mediated determinants. Again, thus is the case for guinea pigs since Bergstrand (1972, 1973) has shown that at least eight antigenic determinants for cell mediated immunity including the tryptophan region, exist in the bovine BP when studied in the migration inhibition (MI) assay using sensitized guinea pig lymphocytes (lymph node cells).

It is important to note, however, that while the minimum length limit of the tryptophan determinant is nine residues, that the conformation of the nonapeptide may not fit precisely that of a larger peptide segment, or the intact BP molecule. Recent studies indicate that a larger peptide, res. 89-169, may be more consistently active in inducing EAE than the shorter fragments (Driscoll et al, 1976). Nonetheless, it is remarkable that a small nonapeptide should contain both the hapten and carrier specificity required for immunogenicity (Gell, 1970). Thus the conformation of the nonapeptide must not be too far removed from the same region of the intact BP since cells sensitized to the nonapeptide recognize the same region in BP (Eylar, 1972).

2. Other Possible Sites. All studies in the disease-inducing site of BP active in guinea pigs agree that the tryptophan region is the major, perhaps the only, encephalitogenic determinant. The tryptophan residue is essential as confirmed by Hashim and Sharpe (1975) who substituted tyrosine for tryptophan and found inactivity (Table II). They also reported that the Gly-Gly for Phe-Ser substitution (just preceeding tryptophan) led to inactivity, whereas we found Ala for Ser was still active. Interestingly, Lamoureux et al. (1972)

found in a study of synthetic peptides that the Phe-Ser- sequence at the COOH-terminus was unnecessary for activity. This result contradicts our early findings (Eylar and Hashim, 1968) and those of Lennon et al. (1970) that the peptic peptide, which lacks Phe and begins with Ser-TRP-etc., was inactive. A reasonable explanation for this disagreement is that Lamoureux et al injected 200 ug of peptide whereas our peptides were generally highly active at 1 ug or less, and even the deaminated peptide (#12, Table II) was marginally active at 3 ug histologically. These results emphasized the importance of studies at several different quantities of test material since the EAE assay is so difficult to quantitate.

It is also of interest that Hashim and Sharpe found that the Gly-Gly substitution for Ala-Glu led to inactivity (Table II). These results indicate that the alanine residue may be important since we had found that the glutamic acid residue could be replaced with isoleucine.

It has been reported (Shapira et al, 1971) that Peptide 43-88 (Table I), active in rabbits, is also mildly active in guinea pigs, but we (Eylar et al, 1971) could not confirm this result. There is some similarity between this peptide at the tyrosine locus and the tryptophan region. However, tyrosine will not substitute for tryptophan in the nonapeptide (Table II). When tryptophan is blocked by reaction of BP with 2-hydroxy-5-nitrobenzylbromide (HNB), the modified BP product is essentially inactive in guinea pigs (Hashim and Eylar, 1969b). If the tyrosine region of Peptide 43-88 were active, it should have been expressed.

It can be concluded, therefore, that the tryptophan region is surely the dominant encephalitogenic determinant active in guinea pig; at least three residues (Trp, Gln, and Lys or Arg) are essential and possibly the alanine residue as well. The tryptophan-to-lysine region spans 7 residues, but activity is much enhanced if two additional residues are present at the NH_2-terminus.

3. Precautions. In determining encephalitogenic activity, the assay is often variable and difficult to quantitate. For this reason, and because of the high sensitivity of guinea pigs to EAE, it is essential that only peptides of high purity be used. A slight contamination can easily lead to an erroneous result as shown by recent work in which the presence of contaminating tryptophan peptides were found by fluorescence but missed by other criteria (Driscoll et al, 1976). Thus peptides 1-36 and 1-88 showed some encephalitogenic activity at high doses, probably because of slight contamination with tryptophan-containing peptides. For this reason, peptides which show low activity relative to BP itself must be looked upon with suspicion, i.e., the 20 residue NH_2-terminal peptide from human BP, res. 1-19, claimed to be active in guinea pigs, may be, in fact, inactive. The analagous peptide derived from bovine BP is inactive (Hashim and Eylar, 1969c). Moreover, a peptide should induce the same signs of disease as BP; milder signs may arise from traces of contaminants. Thus the finding that Peptide 43-88 at 500 ug induced only mild

histologic signs in one of three monkeys tested must be considered questionable (Shapiro et al, 1971). These workers also reported that this peptide produced weight loss at 5 ug in guinea pigs, but this is not sufficient evidence for encephalitogenicity. Other studies (Driscoll et al, 1976), using highly purified material, have in fact found Peptide 43-88 to be inactive in guinea pigs (Eylar et al, 1971).

Difficulties may be encountered in other directions as well since, for example, peptides may deaminate at glutamine or asparagine residues. Particularly the synthetic peptides as shown in Table II, often purified by chromatography in acid media, may suffer deamination and thus show low activity. We have noted loss of the amide group in synthetic peptides stored at -20° when lyophilized from acidic media. Deamidation is easily detected by paper electrophoresis at pH 4.6 because of the retarded migration of the degraded peptide. Mixtures of peptides also may mask encephalitogenic activity. Both tryptic peptides, derived from BP, containing the tryptophan region, are much less active as part of the digestion mixture of BP than when given alone (Hashim and Eylar, 1969). This phenomena caused considerable confusion historically since mixtures of peptides were generally tested rather than the purified peptides.

D. THE TRYPTOPHAN REGION. Data accumulated over the past few years emphasize the importance of the tryptophan region as the dominant determinant eliciting EAE in the guinea pig. Firstly, the isolated peptides are roughly comparable in encephalitogenic activity to BP on a molar basis, inducing both clinical signs and histologic signs of EAE identical to that found with intact BP. Although it is difficult to obtain quantitative results by the EAE assay, it is apparent that on a weight basis, the peptic peptides (Table I) are nearly as active as BP on a molar basis shown by results from two different laboratories (Eylar and Hashim, 1968; Lennon et al, 1970). In our experience, over 90% of guinea pigs show histologic signs of EAE when given 1 ug of BP (any mammalian species); the peptic peptides are positive in most animals down to 0.33 ug. As a rough approximation, the peptic peptides are about 50% as active as BP, with the tryptic nonapeptide somewhat less so. However, because of the variability in the assay, considerable deviation may be found in any particular experiment. Although it is important to use a statistically significant number of guinea pigs for assay, it is often impractical to use a large number of guinea pigs in routine assays. Secondly, the amino acid sequence in the tryptophan region shows a phylogenetic correlation with encephalitogenic activity (Eylar et al, 1974). The BP from all mammalian species tested in the guinea pig were equally encephalitogenic; these include human, bovine, monkey, guinea pigs, rabbit, horse, dog, rat, mouse and sheep. In each of these species, the critical residues (tryptophan, glutamine, lysine or arginine) in the tryptophan region are preserved. Significant changes in sequence occur only in the chicken and turtle proteins, both of which are relatively non-encephalitogenic. The chicken

BP does not induce clinical signs, but does induce mild perivascular cuffing; it is about 1/100 as active as mammalian BP. The turtle BP does not induce clinical or histologic signs. Two substitutions in the active tryptophan region occur in the chicken sequence; alanine to glycine and glutamine to histidine, as shown: Phe-Ser-Trp-Gly-GLY-Glu-Gly-HIS-Lys. It is the latter change which likely accounts for the major loss of encephalitogenic activity, because of the importance of the glutamine residue, but as shown in Table II, the Gly for Ala substitution may also be important. In the turtle BP, many changes from the mammalian BP sequence are apparent from the composition of the peptide which was not sequenced. All these data suggest a strict correlation between the essential amino acid residues of the tryptophan region in BP from different species and their encephalitogenic activity.

Thirdly, chemical modifiction of the single tryptophan residue is specifically achieved by reaction with 2-hydroxy-5-nitrobenzylbromide (HNB). The resulting HNB-BP molecule is essentially inactive. Even at a 150 ug doses, no clinical signs of EAE were observed although sparce histologic signs are sometimes present. We concluded from these data that the tryptophan residue is clearly essential for activity, in keeping with the synthetic peptide data, since the modified protein was several hundredfold less active than the untreated protein, and that other regions were inactive. These results have subsequently been confirmed in other laboratories (Chao and Einstein, 1970).

Fourthly, peptides derived from regions other than the tryptophan region appear inactive. We tested a large number of peptides derived from BP obtained from tryptic and peptic digests; all were inactive. Two other peptides, referred to as Peptide L and T, were derived by cleavage of the COOH-tryptophanyl linkage with BNPS-skatole (Burnett and Eylar, 1971). Both peptides were at least one hundredfold less active than BP.

Fifthly, further proof for the required residues in appropriate positions of the nonapeptide sequence are provided by the rat small basic protein (SBP) where the sequence is:

Phe-Ser-Trp-Gly-Arg-Asp-Ser-Arg-Ser-etc.

Following the glycine residue, it is apparent that this sequence differs greatly from that in mammalian BP including replacement of the glutamine-lysine (arginine) sequence by Arg-Ser. The SBP protein is essentially nonencephalitogenic in the guinea pig (Martenson et al, 1972).

E. MONKEY. The major stimulus for present day work on EAE came from the classic studies on EAE in the monkey by Kabat et al, (1947) who first used CNS tissue in FCA. Our first objective was to evaluate the ability of the purified BP to induce EAE. We found that rhesis monkeys develop an acute fatal form of EAE, when given 5 mg BP, in 100% of the animals (Jackson et al, 1972). Clinical signs of EAE, which become evident on days 14-30 following sensitization, included anorexia initially followed by loss of alarm reaction and lethargy. Weight loss, ataxia, reduction in visual acuity, leg and/or arm weakness and paralysis were also characteristic. Finally, the animal becomes semiconscious, sometimes developing severe paralysis and tremors, and generally expires 1-4 days after appearance of the first definite signs. The human, bovine, rabbit and monkey BP all appeared equally effective for EAE induction.

Histologic examination prior to or during the clinical response revealed numerous lesions consisting of perivascular mononuclear cells in the forebrain, cerebellum, choroid plexis, meninges, pons, optic tract and spinal cord. In most cases, there were also large areas of infiltration by polymorphonuclear cells, and in some cases, necrosis, hemorrhage and lipid-laden macrophages. Macroscopic observation of the brain often showed visible scattered loci (large and small), usually hemorrhagic. The clinical and histologic picture is not significantly different from that described 25 years ago by Kabat et al, and reported by Rauch & Einstein (1971), who found a similar response when EAE was induced with whole monkey CNS tissue, or bovine or guinea pig BP.

It became apparent that the chemical grouping responsible for EAE in the guinea pig was inactive in the monkey. The AMS-derivative of BP, in which the carboxyl groups are converted into the aminomethane sulfonic acid form, induced EAE in the monkey but not in the guinea pig (Eylar, 1972). Thus carboxyl groups are not an essential feature of the region active in the monkey. However, glutamic acid-118, which is found in the middle of the tryptophan region, while not essential for activity in the guinea pig, may be converted into a bulky group which interferes with the essential tryptophan-glutamine-lysine relationship.

The species difference in the encephalitogenic response was emphatically confirmed when it was found that the HNB derivative (inactive in the guinea pig) was active in the monkey, and the tryptophan-containing nonapeptide was inactive in the monkey, even at doses of 1 mg. (Jackson et al, 1972; Eylar, et al, 1972a). We conclude therefore that the tryptophan region is not encephalitogenic in the monkey. It was apparent however, that whatever antigenic region(s) elicits in EAE in the monkey, it was present in BP of each species tested including bovine, rabbit, human, monkey, and guinea pig (Jackson et al, 1972; Eylar et al, 1972).

In order to determine whether EAE induction in the monkey might be ascribed to a restricted domain of the BP polypeptide chain we followed the same strategy as in the guinea pig studies. Various peptides obtained by cleavage with BNPS-skatole and peptic digestion of BP, were tested as shown in Table I. The clinical signs paralleled the histologic signs except for Peptide 1-116 which showed mild histologic signs in two out of four monkeys but not clinical signs. It is uncertain whether this peptide has a small intrinsic activity, or is slightly contaminated with BP. Peptide 117-169, which is inactive in the guinea pig, was fully as active as BP on a molar basis. The localization of a major encephalitogenic determinant in the COOH-terminal region of the BP molecule was confirmed when Peptide 133-169, which contains the 37 residues of the COOH-region, was found to be highly encephalitogenic.

Peptide 133-169 was first derived from bovine BP by hydrolysis of the aspartic acid-tyrosine linkage (res. 132-133) with pepsin, and was purified by subsequent fractionation of Cellex P (Eylar et al, 1972a). It appeared from these data that a major disease-inducing site, active in the monkey, existed within the 37 residue COOH-terminal region of the BP molecule. The region of Peptide 133-169 which is most potent is defined by Peptide 153-169, a 17 residue segment from COOH-terminus (Karkhanis et al, 1975). Removal of the final three residues by CNBr treatment does not destroy activity (Table I). If the Asp-Ser linkage of Peptide 153-169 is cleaved by mild acid treatment however, then activity is lost. A synthetic peptide identical to the 13 residue N-terminal region of Peptide 133-169 was inactive.

It should be stressed that the clinical and histologic characteristics of EAE in the monkey, induced by these peptides, appear indistinguishable from that induced by BP. While the Peptide 153-169 region appears to contain the major encephalitogenic region of the BP molecule active in monkeys, there may be other peptide segments with minor activity. In this regard, Peptide 1-116, which covers a large portion of BP, has a low detectable activity as shown by histologic lesions. Interestingly, Peptide 44-89 also appears slightly encephalitogenic in our hands, approximately 10% as active as Peptide 133-169. Only at 5 mg doses of Peptide 44-89 was EAE observed, and onset was often delayed (Eylar et al, 1972a). Although a minor determinant may exist in Peptide R, cautious interpretation is necessary because slight contamination could give misleading results. The report (Shapira et al, 1971) that Peptide 44-89 is a major encephalitogen in the monkey needs further documentation, since it was not compared on a molar basis with intact BP, and of just three animals used, only one showed histologic signs. Additionally, Peptide 1-42, derived from BP by liver cathepsin D, was also mildly active in monkeys and could represent a minor determinant (Brostoff et al., 1974).

F. RABBIT. Historically the study of EAE in the guinea pig dominated that of other species, but the studies of Kibler et al. (1969) used the rabbit to advantage since they were able to isolate an encephalitogenic peptide fragment from CNS tissue, res. 43-89, derived by proteolysis of BP during acid extraction (Table I). This peptide induces EAE in the rabbit, but not in the guinea pig. We confirmed these results using the same peptide derived directly from BP by the action of pepsin (Eylar, et al, 1971). The active portion of this peptide was reported to be the 10 residue peptide, res. 65-74, which was synthesized (Table III). This peptide contains a tyrosine residue in the precise relationship as tryptophan (in res. 113-121) to the important Gln-Lys sequence. Hashim and Sharpe (1974) also synthesized this peptide and showed that it was very encephalitogenic in rabbits, but not guinea pigs, and elicited a strong delayed-type skin reaction in rabbits as well.

TABLE III

OTHER SYNTHETIC ENCEPHALITOGENIC PEPTIDES

Res. No. In Bovine BP	Sequence	Active in	Ref.
64-73	Thr-Thr-His-Tyr-Gly-Ser-Leu-Pro-Gln-Lys	Rabbit	Shapira et al 1971
68-83	Gly-Ser-Leu-Pro-Gln-Lys-Ala-Gln Gly-His-Arg-Pro-Gln-Asp-Glu-Asn	Rat (very weak)	Hashim 1977
68-83 (minus 76-77)	" (Gly-His) deleted "	Rat (potent)	Hashim 1977
74-81 (Guinea pig BP)	Ser-Gln-Arg-Ser-Gln-Asp-Glu-Asn	Rat	Hashim 1977a
74-81 (Bovine BP Sequence)	Ala-Gln-(Gly-His)-Arg-Pro-Gln-Asp-Glu-Asn		

The tryptophan peptide is also active in the rabbit. It is clear that the tyrosine region is not the sole encephalitogenic site active in the rabbit since nitration of the tryosine residues does not severly limit the encephalitogenic activity of BP (Eylar, unpublished). Alternately, the HNB-BP is quite active in the rabbit; thus the tryptophan region is not overly dominant in the rabbit as it is in the guinea pig (Einstein et al., 1972). Bergstrand (1972a) has found another site active in the rabbit that differs from the tyrosine or tryptophan regions. This region is contained in Peptide 134-169, the 36 residue peptide so active in the monkey. Both peptides 134-150 and 151-169 are also active; the latter is of interest since it is this peptide which induces EAE in the monkey. Removal of the terminal Ala-Arg-Arg with CNBr (with conversion of methionine to homoserine) reduces activity in the rabbit but not in the monkey. It can be concluded, therefore, that at least three major encephalitogenic determinants exist in BP that are active in the rabbit. It was also found that several peptide regions of BP behave as antigenic sites for cell-mediated immunity using rabbit lymph node cells in a transformation test (Bergstrand and Kallen, 1974); these include the encephalitogenic regions.

G. THE RAT. In contrast to most strains, the Lewis rat is highly susceptible to EAE, and has, therefore, been a popular strain for studies of encephalitogenic activity (Martenson et al, 1972). The guinea pig BP is the most encephalitogenic of all species of BP in the Lewis rat, being 25 times more active than bovine, human, or rabbit BP and 10 times more active than rat BP (Table IV). This finding contrasts with EAE in guinea pig where all mammalian species are about equally active. Even at 5 μg of BP per guinea pig, class-

TABLE IV

RELATIVE ACTIVITY OF THE PEPTIDES
PRODUCING EAE IN THE RAT*

Peptide	Clinical signs (animals positive) / (animals tested)	Dose (µg)
BP (bovine)	1/6	100
BP (guinea pig)	5/5	1
63-83 (bovine)	3/6	100
63-83 (bovine) minus Gly-His (77-78)	6/6	25
	3/6	2.5
	1/6	0.5
74-81 (guinea pig)	3/6	2.5
	2/6	0.5

*Hashim, G., personal communications; Martenson et al, 1974

ical clinical (and histologic) signs appear in a high percentage of animals, but in the Lewis rat, 50 µg of many mammalian BP do not produce clinical signs whereas 1-2 ug of guinea pig BP elicits clinical signs (McFarlin et al, 1973). BP from chicken, turtle, and frog, all relatively inactive in the guinea pig, are mildly encephalitogenic in the Lewis rat (Martenson et al, 1972). It is obvious, therefore, that the situation in the rat differs from that in the guinea pig and other species. Further differences between rats and guinea pigs are shown by the equal activities of rat BP and SBP in Lewis rats, whereas SBP is essentially inactive in guinea pigs. Thus, the encephalitogenic determinants in the rat SBP is not affected by the 45 residue deletion from BP. Finally, the tryptophan region, responsible for EAE in guinea pigs, is not active in rats since the HNB-derivative of BP, in which the tryptophan residue is modified, is fully active.

All of the above data vividly show that the disease-inducing site of BP active in the rat must be an entirely different region from the guinea pig. The encephalitogenic site for the rat must also differ from that active in rabbits and monkeys since these species show an equal response to the bovine, human, and guinea pig BP. What then is the region active in rats? With knowledge of the primary sequence, and the isolation of many peptic and tryptic peptides, the matter should be easily resolved. However, until recently, considerable disagreement prevailed. McFarlin et al (1973) reported that bovine peptide 43-87 was inactive, whereas the guinea pig peptide was active. Martenson et al (1975) reported in an extensive study that bovine peptic peptides with residues 1-42 and 37-88 were both active whereas peptides 1-36 and 43-88 were inactive; thus a major encephalitogenic site seemed to exist between the overlapping residues 37-42, or Asp-Ser-Leu-Gly-Arg-Phe. A weaker activity was found in a bovine peptide having residues 88-153, and was proposed to reside within residues 107-118. Residues 109-113 were emphasized because this sequence, Ser-Leu-Ser-Arg-Phe, compares closely with residues 37-42. Thus, the weakly active bovine BP was claimed to have two encephalitogenic sites, one stronger, defined by residues 37-42 and a weaker site at res. 109-113.

It seems reasonable that the same region of the guinea pig BP, which is much more active in rats than bovine BP (Table IV) should be the major determinant in the Lewis rat. However, peptides 37-88 and 43-88 of guinea pig BP were both as active as the original guinea pig BP (McFarlin et al, 1973) and confirmed by Martenson et al. These data suggest that the major disease-inducing site in Lewis rats must reside within residues 43-88 and not in the overlap region. Such a result was also found by Chou et al, who isolated several peptic peptides from guinea pig BP, and found that chymotryptic peptide 69-89 was highly active. The only difference is sequence between the guinea pig and rat peptide (10 times less active) is a Ser (guinea pig) for Thr (rat) substitution at position 80. It appeared highly probable therefore that the major determinant for rats is localized in res. 69-89 of guinea pig BP, and includes res. 80 and not in res. 37-42. The bovine, human and rabbit sequence contrast considerably with guinea pig sequence in this region, and thus, the species may be accounted.

1. Synthetic peptides. The recent impressive work of Hashim and coworkers has now elegantly resolved the problems of the encephalitogenic determinant active in the rat. The Peptide 68-83 of the bovine BP sequence was synthesized with and without the Gly-His (res. 76-77) region present; it is this segment which is deleted in guinea pig BP (Table III). The activity was approximately 50 times greater in the deleted peptide (Table IV), thus demonstrating that the reason for the difference in activities of the bovine and guinea pig BP was the presence of the Gly-His segment in the encephalitogenic determinant of the bovine BP.

Hashim (1972a) further defined the disease-inducing determinant by synthesis of the octapeptide 74-81 based on the guinea pig BP sequence. This octapeptide is an extremely potent inducer of EAE in the Lewis rat although not as active as guinea pig BP itself (Table IV).

These results are analagous to the situation in the guinea pig; in both cases the active determinant is localized to a small domain of 8-9 amino acid residues. It is remarkable that the synthetic peptides are so strongly encephalitogenic and supports the early evidence showing that the conformation of these regions must be similar whether in intact BP or in sythetic peptides. The use of synthetic peptides to elucidate the disease-inducing determinants in the rat and guinea pig is powerfully illustrated by these studies.

TABLE V

THE COMPLETE AMINO ACID SEQUENCE
OF THE BOVINE BP

```
                                                          10
N-Ac-Ala-Ala-Gln-Lys-Arg-Pro-Ser-Gln-Arg-Ser-Lys-Try-Leu-Ala-
                  20                                          30
Ser-Ala-Ser-Thr-Met-Asp-His-Ala-Arg-His-Gly-Phe-Leu-Pro-Arg-His-
                                        40
Arg-Asp-Thr-Gly-Ile-Leu-Asp-Ser-Leu-Gly-Arg-Phe-Phe-Gly-Ser-Asp-
          50                                          60
Arg-Gly-Ala-Pro-Lys-Arg-Gly-Ser-Gly-Lys-Asp-Gly-His-His-Ala-Ala-
                              70          SER
Arg-THR-THR-HIS-TYR-GLY-SER-LEU-PRO-GLN-LYS-Ala-GLN-(Gly-His)-
    SER 80                                          90
ARG-Pro-GLN-ASP-GLU-ASN-PRO-VAL-Val-His-Phe-Phe-Lys-Asn-Ile-Val-
                        100                  (CH3)
Thr-Pro-Arg-Thr-Pro-Pro-Pro-Ser-Gln-Gly-Lys-Gly-Arg-Gly-Leu-Ser-
110                                     120
Leu-Ser-Arg-PHE-SER-TRP-GLY-ALA-GLU-GLY-GLN-LYS-Pro-Gly-Phe-Gly-
            130                                         140
Try-Gly-Gly-Arg-Ala-Ser-Asp-Tyr-Lys-Ser-Ala-His-Lys-Gly-Leu-Lys-
                                150
Gly-His-Asp-Ala-Gln-Gly-Thr-Leu-Ser-Lys-Ile-PHE-LYS-LEU-GLY-GLY-
        160                                 169
ARG-ASP-SER-ARG-SER-GLY-SER-PRO-MET-Ala-Arg-Arg-COOH
```

H. SPECIES VARIATION IN ENCEPHALITOGENIC SITES. One of the striking findings in the study on encephalitogenic determinants of BP is the species variation. When each animal species is presented with the same highly open BP molecule, it is a different peptide domain which serves as the disease-inducing site (see Table V). This preference in the encephalitogenic response of the guinea pig, monkey, rabbit and rat to dissimilar regions of the BP molecule might reasonably be explained in terms of both genetic and anatomical factors. Genetically, it is known that different strains of mice respond to different chemical groupings in a given complex synthetic polypeptide. Thus, based on genetic factors, different animals species may respond preferentially to certain antigenic determinants but show nonresponsiveness to others. However, this explanation is not complete since we know that the guinea pig and rabbit show a cell-mediated immune response to many antigenic sites on the BP molecule (Bergstrand, 1972, 1973; Burnett, and Eylar, 1971) including the disease-inducing sites. Why then is only one or two of the antigenic sites also encephalitogenic? Discrimination at the target site offers one explanation. When lymphocytes, sensitized to many sites on the BP molecule, migrate to the guinea pig brain, they may not find the antigenic site on the BP molecule in situ in the appropriate conformation, except for the tryptophan region. The BP undoubtedly exists in myelin in a partially buried state where it strongly interacts with lipids such as cerebroside sulfate (London et al, 1973; Eylar, 1976). Therefore the conformation and accessibilty of many antigenic sites may be altered from that in the isolated BP used for sensitization. A combination of genetic and anatomical factors thus may account for the small number of disease-inducing determinants on the BP molecule for a given species.

It is evident that the synthetic peptides have provided a powerful tool in delineating the essential residues of the encephalitogenic determinants. For the rat, rabbit and guinea pig, the size of the disease-inducing site, 8-10 residues, is close to that found for antigenic sites in synthetic polypeptides. It is remarkable that these peptides themselves elicit disease. Although less potent than BP on a molar basis, they are effective encephalitogens reproducing essentially the same clinical and histologic signs of disease as the BP molecule.

The structures of the encephalitogenic sites are shown as part of BP in Table V. It is interesting to note that in each case a proline residue is found near the end of the active sequence. The 10 residue tyrosine region (64-73) is the major determinant for the rabbit and is not active in the guinea pig, rat or monkey.

The 8 residue region (74-85; Gly-His deleted in the guinea pig BP sequence) comprises the major encephalitogenic determinant for the rat. Apparently it is the deletion of the Gly-His segment which explains the relative impotencey of the bovine BP in inducing EAE in the rat. The other substitutions such as Ser for Ala and Ser for Pro are not crucial. The latter change (Ser for Pro) probably accounts, however, for the greater activity of the guinea pig BP over the rat BP since that is the only difference in their BP sequences in that region.

The tryptophan region, 9 residues (113-121) is the major determinant for the guinea pig and is quite active in the rabbit. It is not encephalitogenic, however, in the rat or monkey.

The 14-residue region (153-166) is the major encephalitogenic determinant active in the monkey. It serves as a minor determinant for the rabbit as well. It is quite likely that the length of this determinant is shorter than 14 residues, but appropriate synthetic peptides have not yet been prepared to define this region more precisely. It is also possible that other regions such as Peptide 1-42 and 43-89 contain minor determinants active in the monkey.

One question which arises from this study concerns the encephalitogenic determinant for EAE in humans. It is known that rabies post-vaccinal encphalomyelitis may arise when the vaccine is prepared from guinea pig, rabbit or mouse tissue. Presumbably, EAE is induced because of BP present in CNS tissue contaminating the virus preparation. It may be possible by indirect means using peptides from the human BP to evaluate the reactivity of T lymphocytes in such patients.

One of the likely encephalitogenic determinants in humans is the antigen of the Peptides 133-169 active in the monkey. Recently Sheremata and Eylar, 1975 found that circulating lymphocytes from multiple sclerosis patients responded to Peptide 116-169, but not to Peptide 1-116. Thus it is possible that sensitization to the disease inducing site active in monkeys may play a role in multiple sclerosis, and suggests a similarity between EAE and the human disease. For the future it is possible that peptides modeled on the BP sequence might serve an important purpose diagnostically or otherwise in human demyelinating diseases.

Adendum: Some relevent data was inadvertently omitted in the text. With regard to the crucial residues of the tryptophan domain of the BP (Table II), the disease-inducing site active in guinea pigs, it was first shown by Nagai et al (1973) that the alanine residue was required, since substitution by glycine led to inactivity. The following peptide, showing an Ala to Gly substitution, was inactive at 0.1 mg doses: Arg-Phe-Ser-Trp-Gly-Gly-Glu-Gly-Gln-Arg

Thus at least 4 residues are crucial for induction of EAE in guinea pigs: Trp, Ala, Gln and Lys (Arg). It should also be noted, that under certain circumstances, the seven residue peptide: Trp-Gly-Ala-Glu-Gly-Gln-Arg induced disease in guinea pigs. For activity of this heptapeptide, it was necessary to use snythetic N-acetylmuramyl-L-alanyl-D-isoglutamine instead of mycobacteria in the adjuvant. This remarkable finding (Nagai et al, 1978) shows that a seven residue segment may constitute the smallest encephalitogenic fragment. The nonapeptide, rather than the heptapeptide, is the smallest active fragment when regular FCA is used to induce EAE. The muramyl dipeptide is of special interest therefore. Only 5 μg are required with 5 μg of the nonapeptide to induce a high level of EAE in most guinea pigs whereas 90-100 μg are required with 50 μg of the heptapeptide. Thus, even with the muramyl dipeptide replacing the mycobacteria, the nonapeptide is much more active than the heptapeptide, but the latter appears to contain the essential residues.

With regard to the encephalitogenic determinant active in the rat, a major clue was provided by Martenson et al (1977) prior to the synthetic peptide work of Hashim (1977, 1977a). It was found that peptide 72-84 was active at 2.5 n mole, and while not as active as peptide 61-88 (active at 0.02 n mole), clearly contains the elements essential for encephalitogenic activity in the rat. The corresponding peptide derived from bovine BP, where Gly-His (res. 76-77) is deleted, is inactive. It is of interest that the localization of the encephalitogenic determinant active in the rat into a small peptide domain was accomplished using proteolytic enzymes alpha-protease and thermolysin (Nomura et al, 1977). The resulting peptides were purified; the animal studies were then possible.

REFERENCES

Alvord, E., Shaw, C.-M., Hruby, S., and Kies, M., (1965). Ann. N.Y. Acad. Scie. 122, 333.
Appel, S., Almon, R., and Levy, N., (1975). N. Engl. J. Med. 293, 760.
Arnason, B., Asbury, A., Astrom, K., Adonis, R., (1968). Trans. Amer. Neur. Assoc. 93, 133.
Arnon, R., Sela, M., Yaron, A. and Sober, H. (1965). Biochemistry 4, 948.
Ben-Efraim, S., Fuchs, S. and Sela, M. (1963). Science 139, 1222.
Bergstrand, H. (1972), Europ. J. Biochem. 27, 126.
Bergstrand, H. (1972a), FEBS Lett. 23, 195.
Bergstrand, H. (1973), Immunochem. 10, 611.
Bergstrand, H. and Kallen, B. (1974). Neurobiol. 4, 328.
Brostoff, S., and Eylar, E. H. (1971). Proc. Nat. Acad. Sci. USA 68, 769.
Brostoff, S., Burnett, P., Lampert, P. and Eylar, E. H., (1972). Nature New Biol., 235, 210.
Brostoff, S., Reuter, W., Hichens, M., and Eylar, E. H. (1974). J. Biol. Chem. 249, 559.
Burnett, P. and Eylar, E. H. (1971). J. Biol. Chem. 246, 3425.
Carnegie, P. (1969). Biochem. J. III, 240.
Chao, L.-P. and Einstein, E. (1970). J. Neurochem. 17, 1121.
Chou, C.-H., Chou, F., Kowalski, J., Shapira, R., and Kibler, R., (1977). J. Neurochem., 28, 115.
Driscoll, B., Kies, M. and Alvord, E., (1975). J. Immunol. 112, 392.
Driscoll, B., Kies, M. and Alvord, E., (1976). J. Immunol. 117, 110.
Einstien, E., Csejtye, J. and Marks, N. (1968). FEBS lett. 1, 191.
Einstien, E., Chao, L.-P., Csejtey, J., Kibler, R. and Shapira, R. (1972). Immunochem. 9, 73.
Epand, R., Moscarello, M., Zierenberg, B. and Vail, W. J. (1974). Biochem. 13, 1264.
Eylar, E. H., and Hashim, G., (1968). Proc. Nat. Acad. Sci. USA 61, 644.
Eylar, E. H., Salk, J., Beveridge, G., and Brown, L. (1969). Arch. Biochem. Biophys. 132, 34.
Eylar, E. H., and Thompson, M. (1969). Arch. Biochem. Biophys. 129, 468.
Eylar, E. H., Caccam, J., Jackson, J., and Robinson, A., (1970). Science, 168, 1220.
Eylar, E. H., Westall, F. and Brostoff, S. (1971). J. Biochem.,246, 3418.
Eylar, E. H., Brostoff, S., Hashim, G., Caccam, J. and Burnett, P. (1971a). J. Biol. Chem. 246, 5770.
Eylar, E. H., Jackson, J., Rothenberg, B. and Brostoff, S. (1972). Nature, 236, 74.
Eylar, E. H., (1972). In Multiple Sclerosis (Wolfgram, F., Ellison, G., Stevens, J. and Andrews, J., eds.) p449, Acad. Press, New York.

Eylar, E. H., Brostoff, S., Jackson, J. and Carter, H., (1972a). Proc. Nat. Acad. Sci. USA, 69, 617.
Eylar, E. H., Jackson, J., Bennett, C., Kniskern, P., and Brostoff, S., (1974). J. Biol. Chem. 249, 3710.
Eylar, E. H., in Structure of Biological Membranes (Abrahamsson, S. and Pascher, I. eds.). (1976). Plenum Pub. Corp. New York, p.157.
Gell, P. (1970). N. Y. Acad. Sci. 169, 245.
Gill, T. and Doty, P. In Polyamino Acids, Polypeptides, and Proteins (Stahmann, M., ed.). p. 367 (1962). Univ. of Wisconsin Press, Madison.
Hagopian, A., Whitehead, J., Westall, F. and Eylar, E. H. (1971). J. Biol. Chem. 246, 2519.
Hagopian, A., Jackson, J., Carlo, D., Limjuco, G., and Eylar, E. H. (1975). J. Immunol. 115, 1731.
Hashim, G. and Eylar, E. H. (1969). Arch. Biochem. Biophys. 129, 635.
Hashim, G. and Eylar, E. H. (1969a). Arch. Biochem. Biophys. 129, 645.
Hashim, G. and Eylar, E. H. (1969b). Arch. Biochem. Biophys. 131, 215.
Hashim, G. and Eylar, E. H. (1969c). Arch. Biochem. Biophys. 135, 324.
Hashim, G. and Sharpe, R. (1974). Immunochem. II, 633.
Hashim, G. and Sharpe, R. (1975). Nature 255, 484.
Hashim, G. Science 196, 1219. (1977)
Hashim, G. Adv. Exp. Biol. Med. (in press) (1977a).
Jackson, J., Brostoff, S., Lampert, P. and Eylar, E. H. (1972). Neurobiol. 2, 83.
Jackson, J., Hagopian, A., Carlo, D., Limjuco, G. and Eylar, E. H. (1975). J. Biol. Chem, 250, 6140.
Kabat, E., Wolf, A., and Bezer, A. (1947). J. Exp. Med., 85, 117.
Karkhanis, Y., Carlo, D., Brostoff, S., and Eylar, E. H., (1975). J. Biol. Chem., 250, 1718.
Kibler, R., Shapira, R., McKneally, S., Jenkins, P., Selden, P., and Chow, F. (1969). Science, 164, 577.
Lamoureux, G., Thibeault, G., Richer, G. and Bernard, C. (1972). Union Med. Can. 101, 674.
Lennon, V., Wilks, A., and Carnegie, P. (1970). J. Immunol. 105, 1223.
London, Y. and Vossenberg, F. (1973). Biochim. Biophys. Acta. 307, 478.
Lumsden, C., Robertson, D. and Blight, R. (1966). J. Neurochem. 13 127.
Martenson, R., Levine, S. and Sowinski, R. (1975). J. Immunol. 114, 592.
Martenson, R., Deibler, G., Kies, M., Levine, S. and Alvord, E. (1972). J. Immunol. 109, 262.
McFarlin, D., Blank, S., Kibler, R., McKneally, S., and Shapira, R. (1973). Science 179, 478.

Martenson, R., Nomura, K., Levine, S. and Sowinski, R. (1977). J. Immunol. 118, 1280.
Nagai, Y., Yasuda, T., Suzuki, K., and Yonezawa, T. in The Etiology and Pathogenesis of Demyelinating Diseases (Shiraki, H., Yonezawa, T. and Kuriowa, Y., Eds.), Sym. held in 1973, Jap. Soc. Neuropath. (1976), p. 171.
Nagai, Y., Akiyama, K., Suzuki, K., Kotani, S., Watanabe, Y., Shimono, T., Shiba, T., Kusumoto, S., Ikuta, F., and Takeda, S. (1978). Cell. Immunol., in press.
Nomura, K., Martenson, R., and Deibler, G. (1977). J. Biol. Chem. 252, 1723.
Oshiro, Y. and Eylar, E.H. (1970). Arch. Biochem. Biophys. 138, 606.
Patrick, J. and Lindstrom, J. (1973). Science 180, 871.
Rauch, H. and Einstein, E. (1971). Fed. Proc. 30, 306.
Rivers, T., Sprunt, D., and Berry, G. (1933). J. Exp. Med. 58, 39.
Rose, N. and Witebsky, E. (1968). In Textbook of Immunopathology (Miescher, P. and Muller-Eberhardt, H., Eds.). New York, Grune and Stratton 1, 150.
Sage, H., Deutsch, G., Fasman, G. and Levine, L. (1964). Immochem. 1, 133.
Salvin, S. and Liauw, H. (1967). J. Immunol. 101, 33.
Shermata, W., Colby, S., Karkhanis, Y. and Eylar, E.H. (1975). Can. J. Neurol. Sci. 2, 87.
Shermata, S., Eylar, E.H., and Cosgrove, J. Br., (1977). J. Neurol. Sci. 32, 255.
Spitler, L., von Muller, C., Fudenberg, H. and Eylar, E. H. (1972). J. Exp. Med. 136, 156.
Toyka, K., Drachman, D., and Pestronk, A. (1975). Science 190, 397.
Westall, F., Robinson, A., Caccam, J., Jackson, J., and Eylar, E.H. (1970). Nature 168, 1220.
Wisniewski, H., Brostoff, S., Carter, H. and Eylar, E.H. (1974). Arch. Neurol. 30, 347.

MECHANISMS OF TOLERANCE TO HGG INDUCED IN NEONATAL AND ADULT MICE

D. C. Benjamin

Department of Microbiology, School of Medicine
University of Virginia

In 1973 we repeated some of the experiments initially carried out by Chiller, Weigle, and their colleagues (Chiller et al., 1974) by attempting to terminate the tolerant state to human γ-globulin (HGG) induced in adult A/J mice by reconstitution with normal or immune lymphocytes or by the injection of crossreacting γ-globulin. We found the same results, i.e. that it was nor possible to terminate this tolerant state by either method. One would have thought that if clonal deletion was the sole mechanism responsible for this tolerance, that by providing the missing specific lymphocyte, these mice could be reconstituted to a fully normal status. Both of these methods were highly successful in terminating the tolerance to bovine serum albumin (BSA) induced in neonatal rabbits (Benjamin and Weigle, 1970; Benjamin, 1974). The results obtained in the attempts to terminate this HGG tolerance with heterologous γ-globulins made us suspect that there was much more involved than the simple deletion of HGG-specific clones. The data shown in Table I illustrate this point quite well. Adult A/J male mice that had been injected with 2.5 mg deaggregated HGG (DHGG) do not respond to subsequent injections of aggregated HGG (AHGG) (Group 2), nor is this tolerant state terminated by the injection of aggregated bovine γ-globulin (ABGG) (Group 3). In fact the response of such HGG tolerant mice to the specific determinants on BGG is much reduced (compare the BGG response of Groups 3 and 4 - Table I). The reverse is also true, i.e. mice tolerant to BGG do not respond well to HGG specific determinants. Ruben et al. (1973) attributed this lack of response to non-crossreacting determinants to the loss of crossreactive T-helper cells in these HGG tolerant mice. However, it seemed to us that it could also have been due to the presence of crossreactive suppressor cells induced by the injection of tolerogen.

TABLE I

CAPACITY OF CROSSREACTING γ-GLOBULINS TO TERMINATE ADULT-INDUCED TOLERANCE TO HGG*

Group	Tolerogen	Immunogen	Indirect PFC/10^8 Spleen Cells	
			HGG	BGG
1	Nil	AHGG	17,000**	500
2	DHGG	AHGG	700	-
3	DHGG	ABGG	0	4,800
4	Nil	ABGG	1,700	24,700
5	DBGG	ABGG	-	1,700
6	DBGG	AHGG	100	100

* Immunizations were initiated 35 days after the induction of tolerance.

** Mean of 6-14 mice individually assayed.

Our first real indication that suppressor cells were probably involved came about as the result of transferring tolerant spleen cells into normal adult A/J recipients and challenging with AHGG. These mice failed to respond to this challenge (Benjamin, 1975). This suppression of the HGG response was specific since similarly treated mice responded normally to goat erythrocytes. Chiller and Weigle (Chiller and Weigle, 1973) had been unsuccessful in their attempts to demonstrate suppressor activity in this system by adoptive transfer techniques. At about the same time that we had completed the termination experiments, a report appeared in the literature (Herzenberg et al., 1973) demonstrating that following the transfer of spleen cells from allotypically suppressed mice (with or without normal spleen cells) a burst of synthesis of the suppresed allotype was seen. It was only after several weeks that full suppression was reinstated. This indicated to us that when attempting to assess suppressor cell activity by adoptive transfer method one might need to allow a certain period of time between transfer and challenge for the suppressor cells to exert their influence. We therefore repeated the mixed adoptive transfer experiments of Chiller and Weigle (1973) except that we delayed challenge for various periods of time after transfer. The protocol we used for these experiments is shown in Figure 1. Tolerant spleen cells, taken at various times after the induction of tolerance, were transferred either alone or with normal spleen cells into irradiated syngeneic recipients. These recipients were challenged with AHGG either immediately or beginning several weeks after cell transfer. The results of these adoptive cell transfer studies are shown in

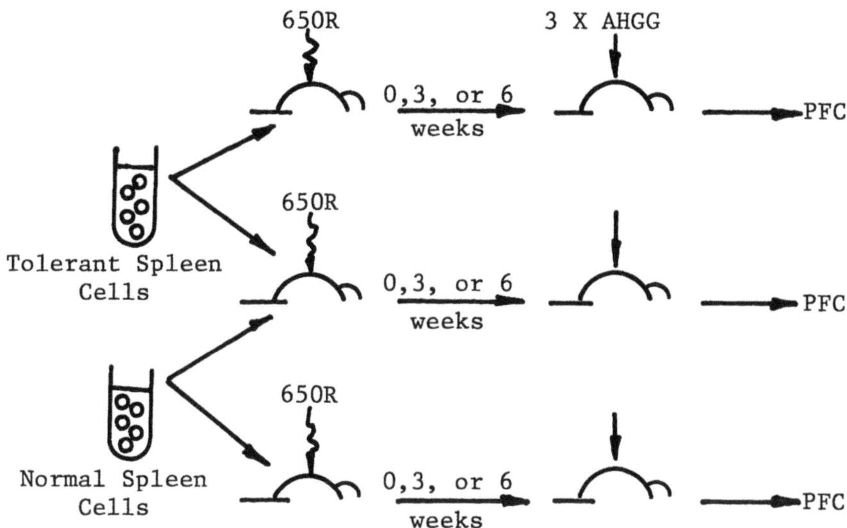

Figure 1. Protocol for Adoptive Transfer Studies. Tolerant mice received a single injection of 2.5 mg DHGG i.p. At various times thereafter spleen cells were removed and co-transferred with normal spleen cells into irradiated syngeneic recipients. Each recipient was given three injections of 400 μg AHGG spaced 10 days apart either immediately after, or beginning 3 or 6 weeks after, cell transfer. Recipient spleens were individually assayed for PFC five days after the last injection of AHGG.

Figure 2. Suppressor cell activity was observed in tolerant spleen cells as early as 10 days after the induction of tolerance and was present for as long as 56 days if challenge was initiated immediately after cell transfer. Much more effective suppression was observed if challenge was delayed. This suppression was both HGG specific and sensitive to anti-Thy.1 plus complement. These kinetics demonstrated that suppressor activity was present in spleen cells of HGG tolerant mice at a time after HGG-specific B-cells had recovered from tolerance (Weigle et al., 1971) but not quite as long as tolerance in the T-cell compartment. We suggested (Benjamin, 1975) that the presence of such suppressor cells could well be responsible for the extended T-cell tolerance and that only when the suppressor activity had waned could new HGG-specific T-helper cells be formed from precursor cells. Basten (1974) had also demonstrated HGG specific suppressor cells in a system using HGG as carrier for an immune response to DNP. More recently, several other laboratories (Doyle et al., 1976a, 1976b; Jones and Kaplan, 1977) have also shown HGG specific suppressor cells in spleens of HGG Tolerant mice.

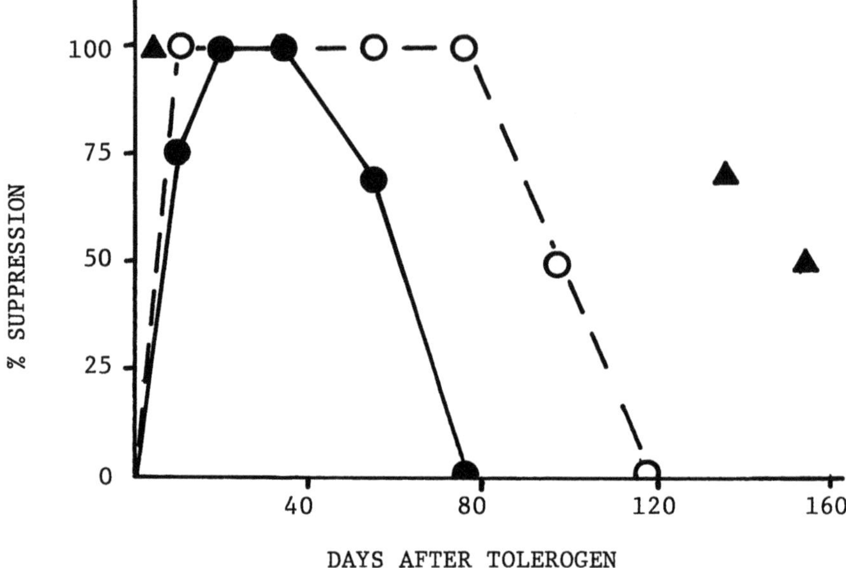

Figure 2. Suppression of the Response of Normal Spleen Cells to AHGG by Spleen Cells from Mice Given 2.5 mg DHGG. Adult mice were injected with 2.5 mg DHGG on day 0. At various times thereafter spleens were removed and adoptive cell transfers were performed as shown in Figure 1. The percent suppression of the HGG-specific PFC response was calculated relative to the response of recipients of normal spleen cells alone. ●—●, immediate challenge; O—O, delayed challenge; ▲, thymus cell tolerance from Weigle et al. (1971).

The results of Jones and Kaplan (1977) confirmed the kinetics of suppressor cell activity shown above. In addition, they were able to demonstrate an HGG specific suppressor factor, of 50,000 molecular weight, in lysates of spleen cells taken from HGG tolerant A/J mice. The kinetics of the presence of this factor in the spleen cell lysates was quite similar to the kinetics of T-cell tolerance reported by Weigle et al. (1971). This factor was removed from the lysates by passage over a HGG immunoadsorbent column but not by passage over an anti-HGG column. These results have reinforced our hypothesis that suppressor cells are responsible for the extended kinetics of T-cell tolerance.

We next returned to the question of why HGG tolerant mice do not respond to the specific determinants on BGG when challenged with the immunogenic for of that antigen. Ruben et al. (1973) had suggested that this lack of a specific response was due to extensive crossreaction at the helper T-cell level and that injection of DHGG had simply eliminated most of the helper T-cells that could function when challenge was with ABGG. Since we were successful in demonstrating suppressor cells in such mice, we thought that the lack of response to these heterologous γ-globulin specific determinants could well have been due to crossreaction at the suppressor T-cell level. We therefore repeated the adoptive transfer experiments as above but also included several groups of mice that had HGG tolerant plus normal spleen cells and were challenged with the crossreacting antigen ABGG. Our previous results (Table I) had shown that the response of HGG tolerant mice to ABGG was reduced by as much as 80% and that HGG and BGG were crossreactive at the B cell level only to the extent of 10% or less. The results shown in Table II demonstrated that, indeed, spleen cells from HGG tolerant mice, taken 35 days after the induction of tolerance, were quite effective in suppressing the response of normal spleen cells not only to AHGG but also to ABGG. Thus suppressor cells can be crossreactive.

It is not known what fraction of the total HGG induced suppressor cells are crossreactive since the results shown in Table II could have resulted from cells recognizing only a few crossreactive determinants on the BGG molecule. However, these results do show that the potential for stimulating such crossreactive suppressor cells may provide a mechanism for control of immune responses to classes of antigens.

We were also interest in what mechanisms might be responsible for the long term maintenance of tolerance to self antigens in the

TABLE II

SUPPRESSION OF THE RESPONSE TO BGG BY SPLEEN CELLS FROM HGG TOLERANT MICE

Group	Spleen Cells[a] Transferred	Immunogen	$PFC/10^6$ Spleen Cells HGG	BGG
1	N + T	AHGG	9	-
2	N	AHGG	191	-
3	N + T	ABGG	-	76
4	N	ABGG	-	498

[a] T, tolerant - spleen cells taken 35 days after the induction of tolerance. N, 8-10 week old normal mice.

natural situation. Because of the extended kinetics of suppressor cell activity seen as the result of only a single injection of DHGG we thought it would be possible that continued stimulation of suppressor cells by self antigen might be responsible for maintaining tolerance in the helper T-cell compartment. If true then reinjection of tolerogen into tolerant mice after suppressor activity had waned, but before competence in the T-cell compartment had returned, should result in the reappearance of suppressor cells which would then extend the duration of T-cell tolerance. The experiment we designed to test this hypothesis was as follows: adult mice were injected with DHGG tolerogen, 80 days later (a time when suppressor activity had waned as assessed by adoptive transfer and immediate challenge) these mice were reinjected with another dose of tolerogen. 10 or 20 days after this second injection, spleen cells from these mice were co-transferred with normal cells into irradiated recipients. Challenge with AHGG was initiated immediately. The results of this experiment are shown in Figure 3. It

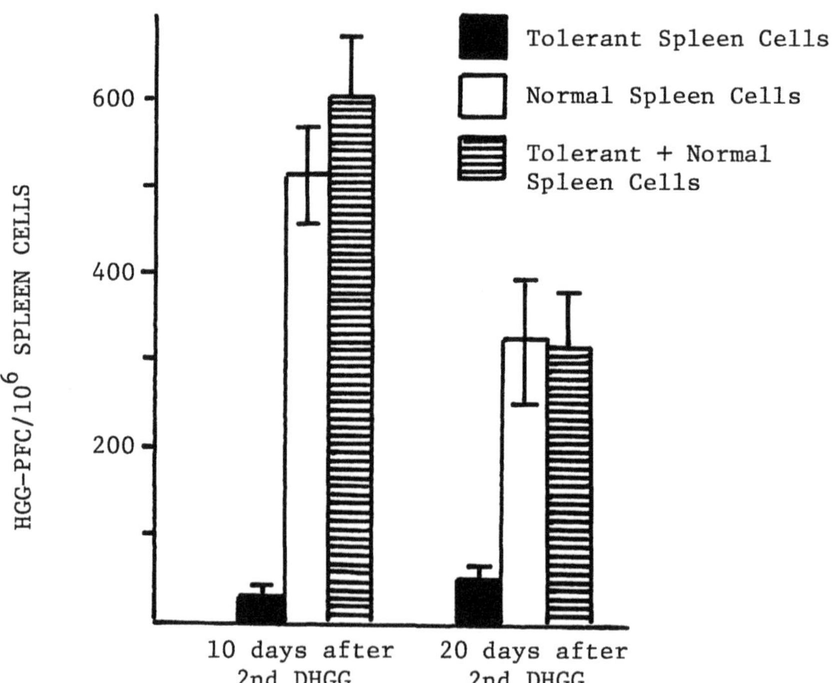

Figure 3. Failure to Reinduce Suppressor Cells in HGG Tolerant Mice. HGG tolerant mice were reinjected with a second dose of tolerogen. 10 or 20 days after this second injections their spleen cells were examined for suppressor activity by adoptive transfer with normal spleen cells and immediate challenge with AHGG.

was apparent that suppressor activity could not be reactivated. Recipients of tolerant cells alone did not respond to challenge with AHGG demonstrating that they were tolerant. Recipients of a mixture of tolerant and normal cells responded as well as recipients of normal cells alone. Delay of challenge after transfer did not result in suppression above that predicted to occur from delayed challenge if such tolerant donors had not been reinjected with tolerogen. Thus it would appear that T-suppressor cells do not possess memory. A similar lack of memory in T-suppressor cells has been reported by Benaceraff et al. (1975) in their studies on GAT specific suppressor cells in non-responder mice. These results also suggest that HGG specific suppressor cells had not been replenished from a precursor cell, at least not in numbers sufficient to be stimulated and observed. It is possible that suppressor cells and helper cells have a common precursor with specific receptors and that this common precursor can be tolerized as easily as are helper T-cells. Suppressor T-cells would then be activated and function for a limited period of time. In the absence of further contact with tolerogen both new helper T-cells and new suppressor T-cells would appear with time. Only then would contact with the tolerogenic form of an antigen result in the reappearance of suppressor activity. It would be interesting to determine whether suppressor activity is recovered at the same time as helper T-cell activity.

Weigle et al. (1971) have shown that not only are the kinetics of tolerance in the B-cell and T-cell compartments different but that there is a difference in the threshold doses of tolerogen that are required for the induction of tolerance in these two classes of lymphocytes. The injection of low doses of tolerogen can result in tolerance only in the T-cell compartment. We decided to determine whether there was a suppressor cell component in this low dose tolerance to HGG. Tolerance was induced by the injection of 100 μg of DHGG. At various times, thereafter, spleen cells from such tolerant mice were transferred either alone or with normal spleen cells into irradiated recipients. Challenge with AHGG was either initiated immediately or several weeks after transfer. The results shown in Table III demonstrate that this procedure did induce tolerance in these mice but did not activate suppressor cells. Indeed, delay of challenge after transfer did not enhance suppressor activity as in the high dose tolerance experiments reported above (Benjamin, 1977). Similar results were obtained using cell ratios of 1:1, 2:1, or 4:1 (tolerant:normal). These results demonstrate that there may be a dose dependency for the stimulation of suppressor T-cells. They also show that tolerance in T lymphocytes can be induced in the absence of apparent suppressor T-cells presumably by a clonal deletion and/or clonal abortion mechanism. Tolerance to HGG in B-cells can also be induced in the absence of T-cells (Chiller et al., 1974) and therefore presumably in the

TABLE III

ABSENCE OF SPECIFIC SUPPRESSOR CELLS IN LOW DOSE TOLERANCE

Group	Time of Transfer[a]	Source of Cells[b]	Indirect PFC/10^6 Spleen Cells
1	7 days	T + N	157[c]
2	7 days	nN + N	166
3	21 days	T + N	271
4	21 days	nN + N	177
5	3 days	T	21
6	21 days	T	4

[a] Days after the injection of 100 μg DHGG that spleens were removed for cell transfer.

[b] T, tolerant; N, normal eight week ol donors; nN, age-matched normal mice.

[c] Mean of five to ten mice individually assayed.

absence of suppressor T-cells. What then is the role of T-suppressor cells in tolerance induction and maintenance? They apparently are not required for induction of tolerance. We have proposed two roles for such suppressor cells: a) a failsafe mechanism preventing the activation of T-helper cells such that tolerance might be more easily induced in both B-cells and in T-cells; and b) partially responsible for the long term maintenance of tolerance in the T-cell compartment (Benjamin, 1977).

A number of laboratories (e.g. Cambier et al., 1976; Metcalf and Klinman, 1976) have demonstrated a differential susceptibility of mature and immature B-lymphocytes to tolerance induction. Although model tolerance systems involving the induction of tolerance in adult mice may help us understand some of the mechanisms involved in the control of immune responses, can we extrapolate our findings in such adult systems to the natutal tolerance resulting from contact with self antigen early in life when the immune system is developing. We therefore decided to compare the cellular parameters involved in tolerance to HGG in neonatal A/J mice with those seen in the adult-induced tolerance system. The protocol for inducing tolerance in neonatal mice is shown in Figure 4. Female mice were injected with 20 mg DHGG within 24 hours of delivery of a litter. We have shown that this DHGG enters the colostrum of the mother and is absorbed intact across the gut of the suckling mice (Halsey and Benjamin, 1976). The offspring of such treated mothers

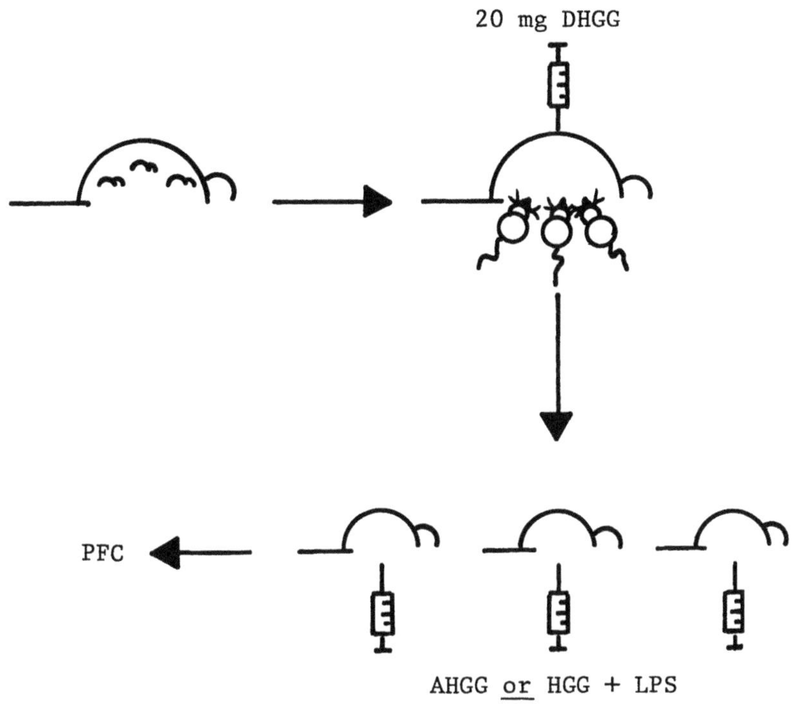

Figure 4. Protocol for Induction of HGG-Specific Tolerance in Neonatal Mice.

do not respond to immunogenic HGG for as long as 18-20 weeks after birth (Figure 5). Offspring of normal mice (i.e. not injected) do not respond during the first few weeks of life but attain adult potential by 8-10 weeks of age. This lack of response of young, normal mice is non-specific since they also fail to respond to control non-related antigens (Mosier and Johnson, 1975; Benjamin, 1977a). However, the failure of tolerant mice to respond to AHGG is specific in that they do respond normally to non-related T dependent antigens. This neonatally induced tolerance to HGG is also stable upon adoptive cell transfer to irradiated recipients.

To assess the B-cell potential in this neonatally-induced tolerant state we challenged such mice with a mixture of lipopolysaccharide and HGG. Chiller et al. (1974) have shown that such an immunization protocol results in direct stimulation of B-cells from normal and HGG tolerant mice (made tolerant as adults) and that the response to subsequent challenge with AHGG is T-cell independent.

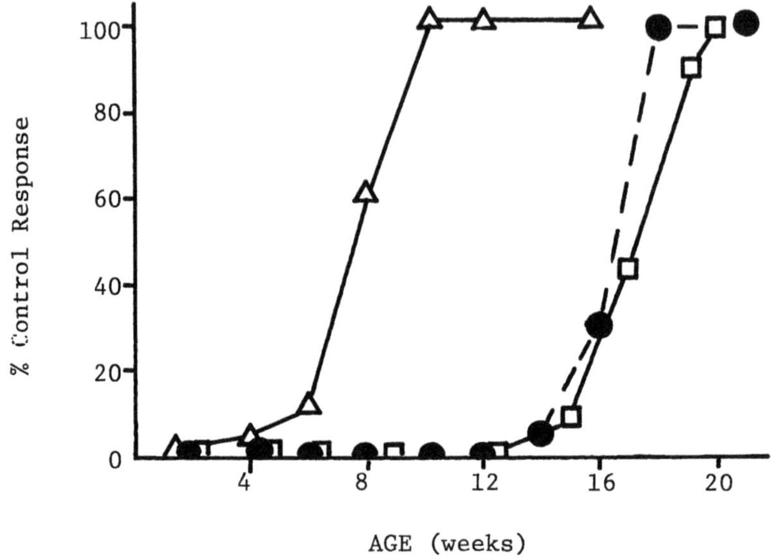

Figure 5. Duration of Neonatally Induced Tolerance to HGG. The method of induction of tolerance is shown in Figure 4 and is described in the text. At various times after birth such treated mice and age-matched normal control mice were immunized with AHGG or with LPS + HGG. The response to these injections was measured by the hemolytic plaque assay. △—△ , Normal mice immunized with AHGG; ● - ●, Tolerant mice immunized with AHGG; □—□ , Tolerant mice immunized with LPS + HGG.

Normal mice responded quite well to the LPS + HGG challenge even at two weeks of age. Mice that had received tolerogen in the colostrum from DHGG injected mothers, however, did not respond at all until 18-20 weeks of age (Figure 5). Thus the duration of neonatally induced tolerance in the B-cell population was identical to that of tolerance in the intact animal assessed by challenge with AHGG. This is in direct contrast to the results reported by Weigle et al. (1971) in the adult-induced tolerance system where B-cell competence has completely returned by 7 weeks after the induction of tolerance. Thus the induction of tolerance in neonatal mice results in the extended duration of tolerance in the B-cell population.

Although our attempts to demonstrate suppressor cell activity in the neonatal tolerance system is hampered by the presence of naturally occuring, non-specific suppressor cells, present early in life (see Figure 5 for the response of normal mice to AHGG during the first 6 weeks of life), we have not been able to demonstrate a specific suppressor component in this tolerance system (Benjamin, 1977a). This lack of specific suppressor cells is also in direct contrast to our results with adult-induced tolerance to HGG.

Any attempts to examine tolerance in the T-cell compartment of these neonatal mice is also hindered by the presence of such non-specific suppressor cells. However we have carried out several experiments, using eight week old mice that had been made tolerant as neonates. The first such experiment was an attempt to determine whether HGG specific helper T-cells could provide carrier function for a response to DNP coupled to HGG. Eight week old tolerant mice and age-matched normal control mice were injected two times with DNP-HGG in complete Freund's adjuvant, spaced four weeks apart. Seven days after the second injection these mice were exsanguinated and their serum examined both for anti-DNP antibody and anti-HGG antibody. Similar groups of mice were injected either with HGG or DNP-KLH in complete Freund's adjuvant. The results shown in Figure 6 demonstrate that tolerant mice do not respond to immunization with the immunogenic form of the tolerogen, nor do they respond to HGG determinants when presented in the form of carrier for the DNP hapten. In contrast, such tolerant mice produce normal quantities of anti-DNP when challenged with DNP-HGG or with the control antigen, DNP-KLH (Figure 6). This would seem to suggest that although tolerance was induced in HGG specific B-cells (see Figure 5) it was not induced in HGG specific T-cells. However, since the HGG specific response to DNP-HGG by normal mice was less than that to immunization with HGG alone, it seemed possible that conjugation with DNP had altered the HGG carrier. The normal anti-DNP response of the tolerant mice may then have been due to the interaction of DNP specific B-cells and T-cells recognizing altered (non-HGG) determinants on the DNP-HGG immunogen.

Another type of experiment was then carried out to determine the HGG-specific T-cell potential in these neonatally tolerized mice. This experiment was an attempt to reconstitute irradiated mice with normal B-cells and T-cells from tolerant mice. The source of normal B-cells was eight week old normal spleen cells that had been treated with anti-Thy.1 plus complement. The source of T-cells (tolerant or normal) was thymocytes from eight week old mice. Control mice received either normal spleen cells, normal B-cells, tolerant spleen cells, or a mixture of normal B-cells and normal T-cells. All mice were then challenged with AHGG and their response assessed using the hemolytic plaque assay. The results shown in Table IV demonstrate that tolerant thymocytes were as effective as normal thymocytes in providing T-helper function for an anti-HGG response. This confirmed the results presented above and showed

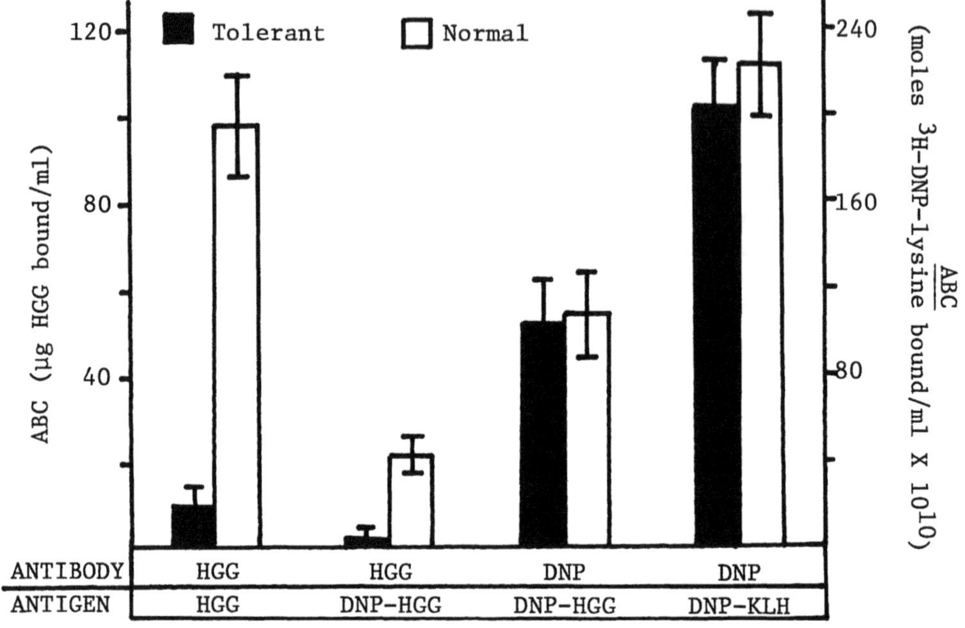

Figure 6. HGG-specific T-cell Carrier Function in Neonatally Induced Tolerance. Mice made tolerant as neonates and normal control mice were immunized with HGG, DNP-HGG, or with DNP-KLH at eight weeks of age. Two injections were given spaced four weeks apart. These mice were bled seven days after the second injection and their sera assayed for antibody to HGG and to DNP.

TABLE IV

NORMAL T-CELL FUNCTION IN NEONATALLY-INDUCED TOLERANCE

Group	Cells Transferred[a]	HGG-PFC/10^6 Spleen Cells
1	5×10^7 Norm. Spleen	176
2	5×10^7 Norm. B-cells	17
3	5×10^7 Norm. B-cells + 5×10^7 Norm. T-cells	291
4	5×10^7 Norm. B-cells + 5×10^7 Tol. T-cells	245
5	5×10^7 Tol. Spleen	16

[a] B-cells, anti-Thy.1 + complement treated normal spleen cells; T-cells, thymocytes; tolerant donors were 8 weeks of age.

that tolerance induced in neonatal mice by our methods did not result in tolerance in HGG-specific T-cells.

Another experiment was an attempt to reconstitute the response of these tolerant mice by supplementation with normal spleen cells. Reconstitution of rabbits made tolerant to BSA as neonates with normal sibling thymocytes restored their capacity to respond to immunogenic BSA (Benjamin, 1974). Reconstitution with BSA tolerant thymocytes did not. In contrast, reconstitution of mice, made tolerant to HGG as adults, with either normal spleen cells, normal thymocytes, or immune spleen cells did not restore the capacity to respond to AHGG (Chiller et al., 1974; Benjamin, 1975). Similar reconstitution experiments were therefore carried out using either normal eight week old mice or eight week old mice that were made tolerant to HGG as neonates as recipients of normal spleen cells. Some groups of recipients received light irradiation, i.e. 200R whole body, prior to cell transfer. Challenge with AHGG was initiated immediately after transfer and the response was assessed by the hemolytic plaque assay. Similarly treated mice were challenged with aggregated turkey γ-globulin as a control antigen. Tolerant mice that did not receive normal spleen cells (with or without irradiation) did not respond to challenge with AHGG although they produced a normal response to TGG (Figure 7). Normal control mice however responded quite well. In contrast, tolerant recipients of normal spleen cells did respond to AHGG whether or not they received irradiation. These results again are in direct contrast to the results of similar experiments carried out in adult-induced tolerance. However, they do agree with our previous success in terminating neonatally induced tolerance to BSA in rabbits. They also demonstrate that suppressor activity was not present in these eight week old tolerant recipients.

It is possible that tolerance was induced in the T-cell compartment. The experiments above were all carried out using eight week old tolerant mice. It is possible tolerance in T-cells was induced but that its duration was relatively short (i.e. less than eight weeks after birth). Although the serum concentration of the tolerogenic DHGG during the first week of life was found to be equivalent to that in the adult-induced tolerance (Halsey and Benjamin, 1976) we are not sure of the absolute quantity of DHGG received by these suckling neonates. It may be that the quantity (and concentration) of DHGG was sufficiently large to induce tolerance in B-cells but not in T-cells especially if the maturation of competent T-cells begins later than that of B-cells. Indeed, Cantor and Boyse (1975) have demonstrated that few, if any, T-cells with the helper T-cell phenotype (i.e. $Ly\text{-}1^{+}$, $Ly\text{-}2^{-}3^{-}$) are present during the first two weeks of life and do not reach adult levels until 5-8 weeks of age. Thus the quantity of DHGG received in the colostrum may have decreased to levels insufficient to induce tolerance

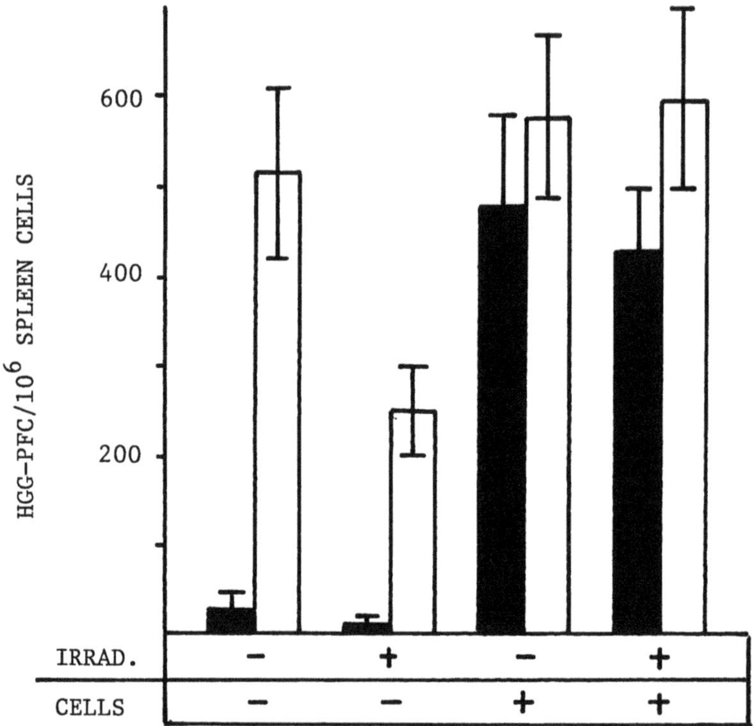

Figure 7. The Termination of Neonatally-Induced Tolerance to HGG by Reconstitution with Normal Spleen Cells. Eight week old normal mice and eight week old tolerant mice were injected with normal spleen cells and and challenged with AHGG. Some recipient mice received light irradiation prior to cell transfer. ■ = Tolerant mice; □ = Normal mice.

in T-cells arising later during neonatal life. The continued presence of self antigen, however, would be expected to induce tolerance in these newly arising T-cells. The absence of suppressor cells in this neonatal system may have been due to a delayed appearance of competent T-cells. It would be interesting to determine whether tolerance induced in two or three week old mice did result in T-cell tolerance and stimulation of suppressor cells.

This type of tolerance, i.e. in B-cells but not T-cells, may result naturally from contact with self antigens which become sequestered early. This presumably would lead to a highly dangerous immunologic situation should the host come in contact with a crossreacting antigen or with the sequestered antigen as the result of injury. Such contact could result in the production of a cytotoxic or delayed type hypersensitivity response to self antigens. This is in contrast to the situation which we are all used to considering, i.e. that where T-cells may be tolerant but B-cells normal. In this latter situation, contact with the sequestered antigen would not be expected to result in an immune response (if it is a T dependent antigen) and contact with a crossreacting antigen may not result in an immune response because of the presence of crossreacting suppressor cells.

Before going on to the last experiment I would like to discuss, let me summarize the results on HGG tolerance so far. Tolerance in T-cells and in B-cells does not require the presence of specific suppressor cells and presumably is occuring by a clonal deletion and/or clonal abortion mechanism. Adult-induced tolerance to HGG is characterized by B-cell tolerance of short duration and T-cell tolerance of long duration. Tolerance induced to high doses of tolerogen in adult mice also has a suppressor component which may function by preventing activation such that tolerance might be more easily induced and may also function by prolonging T-cell tolerance. The reverse seems to be true for tolerance induced in neonatal mice as the result of a single contact with tolerogen. Here, tolerance in B-cells is of long duration and tolerance in T-cells is either of short duration or non-existent. Non-specific, naturally occuring, suppressor T-cells are quite evident soon after birth, but specific suppressor cells do not seem to be induced. These results point out that we should be very careful before extrapolating the results from adult-induced tolerance experiments to the natural situation where tolerance is first induced in a maturing immunological system.

Although such studies as those described above have given us greater insight into some of the mechanisms of tolerance, the use of such a complex protein as HGG as tolerogen has restricted the type of questions that can be asked. This is especially true with regard to the genetic potential of such tolerant mice upon spontaneous recovery from tolerance. What is needed is a model system in which specific probes can be used to follow the expression of certain B-cell clones during the induction and loss of tolerance. The use of such a system would then permit the circumvention of many of the restrictions imposed by the use of complex protein tolerogens. The anti-azobenezenearsonate (Anti-Ars) idiotypic system in A/J mice as described by Nisonoff and his colleagues (Kuettner et al., 1972; Hart et al., 1972) seemed to be ideal for such studies. All normal A/J mice injected with p-aminobenzenearsonate (Ars) conjugates of KLH (Ars-KLH) respond by producing anti-Ars antibody of which 20-70% bear a crossreactive idiotype. Thus the anti-Ars response of these mice can be grossly divided into two categories, i.e., those anti-Ars antibodies bearing the crossreactive idiotype and those without it.

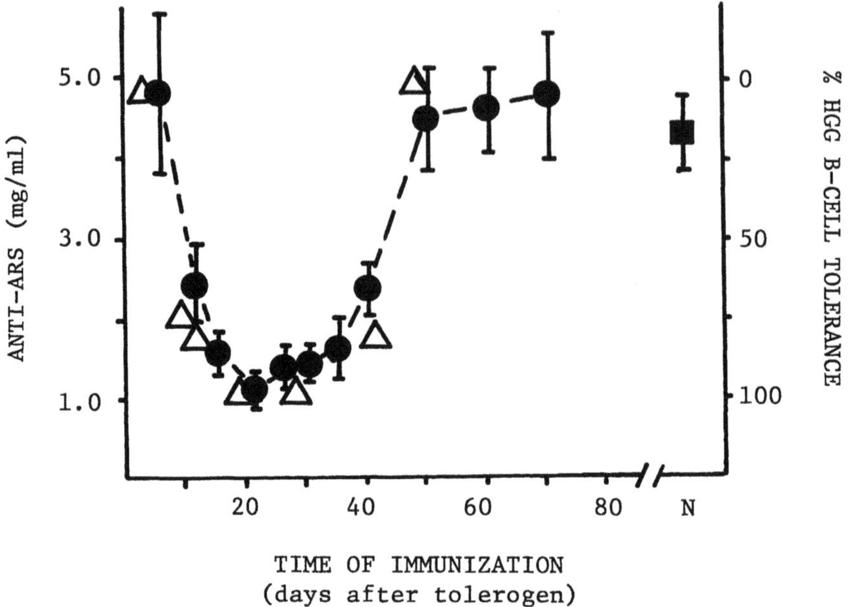

Figure 8. Kinetics of Tolerance Induced to the p-Aminobenzene-arsonate Hapten in Adult A/J Mice. Adult A/J mice were injected with Ars-DHGG on days 0, 3, and 6. On day 7 or later these mice were immunized with Ars-KLH and their sera assayed for anti-Ars antibody. ●– –●, mg anti-Ars/ml serum; △ , B-cell tolerance to HGG - adapted from results of Weigle et al. (1971). ■ normal anti-Ars, mean of 33 mice individually assayed.

We have used such an anti-idiotype to determine the effect of the injection of deaggregated conjugates of Ars and HGG (Ars-DHGG) on the subsequent response of A/J mice to immunization with Ars-KLH. Adult A/J mice were given three injections of 5.0 mg Ars-DHGG each on days 0, 3, and 6. These three injections were necessary due to the short half-life of the conjugate in the circulation of adult mice (approximately 24 hours). On day 7 or later, immunization with Ars-KLH was begun. This consisted of 5 injections, spaced two weeks apart, of 500 μg Ars-KLH i.p. The first two injections were given in complete Freund's adjuvant and the remaining 3 in incomplete Freund's adjuvant. These mice were bled from the retroorbital sinus 7 days after the second injection and/or 7 days after the last injection. Control mice received either DHGG alone or saline prior to immunization. Other control mice were similarly injected but were immunized with DNP-KLH. The results shown in Figure 8 demonstrate that although a complete tolerant state was not established, a definite hyporesponsiveness was induced with as much as an 80% reduction in the total anti-Ars produced. The kinetics of this hyporesponsiveness was compared to those of B-cell tolerance to HGG (Weigle et al., 1971) and found to be identical. Thus it would seem that the host immune system was seeing the Ars hapten, on the HGG carrier, to be just another HGG determinant. The response of normal mice injected with DHGG and immunized with Ars-KLH was normal. The response of Ars- tolerant mice to challenge with DNP-KLH was also normal. None of the Ars-DHGG treated mice responded either to HGG or to Ars-HGG in CFA demonstrating that they were carrier tolerant. Thus a specific hyporesponsive state can be induced to the Ars hapten by these methods in adult A/J mice. We have also succeeded in inducing tolerance to the Ars hapten in neonatal mice by the same method used with HGG above. These studies are as yet incomplete but have demonstrated that B-cell tolerance to Ars induced in neonatal mice last for at least 11 weeks.

We prepared an anti-idiotype to purified anti-Ars from normal A/J mice as described by Kuettner et al. (1972). The specificity of this anti-idiotype(Ars) was demonstrated in that it was not inhibitible by either normal A/J serum, by anti-Ars from which the anti-Ars antibody had been removed on an immunoadsorbent, nor by antisera directed against non-related haptenic determinants (i.e. anti-DNP). This anti-idiotype was shown to be partially site-specific in that it could be partially inhibited by the Ars hapten.

We then used this anti-idiotype(Ars) to determine the relative proportion of the total anti-Ars in the serum of Ars-tolerant mice that carried the crossreactive idiotype. This was carried out using an inhibition assay (Kuettner et al., 1972) containing 30 ng ^{125}I-anti-Ars and sufficient anti-idiotype(Ars) to bind 50% of the labele. Varying amounts of tolerant or normal anti-Ars antisera were added as inhibitors of this reaction and the nanograms of anti-Ars required to give 50% inhibition of the standard reaction was thus determined. The results are expressed as the ratio of tolerant anti-Ars:normal anti-Ars required to give this 50% inhibition. The results are shown in Figure 9. As can be seen the injection of Ars-DHGG resulted in the preferential loss of antibody bearing the crossreactive idiotype. Although such treatment with Ars-DHGG resulted in a four fold reduction in total anti-Ars, it resulted in as much as a 285 fold reduction in anti-Ars bearing the crossreactive idiotype. Mice immunized 1 day after the last injection of Ars-DHGG made a normal total anti-Ars response but produced a 23 fold lower quantity than did normal mice. Similarly mice which had recovered from tolerance, as assessed by their total anti-Ars response, still produced 10-25 fold less of the crossreactive idiotype. Indeed three wekks after the capacity to produce normal levels of total anti-Ars had returned the capacity to produce anti-Ars bearing the crossreactive idiotype was still ten fold less than normal.

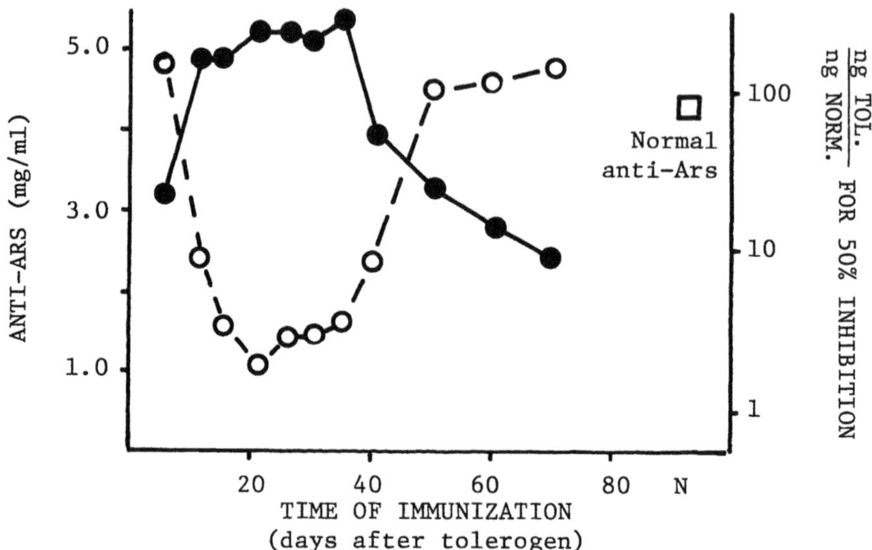

Figure 9. Preferential Loss of the Major Normal Crossreactive Idiotype during Tolerance to Ars Hapten. Conditions of the experiment were the same as in Figure 8, except that the relative proportion of anti-Ars from tolerant mice required to inhibit a standard anti-Ars- anti-idiotype reaction was determined. O--O, mg anti-Ars/ml serum; ●——●, ratio of nanograms anti-Ars from tolerant mice to that from normal mice required to give 50% inhibition of a standard reaction between ^{125}I-anti-Ars and anti-Idiotype(Ars) sufficient to bind 50% of the label.

Thus we have demonstrated a selective loss of the ability to produce a given B-cell clonal product within a given specificity, as the result of pretreatment with the tolerogenic form of an antigen. The selective loss of the ability to produce other forms of antibody have been demonstrated: a) allotype suppression (Herzenberg et al., 1973); b) carrier specific suppression of the ability to produce IgG antibody (Tada and Takemori, 1974); c) a selective loss of the ability to produce antibody of a given specificity in response to antigens bearing multiple, different, haptenic determinants (Stollar and Borel, 1975); and d) the selective loss of a given idiotype as the result of the injection of anti-idiotype (Hart et al., 1973).

What is the mechanism of the induction and maintenance of this hyporesponsive state to the Ars hapten? More specifically, what is the mechanism responsible for the selective loss of the ability to produce anti-Ars bearing the crossreactive idiotype? We do not think it is receptor blockade since Ars-DHGG treated mice that were immunized 1 day after the last tolerogen injection, produce normal quantities of anti-Ars although the do produce reduced level of anti-Ars with the crossreactive idiotype. This is true in spite of the fact that tolerogen has been present for 7 days and was at a greater concentration in the circulation than at later times when reduced total anti-Ars reponses were made. It is probably not due to differences in affinity of B-cells bearing receptors with the crossreactive idiotype as compared to those with receptors with other idiotypic specificities. Kapsalis et al. (1976) have shown that the anti-Ars with the crossreactive idiotype does not differ from other anti-Ars in affinity for the Ars hapten.

Active suppressor mechanisms would not seem to be involved. Indeed carrier HGG-specifc suppressor cells may have been activated as seen in adult-induced tolerance to HGG but their effect would have been by passed by immunization with Ars-KLH. Nonspecific suppressor cells are also ruled out since the hyporesponsiveness we have demonstrated to be specific. Ars-specific suppressor cells may have been induced but one would not expect their activity to be responsible for the selective loss of anti-Ars with the crossreactive idiotype. Idiotype specific suppressor cells remains a viable possibility. Ju et al. (1977) have shown suppressor T-cells to be responsible for anti-idiotype induced suppression in this anti-Ars system. However, the duration of the presence of such idiotype specific suppressor cells is quite different than that for the tolerance seen here and could account for the selective loss of the crossreactive idiotype but not for the reduction in total anti-Ars.

This would seem to leave clonal deletion and/or clonal abortion as possible mechanisms. However, neither of these would be expected to result in the preferential loss of certain clones. Indeed, several mechanisms, acting in concert, may be responsible for the results presented above: a) one resulting in elimination of B-cells regardless of the nature of their anti-Ars product, i.e. clonal deletion and/or clonal abortion; and b) one resulting in the selective loss of certain anti-Ars clones, i.e. idiotypic specific suppressor cells.

In summary we have demonstrated that the cellular parameters involved in tolerance to HGG induced in Adult mice are quite different than those of tolerance induced in neonatal mice. Although in the adult system, we do find specific suppressor cells, they do not seem to be required for the induction of tolerance in T-cells or in B-cells. Thus our results to date support the concept of clonal selection for the discrimination between self and non-self (Burnet, 1959). In addition, our results with the Ars tolerance system leads us to suspect that some very selective control mechanisms may be involved in the induction and maintenance of the tolerant state.

ACKNOWLEDGEMENTS

The excellent technical assistance over the years of Mrs. C.W. Hershey, Mr. E. Daniel Hershey, and Ms. Candace Johnson is gratefully appreciated. This work was supported by Grants AI10225 from the National Institutes of Health and BMS-75-09786 from the National Science Foundation. Dr. Benjamin is the recipient of Research Career Development Award AI00029 from the National Institutes of Health.

REFERENCES

Basten, A. (1974) in Immunological Tolerance: Mechanisms and Potential Therapeutic Applications. Eds. Katz, D.H. and Benacerraf, B. Academic Press, New York, P.107.

Benacerraf, B., Kapp, J.A., Debre, P., Pierce, C.W., and de la Croix, F. (1975) Transplant. Rev. 26, 21.

Benjamin, D.C. (1974) J. Immunol. 113, 1589.

Benjamin, D.C. (1975) J. Exp. Med. 141, 635.

Benjamin, D.C. (1977) J. Immunol. 118, 2125.

Benjamin, D.C. (1977a) J. Immunol. 119, 311.

Benjamin, D.C. and Weigle, W.O. (1970) J. Exp. Med. 132, 66.

Burnet, M. (1959) The Clonal Selection Theory of Acquired Immunity. Vanderbilt University Press, Nashville, Tenn.

Cambier, J.C., Kettman, J.R., Vitetta, E.S., and Uhr, J.W. (1976) J. Exp. Med. 144, 293.

Cantor, H., and Boyse, E.A. (1975) J. Exp. Med. 141, 1376.

Chiller, J.M., and Weigle, W.O. (1973) J. Immunol. 110, 1051.

Chiller, J.M., Louis, J.A., Skidmore, B.J., and Weigle, W.O. (1974) in Immunological Tolerance: Mechanisms and Potential Therapeutic Applications. Eds. Katz, D.H., and Benacerraf, B. Academic Press, New York, P. 373.

Doyle, M.V., Parks, D.E., and Weigle, W.O. (1976a) J. Immunol. 116, 1640.

Doyle, M.V., Parks, D.E., and Weigle, W.O. (1976b) J. Immunol. 117, 1152.

Halsey, J.F., and Benjamin, D.C. (1976) J. Immunol. 116, 1204.

Hart, D.A., Wang, A.L., and Nisonoff, A. (1972) J. Exp. Med. 135, 1293.

Hart, D.A., Pawlak, L.L., and Nisonoff, A. (1973) Eur. J. Immunol. 3, 44.

Herzenberg, L., Chan, E.L., Riblet, R.J., and Herzenberg, L. (1973) J. Exp. Med. 137, 1311.

Jones, T.B., and Kaplan, A.M. (1977) J. Immunol. 118, 1880.

Ju, S.T., Sato, S., and Nisonoff, A. (1977). Eur. J. Immunol. 7, 401.

Kapsalis, A.A., Tung, A.S., and Nisonoff, A. (1976) Immunochem. 13, 783.

Kuettner, M.G., Wang, A.L., and Nisonoff, A. (1972) J. Exp. Med. 135, 579.

Metcalf, E.S., and Klinman, N.R. (1976) J. Exp. Med. 143, 1327.

Mosier, D.E., and Johnson, B.M. (1975) J. Exp. Med. 141, 216.

Ruben, T.J., Chiller, J.M., and Weigle, W.O. (1973) J. Immunol. 111, 805.

Stollar, B.D., and Borel, Y. (1975) J. Immunol. 115, 1095.

Tada, T., and Takemori, T. (1974) J. Exp. Med. 140, 239.

Weigle, W.O., Chiller, J.M., and Habicht, G.S. (1971) in Progress in Immunology. Ed. Amos, B. Academic Press, New York, P.311.

RECOGNITION OF LYSOZYME BY LYMPHOCYTE SUBSETS

Robert J. Scibienski, Vicki Klingmann, Cherry Leung,
Karen Thompson, and Eli Benjamini
From the Department of Medical Microbiology, School of
Medicine, University of California, Davis

ABSTRACT

Extensive studies with antisera from a variety of animals have failed to detect any cross-reactivity between egg white lysozyme and its reduced, S-carboxymethylated (CM-) derivative. In contrast, a number of studies addressing the specificity of T lymphocytes have revealed that these two forms of lysozyme cross-react rather extensively at that level. Preliminary attempts to eliminate this latter cross-reactivity by further denaturation and/or chemical modification have so far proven unsuccessful. In a second line of experimentation the response to CM-lysozyme of mice which are genetically unresponsive to native lysozyme was assessed and found deficient. The implications of these findings are discussed.

INTRODUCTION

Over the course of the past decade there has appeared a significant number of papers which suggest basic differences in the manner in which T and B lymphocytes recognize antigen (Parkhouse and Dutton, 1967; Parish, 1971; Thompson et al., 1972; Dennert and Tucker, 1972; Parish, 1972; Scibienski et al., 1972; Schirrmacher and Wigzell, 1972; Playfair and Marchall-Clarke, 1973; Hoffmann and Kappler, 1973). These studies have all led to the conclusion that cross-reactivities which are weak or absent at the antibody level can be very strongly expressed at the T cell level. However, since the majority of such studies have been carried out with systems in which humoral cross-reactivity was low but not absent it has been difficult to assess whether the cellular cross-reactivities which have been observed are due to an enhanced expression of this minimal cross-reactivity or rather to T cell recognition of epitopes which are not perceived by B cells. This question is of considerable importance in view of its implications for T cell recognition of, and activation by, antigen.

Our own efforts have been concerned with the immune response to egg white lysozyme and its reduced/S-carboxymethylated derivative, CM-lysozyme. Over the past five years we have accumulated a considerable amount of information relative to the cross-reactivity of these two antigens at the B and T cell levels. We present here a synthesis of experiments which illustrate the system we have been studying, our attempts to come to grips with the question of the source of the differences we have observed, and preliminary attempts to more rigorously define and manipulate those differences.

METHODS

All methods utilized in the work presented here have been previously described (Thompson et al., 1972; Scibienski et al., 1972; Scibienski et al., 1974; Scibienski and Gershwin, 1977).

EXPERIMENTAL OBSERVATIONS

A. Serological Studies. Lysozyme and its reduced/S-carboxymethylated derivative, CM-lysozyme, do not cross-react at the serological level. As demonstrated in Figure 1a, murine antibodies specific for CM-lysozyme bind that antigen very well but fail to react with native lysozyme. Furthermore, as shown in Figure 1b, the binding between CM-lysozyme and its antibodies is inhibitable by CM-lysozyme but is not inhibited by native lysozyme even at high molar excesses. A similar picture is seen when one looks at the reverse situation. As shown in Figure 2a, although murine antisera specific for native lysozyme react rather well with CM-lysozyme when one looks at the ability of native and CM-lysozyme to inhibit this binding it becomes clear that in fact it does not represent cross-reactivity between the two antigens. As shown in Figure 2b, the binding between anti-native lysozyme and ^{125}I-CM lysozyme cannot be inhibited by native lysozyme whereas it is very effectively inhibited by CM-lysozyme. It thus appears that anti-native lysozyme contains antibodies which react exclusively with denatured lysozyme. Similar results have been obtained with antisera raised in rabbits and guinea pigs. This observation led us to conclude some years ago that emulsification of lysozyme in Freund's complete adjuvant resulted in some degree of denaturation of the antigen, a suggestion which was strengthened by the finding that antibodies raised against aqueous lysozyme do not bind with CM-lysozyme (Scibienski, 1973). We conclude from these studies that lysozyme and CM-lysozyme do not share any structures which are recognized by circulating antibodies.

B. Cell Mediated Immunity. In contrast to the above, native and denatured lysozyme appear to cross-react rather well at the T

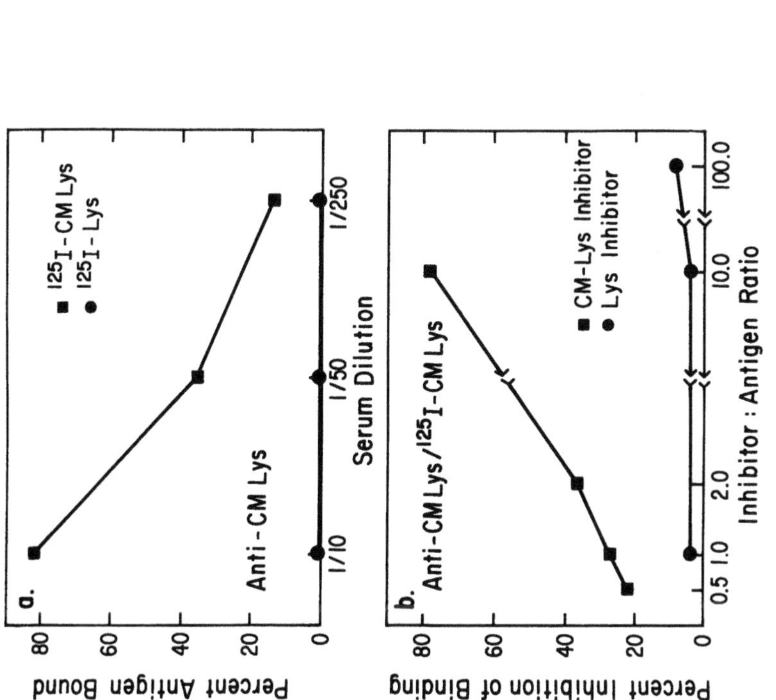

Figure 1. a) Binding of ^{125}I-lysozyme and ^{125}I-CM-lysozyme by mouse anti-CM-lysozyme. b) Inhibition of binding of ^{125}I-CM-lysozyme to anti-CM lysozyme by native and CM-lysozyme.

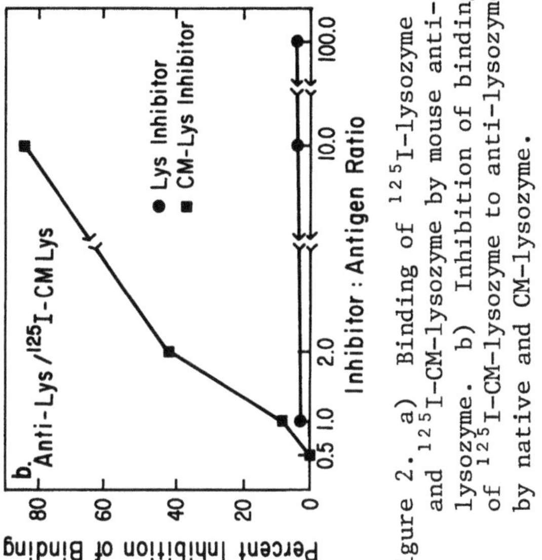

Figure 2. a) Binding of ^{125}I-lysozyme and ^{125}I-CM-lysozyme by mouse anti-lysozyme. b) Inhibition of binding of ^{125}I-CM-lysozyme to anti-lysozyme by native and CM-lysozyme.

cell level. As can be seen in Table I, guinea pigs immunized with native lysozyme give positive skin reactions when challenged with CM-lysozyme, and CM-lysozyme can cause inhibition of *in vitro* migration of peritoneal exudate cells from lysozyme immunized animals. Similar cross-reactivity was observed in guinea pigs immunized with CM-lysozyme and challenged with native lysozyme.

Table I

Cross-Reactivity of Native and CM-Lysozyme at the Level of Delayed Skin Reactivity and Migration Inhibition

Immunogen	Test Antigen	Skin Reactivity[1]	% Inhibition of Migration
Lysozyme	Lysozyme	8/8	60
"	CM-Lys	7/8	44
"	TMVP[2]	0/8	0
CM-Lys	Lysozyme	15/20	69
"	CM-Lys	15/20	73
"	TMVP	0/20	0
TMVP	Lysozyme	N.D.[3]	0
"	CM-Lys	N.D.	0

[1]Ratio of animals showing positive skin reactions (>10 mm).
[2]Tobacco mosaic virus protein, used as control.
[3]Not done.

In a second set of experiments we assessed the ability of the two forms of lysozyme to stimulate DNA synthesis in spleen cells derived from guinea pigs immunized to one or the other. As shown in Table II, cells from animals immunized with either responded equally well to both antigens.

In a third series of experiments we induced tolerance to either native or CM-lysozyme with the aid of cyclophosphamide and then assessed the ability of these animals to respond to either antigen. Lysozyme tolerant mice were found to be unable to respond to CM-lysozyme as well as to lysozyme, and CM-lysozyme tolerant mice were likewise unable to respond to either antigen (data not presented - see Thompson et al., 1972).

Table II

Cross-Reactivity of Native and CM-Lysozyme With Respect to Stimulation of DNA Synthesis by Sensitized Spleen Cells

Immunogen	Test Antigen	Stimulation[1] Ratio
Lysozyme	Lysozyme	4.2
"	CM-Lys	3.9
CM-Lys	Lysozyme	4.0
"	CM-Lys	5.5
TMVP	Lysozyme	1.0
"	CM-Lys	1.0

1 ^{14}C-thymidine counts incorporated in presence of antigen/ counts incorporated in absence of antigen

In a more recent series of experiments we have begun to assess the ability of CM-lysozyme to prime helper T cells specific for native lysozyme. (We have concentrated on CM-lysozyme as a priming antigen since any cross-reactivity in lysozyme primed mice is subject to the criticism of the presence of denatured antigen in FCA emulsions.) In performing these experiments we have taken advantage of the relative radioresistance of primed helper T cell function (Katz and Benacerraf, 1972). Thus, CAF_1 mice primed with native lysozyme in FCA and given 600r one month later do not respond to a second injection of lysozyme. However, as can be seen in Table III, when such animals are supplemented with anti-BAθ treated spleen cells from similarly primed, non-irradiated mice a good secondary PFC response is seen following challenge with lysozyme. A crucial observation is that identically manipulated mice primed with CM-lysozyme also respond well to challenge with native lysozyme.

The above results suggest that CM-lysozyme is capable of priming lysozyme specific helper cells. However, an important question which must be raised at this point is whether in fact the observed cross-priming is due to contamination of the denatured preparation with a serologically non-detectable but immunologically relevant quantity of native lysozyme. A perusual of our accumulated inhibition data reveals that one cannot rule out the presence of less than 1% of native lysozyme determinants in the denatured preparations. It therefore becomes important to determine what the threshold priming dose is for the native and denatured preparations. The results of

Table III

Ability of CM-Lysozyme to Prime Lysozyme Specific Helper Cells

Recipient Priming[1]	B cell Supplement[2]	Lysozyme Specific PFC/10^6 Spleen Cells (IgG)
Lysozyme	+	1811 $\pm$ 591
CM-Lys	+	4437 $\pm$ 1330
FCA	+	17 $\pm$ 5
Lysozyme	-	38 $\pm$ 36

[1]100 μg of the indicated antigen in FCA, administered 1 month prior to irradiation with 600r

[2]5 x 10^7 B cells (anti-mouse brain treated whole spleen from animals primed 1 month earlier with 100 μg lysozyme in FCA) intravenously within 6 hr of irradiation. Challenge with 100 μg aqueous lysozyme one day later, assay five days after challenge.

such a determination are presented in Figure 3. In Figure 3a it can be seen that when one compares the ability of decreasing but equivalent amounts of native and CM-lysozyme to prime lysozyme specific helper cells the activity of CM-lysozyme falls off much more rapidly than that of lysozyme. However, when one compares the priming activity of a given amount of CM-lysozyme with the activity of one percent of that amount of lysozyme (Figure 3b) it can be seen that the priming activity of low amounts of CM-lysozyme cannot possibly be accounted for by contamination with native lysozyme. (An interesting sidelight of these experiments is that as little as one picogram of native lysozyme was capable of priming detectable amounts of T cell help.)

A second line of evidence which rules out contamination of CM-lysozyme by native lysozyme as an explanation of the observed cellular cross-reactivity derives from experiments on neonatally induced tolerance to native lysozyme. As can be seen in Table IV, animals rendered tolerant by neonatal exposure to native lysozyme were also tolerant to CM-lysozyme. In contrast, mice identically exposed to one tenth that amount of lysozyme were not rendered tolerant. This latter finding rules out the possibility that the observed cross-tolerance is due to contamination of the tolerogen with denatured forms since inhibition studies reveal that the maximum possible level of denaturation of native lysozyme is 0.01% (maximum

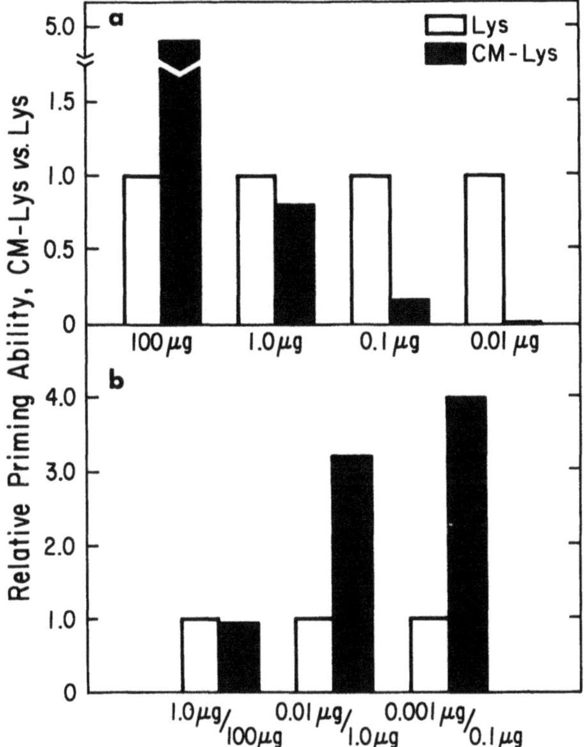

Figure 3. a) Comparison of the ability of equivalent amounts lysozyme and CM-lysozyme to prime lysozyme specific helper cells. b) Ability of several amounts of CM-lysozyme to prime lysozyme helper specific helper cells in comparison to the priming activity of 1% of that amount of native lysozyme.

of 10% inhibition at 1000/1 excess). The tolerance to CM-lysozyme must therefore represent a true cross-reactivity.

From the foregoing it seems clear that T cells can perceive common structure(s) between native and CM-lysozyme which do not elicit circulating antibodies. We have recently begun attempts to determine which region(s) of the molecule is involved by assessing the effect of certain chemical modifications on the cellular cross-reactivity. Presented in Table V are the results of an experiment in which mice were primed with either native or

CM-lysozyme, supplemented with lysozyme primed B cells, and then challenged with either native lysozyme or R-AZO-lysozyme. The rationale for this experiment was that if tyrosine and/or histidine were a component of the cross-reactive site(s) then one would expect to see a diminished secondary response to R-AZO-lysozyme, relative to native lysozyme, in the CM-lysozyme primed animals. In fact, however, there was no difference between the two.

Table IV

Cross-Tolerance Between Lysozyme and CM-Lysozyme

Neonatal[1] Treatment	Immunizing[2] Antigen	Responders[3]	Titer[4]
None	Lysozyme	11/11	16 ± 5
"	CM-Lys	9/9	4 ± 2
0.1 mg/20d	Lysozyme	4/4	6 ± 3
"	CM-Lys	N.D.	-
1.0 mg/20d	Lysozyme	3/10	.5 ± .3
"	CM-Lys	0/11	-

[1]Amount lysozyme administered per day/no. of days administered, commencing on first day of life
[2]100 μg in FCA at six weeks of age, 100 μg aqueous two weeks later
[3]Number animals responding/no. challenged
[4]ABC-33 of responders only, peak response

Table V

Reactivity of R-AZO-Lysozyme with CM-Lysozyme Primed Helper Cells

Priming Antigen (100 μg)	Challenge Antigen	PFC/10^6 Spleen Cells
Lysozyme	Lysozyme	3111 ± 1281
"	R-AZO-Lys	1817 ± 426
CM-Lys	Lysozyme	9978 ± 4362
"	R-AZO-Lys	8020 ± 1065
-	Lysozyme	122 ± 160
Recipient control		5 ± 6

In another experiment, the priming activity of various derivatives of CM-lysozyme, relative to native lysozyme, was assessed. The derivatives used were 1) a preparation which was precipitated from 4% SDS by absolute ethanol, 2) a preparation which was reacted with an equivalent weight of 2-hydroxy-5-nitrobenzyl bromide in 4% SDS and then precipitated as above, 3) a preparation which was reacted with 2-hydroxy-5-nitrobenzyl bromide and then azobenzene arsenate prior to precipitation as above, 4) a preparation which was reacted with an equivalent weight of trinitrobenzene sulfonate in SDS and isolated as above. As can be seen in Table VI, none of these derivatives was significantly reduced in priming activity relative to native lysozyme.

C. Response to CM-Lysozyme of Mice Non-Responsive to Lysozyme. Mice of $H2^b$ histocompatibility type are genetically non-responsive to a number of avian lysozymes, including that of the chicken (Hill and Sercarz, 1975). We therefore thought it would be of interest to assess the responsiveness of such mice to CM-lysozyme. We have performed two types of experiments in this regard. In one of these we asked whether CM-lysozyme is capable of priming lysozyme specific helper cells in $H2^b$ mice. C57Bl/6, A, or B_6AF_1 mice were primed with either lysozyme or CM-lysozyme, irradiated, and supplemented with lysozyme primed B cells derived from B_6AF_1 mice (Skidmore and Katz, 1977). The recipients were then challenged with native lysozyme and their response assessed. As shown in Table VII, both antigens primed lysozyme helper cells in responder A line mice but neither was capable of priming non-responder C57Bl/6 mice.

In another set of experiments we assessed the antibody responsiveness of responder (in this case CAF_1) and non-responder mice to both lysozyme and CM-lysozyme. These animals were primed with

Table VI

Priming of Lysozyme Helper Cells by CM-Lysozyme Derivatives

Priming Antigen	Challenge Antigen	PFC/10^6 Spleen Cells
Lysozyme	Lysozyme	1680 ± 729
SDS-CM-Lys	"	1340 ± 791
HNB-CM-Lys	"	986 ± 711
R-AZO:HNB-CM-Lys	"	870 ± 483
TNP-CM-Lys	"	853 ± 353
-	"	7 ± 2

Table VII

CM-Lysozyme Does Not Prime Lysozyme Helper Cells in Non Responder Mice

Strain	Priming Antigen	B Cell Source	PFC/10^6 Spleen Cells
BAF_1	Lysozyme	BAF_1	356 ± 322
BAF_1	Lysozyme	-	5 ± 9
BAF_1	-	BAF_1	2 ± 2
A	Lysozyme	BAF_1	60 ± 10
A	CM-Lys	BAF_1	127 ± 67
B6	Lysozyme	BAF_1	5 ± 0
B6	CM-Lys	BAF_1	7 ± 10

Table VIII

Response of CAF_1 and C57Bl/6 mice to Native and CM-lysozyme

Strain	Immunogen	Ratio of Animals Responding	Serum Titer[1]
CAF_1	Lysozyme	5/5	690
B6	Lysozyme	1/5	3.1
CAF_1	CM-Lys	5/5	84
B6	CM-Lys	0/10	-

[1]ABC-33 of responders only.

50 μg of antigen in FCA, challenged one month later with 100 μg aqueous antigen, and bled one week later. The results of this experiment are presented in Table VIII, where it can be seen that CAF_1 mice respond nicely to both native and CM-lysozyme, whereas C57Bl/6 respond to neither.

DISCUSSION

There exists a growing body of evidence in favor of the concept that B and T lymphocytes derive their specificity from the same V region pool (Black et al., 1976; Eichmann, 1977; Binz and Wigzell, 1977; Krawinkel et al., 1977). This would suggest that any specificity which is available to one cell line ought to be available to the other. However, it is clear from the evidence presented here that antibodies from a variety of sources fail to perceive any cross-reactivity between lysozyme and CM-lysozyme despite the fact that such cross-reaction is readily demonstrated at the helper T cell level (as pointed out in the introduction, there have been similar findings in a number of other experimental systems). Thus, in contrast to the above, the present data suggest that certain specificities are available to T cells which are not available to B cells. How can we reconcile the two sets of findings? One could argue that use of a common V region pool is not a universal phenomenon, or that the specificity of a particular V region might be altered by its environment. On the other hand it can also be argued that antibodies which recognize the cross-reactive site(s) are potentially available yet are never expressed. Such a situation could easily arise if activated helper cells were restricted in specificity to only one region of an antigen molecule. Viewed mechanistically, this would result in a lack of specific "help" for opposing determinants and thus B cells which recognize the region in question would never be induced. The question therefore reduces to one of how the T cell response might be limited.

We believe that severe strictions might be placed on the apparent T cell specificity of a response by the conditions required for helper cell induction. It is clear that such induction proceeds through presentation of antigen in association with macrophages (Shevach and Thomas, 1977). It also appears that antigen can be considerably degraded and still function in T cell activation (Erb et al., 1976). Given a small protein-like lysozyme it seems possible that only a small, stable "core" structure would escape such degrading, denaturing conditions as might arise during macrophage "processing" of antigen. The result of such an event would be that only those T cells which were specific for this region of the molecule would be induced. Thus, although T cells specific for other regions of the molecule might be available, they would not be activated. With respect to CM-lysozyme, such a stable core would also be expected to survive the denaturing conditions of reduction and alkylation. The end result of such a situation would be that native and CM-lysozyme would share a common determinant but that antibodies specific for this determinant would not be induced.

If the above explanation were true then one might expect to be able to denature CM-lysozyme to the point that it would no longer cross-react with native lysozyme at the T cell level. Two approaches we have taken are to subject the molecule to more rigorous denaturing conditions and/or to subject it to various chemical modifications. In the studies presented here, CM-lysozyme was dissolved in hot 4% SDS and then either directly precipitated by ethanol or chemically modified prior to precipitation. Two of the modifications which we utilized involved use of reagents which attack aromatic amino acids (diazonium salts and hydroxynitrobenzyl bromide). We chose these reagents because aromatic amino acids have been implicated in other studies of T cell specificity (Janeway et al., 1975) and were in fact somewhat surprised that these derivatives were still highly cross-reactive with native lysozyme. With respect to the lack of effect on the cross-reactivity of treatment with SDS, it is possible that the putative "core" determinant is stable to such treatment. An alternative possibility is that we are dealing with a true primary structure determinant. Further studies on this question are currently in progress.

A second, very interesting aspect of the cross-reactivity between native and CM-lysozyme concerns the unresponsiveness of $H2^b$ mice to CM-lysozyme. It has previously been shown that such mice are non-responsive to native lysozyme and that the defect is H2 linked (Hill and Sercarz, 1975). It has also been shown that $H2^b$ mice have functional, lysozyme specific B cells (Hill et al., 1976). In experiments of our own (to be published) we have shown that $H2^b$ mice are capable of responding to lysozyme complexed with LPS, a response which is thymus-dependent in other strains of mice (Scibienski and Gershwin, 1977). These findings raise the possibility that active suppression may be involved in this system, a possibility for which other evidence also exists (E. Sercarz, personal communication). If this possibility can be corraborated then the fact that the non-responsiveness is also expressed for CM-lysozyme may prove to be a very useful finding. For example, one could could then ask whether the same determinant(s) accounts for helper cell activity in responder strains and suppressor cell activity in non-responder strains.

An alternative explanation of the non-responsiveness of $H2^b$ mice to lysozyme has been one in which the phenomenon was attributed to the enzymatic activity of this protein. The possibility existed that $H2^b$ determined carbohydrates, crucial to immune responsiveness, were susceptible to blockage and/or degradation by lysozyme. In view of the fact that CM-lysozyme is enzymatically inactive this possibility would now appear to be untenable.

In conclusion, the data presented here strongly support the notion that there exist certain antigenic structures, as defined by T cell recognition, for which antibodies are never produced. Aside from the implication which this has *vis a vis* the use of antibodies to define molecular relatedness, this finding implies that significant restrictions can be imposed on the specificity of immune responses by the conditions required for their induction. Whether these effects obtain exactly as proposed herein or by some other mechanism remains to be seen. However, it seems clear that in the future such effects should be taken into account when drawing conclusions from studies of immune specificity.

REFERENCES

Binz, H., and Wigzell, H., (1977) J. Supramolec. Structure, Suppl. 1, 222.
Black, S.J., Hammerling, G.J., Berek, C., Rajewsky, K., and Eichmann, K., (1976) J. Exp. Med. 143, 846.
Dennert, G., and Tucker, D.F., (1972) J. Exp. Med. 136, 656.
Eichmann, K., (1977) J. Supramolec. Structure, Suppl. 1, 214.
Erb, P., Feldman, M., and Hogg, N., (1976) Eur. J. Immunol. 6, 365.
Hill, S.W., and Sercarz, E., (1975) Eur. J. Immunol. 5, 317.
Hill, S.W., Yowell, R.L., Kipp, D.E., Scibienski, R.J., and Sercarz, E.E., (1976) Adv. Exp. Med. and Biol. 66, 537.
Hoffmann, M., and Kappler, J.W., (1973) J. Exp. Med. 137, 721.
Janeway, C.A., Cohen, B.E., Ben-Sasson, S.Z., and Paul, W.E. (1975) J. Exp. Med. 141, 42.
Katz, D.H., and Benacerraf, B., (1972) Adv. Immunol. 15, 2.
Krawinkel, U., Cramer, M., Mage, R., Kelus, A., and Rajewsky, K., (1977) J. Exp. Med. 146, 792.
Parish, C.R., (1971) J. Exp. Med. 134, 21.
Parish, C.R., (1972) Eur. J. Immunol. 2, 143.
Parkhouse, R.M.E., and Dutton, R.W., (1967) Immunochem. 4, 431.
Playfair, J.H.L. and Marshall-Clarke, S., (1973) Immunology 24, 579.
Schirrmacher, V., and Wigzell, H., (1972) J. Exp. Med. 136, 1616.
Scibienski, R., Fong, S., and Benjamini, E., (1972) J. Exp. Med. 136, #5, 1308.
Scibienski, R.J., (1973) J. Immunology 111, #1, 1973.
Scibienski, R.J., Harris, L.M., Fong, S., and Benjamini, E., (1974) J. Immunology 113, #1, 45.
Scibienski, R.J., and Gershwin, M.E. (1977) J. Immunol. 119, 504.
Shevach, E.M., and Thomas, D.W., (1977) J. Supramolec. Structure, Suppl. 1, 200.
Skidmore, B.J., and Katz, D.H., (1977) J. Immunol. 119, 694.
Thompson, K., Harris, M., Benjamini, E., Mitchell, G., and Noble, M., (1972) Nature New Biology 238, #79, 20.

DISCUSSION

Marc Feldmann

Imperial Cancer Research Fund
Department of Zoology, University College
London, England

It appears that we have at this meeting two groups of people, both interested in the immunobiology of peptides and proteins, chemists, who are interested in using immunological techniques for knowing much more about the chemistry of antigens and immunologists that want to use chemical tools for knowing much more about the mechanisms of the immune response. And from the discussion or rather the lack of dicsussion so far, we could almost suggest that these two goals are mutually irreconcilable. But I don't think that this is so. What has been missing so far is an awareness of how difficult the problem really is. The first problem discussed yesterday, of how to use immunochemical and chemical approaches to study the structure of determinants. An antigenic determinant is the product of a very complex interaction. The structure of the antigen with some chemical groups exposed, and some not is faced with an animal's recognition system. This recognition system is a product of multiple gene clusters, the immunoglobulin variable genes, the Ir genes of various types. What is going to be recognized as the major determinant is a complex function of that particular function with two sets of variables. The elegant chemical studies which have been performed to define determinants are really only a beginning of such an approach. With outbred rabbits it is possible to identify determinants, but these may be only a part of the whole spectrum of determinants which may be recognized. The use of multiple inbred species is critical to define the role of Ir genes in immune recognition and in defining which are the important determinants as J. Berzofsky has done. The other question that has been discussed several times is the relative specificity of T cells and B cells. What do T cells and B cells recognize? A lot of data has been presented, and there is an enormous literature going back for years Unfortunately, none of the approaches used can focus on the key questions: the types of recognition structures there are on T cells, and their total repertoire. While some approach to knowing the repertoire in B cells has been started, techniques for looking at the repertoire of T cells are still so primitive. For example, there is a lot of evidence now in several systems for cross-reactive idiotypes shared between T cells and B cells. Unfortunately, since we do not know the precise location of idiotypic determinants in these cases we really do not know what these idiotypic cross-reactions really mean. However, all of these idiotypic determinants are linked to allotypes which tells us that both T cells and B cells and presumably all their different subtypes draw their recognition structures from the same total pool of V genes. If we accept this and we know that the B cell pool is very heterogeneous in the absence of having a precise way of measuring specificity of T cell receptors, in most systems all we can measure is the specificity of induction, whereas we measure B cell product specificity, it is not surprising that every possible result has been reported. In most systems only a small number of the total possible clones respond. Thus it is probably surprising that there are examples of identical specificity. With our techniques it is not possible to evaluate the exact repertoire.

What is more interesting, if we accept that the genetic pool from which the receptors are derived is the same for all lymphocytes is to ask what are the differences between the different types of T cells and B cells, and how do these arise. There are rather clear cut differences, which are probably due not so much to receptual sites themselves but to how the different sets of T or B cells are stimulated. There is a literature which has expanded greatly in the last year or two about how the products of the major histocompatibility complex are involved in lymphocyte recognition, and I think here it is important to point out that B cells appear to have minimal direct recognition of MHC structures in the way that the T helper or DHS cells do. Here is immediately important information why there must be a difference in the precise specificity of the recognition function between the various systems but not necessarily of the receptor.

Another problem investigated by immunochemical techniques has been the nature of the mechanisms of induction by using synthetic peptides and antigens. Joel Goodman and others have performed very elegant experiments, using multiple variants of immunogens. The problems of interpreting the results are substantial because the stimulation of most T cell responses requires at least dual recognition. All T cell responses appear to involve interaction between two T cells, and almost always (with one possible exception) macrophages as well. The work of Rosenthal, Shevach and others that indicates that immune specific immune response genes can be expressed in the macrophage. Thus for most T cell recognition systems we are really measuring a complex function of three recognition structures. This is in clear contrast to the observation with B cells assaying antibody, and explains why there is so much conflicting data on the mechanism of stimulation, about what these various chemical approaches tell us, and certainly about the different specificities of the various T cells and B cells. If we can begin to understand the basis of the assays we use, then it should be possible to understand the effect of various biochemical modifications; and this will make the immunobiological approach of importance in the future.

Immunobiology of Protein Conjugates

COMPLEXITY OF CELL INTERACTIONS: ANALYSIS USING ANTIGENS UNDER Ir GENE CONTROL

M. Baltz, P. Erb, M. Feldmann, S. Howie, S. Kontiainen, and A. Torano

ICRF Tumour Immunology Unit, Department of Zoology, University College London, and Institute of Microbiology, University of Basel

ABSTRACT

The properties of three I region associated immunoregulatory factors involved in cell interactions are described. These are antigen specific T helper factor, suppressor factor produced by metabolically active T cells and genetically restricted factor, which is produced by macrophages and is involved in T helper cell induction. The use of these factors to analyse cell interactions is discussed.

INTRODUCTION

The nature of I region control of immune responses is not fully understood and there has been much speculation on the role of Ir (immune response) gene products in the control of immune

---

Abbreviations:

(T,G)-A--L: poly L (Tyr,glu)-poly DL-Ala--poly-L-Lys. (Phe,G)-A--L: poly L (Phe,glu)-poly DL-Ala--poly-L-Lys. (H,G)-A--L: poly(His,glu) -poly DL-Ala--poly-L-Lys. (T,G)-Pro--L: poly(Tyr,glu)-poly-Pro--poly-L-Lys. GLPhe: L-glutamic acid,L-lysine,L-phenylalanine. KLH: keyhole limpet haemocyanin. DNP: dinitrophenyl(ated). AFC: antibody forming cell. HC: helper cell. $HC_{(T,G)-A--L}$: (T,G)-A--L specific helper cell. HF: helper factor. $HF_{(T,G)-A--L}$: (T,G)-A--L specific helper factor. SC: suppressor cell. $SC_{(T,G)-A--L}$: (T,G)-A--L specific suppressor cell. SF: suppressor factor. $SF_{(T,G)-A--L}$: (T,G)-A--L specific suppressor factor. GRF: genetically restricted factor.

responses. We are currently examining I region control as a probe for the greater understanding of the cell interactions involved in antibody production. The soluble mediators of these interactions often bear Ia determinants and/or are partially coded for by the I region of the major histocompatibility complex (MHC). Several factors have been described by us in Erb et al. 1976, Howie and Feldmann 1977, Feldmann and Basten 1972, Kontiainen and Feldmann 1977, Feldmann et al. 1977, and by others (Munro and Taussig 1975, Rich and Rich 1976, Tada et al. 1976, Taniguchi et al. 1976, Schimpl and Wecker 1972, Theze et al. 1977). We will describe here factors produced by T lymphocytes (helper factor, suppressor factor), and macrophages (genetically restricted factor, GRF), and how we are using them to gain a better understanding of Ir gene control. The possibility that some or all of these are the soluble products of Ir genes will be discussed.

MATERIALS AND METHODS

All techniques used have been published elsewhere (Erb et al. 1976, Howie and Feldmann 1977, Kontiainen and Feldmann 1973, 1977).

RESULTS AND DISCUSSION

Helper Factor (HF)

There are several reports on the production of a factor(s) which can specifically circumvent the requirement for T cells to help B cells produce antibody (Howie and Feldmann 1977, Munro and Taussig 1975). Described below are observations on in vitro produced HF (Howie and Feldmann 1977). The majority of our recent work on HF has been done using (T,G)-A--L as an antigen, but HF to GAT, KLH and GLPhe (see below) have also been produced and have analogous properties. Production of such factors has been described in detail elsewhere (Howie and Feldmann 1977, Kontiainen and Feldmann 1977, Baltz et al. submitted); briefly it involves a four-day culture period of normal spleen cells or purified T cells and antigen in Marbrook-Diener flasks, first to produce helper cells and then for a further one-day period with fresh antigen; the cell free supernatant is used as a source of 'helper factor'. The capacity of HF to stimulate primary or secondary antibody responses is tested in a second Marbrook-Diener culture system. Munro and Taussig used a six hour supernatant (HF_{vivo}) produced <u>in vitro</u> from <u>in vivo</u> 'educated thymocytes', which were then injected together with antigen and bone marrow cells into X-irradiated recipients in order to obtain anti-(T,G)-A--L antibody forming cells. They reported that the production of HF was under the control of the I-A subregion, and the response of B cells to $HF_{(T,G)-A--L}$ was also under the control of this region. Since some non-responders made

HF and other non-responders responded to it, two gene control was postulated and proven by complementation experiments, where F_1 crosses of the different types of non-responders yielded responder mice (Munro and Taussig 1975).

We are analysing a similar if not identical factor which is produced entirely _in vitro_ (HF_{VITRO}) and is highly active (Fig. 1). Both factors are Ia positive, can act across allogeneic barriers and do not contain stably bound antigen fragments as judged by the inability of anti-(T,G)-A--L immunoadsorbents to remove the activity (Howie and Feldmann 1977, Mozes et al. 1975). However, the factors contain an antigen binding site (i.e. factors bind to (T,G)-A--L immunoadsorbents but not to other antigens, even if closely related (Isac and Mozes 1977)).

The factors appear to differ in fine antigenic specificity and in some biochemical properties which could reflect technical differences. Isac and Mozes, using HF_{VIVO} found that (T,G)-A--L HF cross reacts with (H,G)-A--L and (Phe,G)-A--L since factors produced in response to any of the three antigens could cooperate with B cells for antibody production to the homologous or the heterologous antigens (Isac and Mozes 1977). Since antibodies to (T,G)-A--L, (H,G)-A--L and (Phe,G)-A--L show cross reactivity, the specificity of HF_{VIVO} appears to be similar to that of antibody. Using HF_{VITRO}, our results show that (T,G)-A--L specific HF will help DNP specific B cells produce antibody if challenged with DNP-(T,G)-A--L, but not if challenged with DNP-(H,G)-A--L or DNP-(Phe,G)-A--L (Table 1). This suggests that HF has a different specificity from that of antibody.

There are many possible reasons for this difference. The one we favour is that factor preparations are relatively oligoclonal, and that depending on the exact spectrum of clones stimulated the cross reactivity varies. Cultured cells may be in a somewhat unfavourable milieu, so that only the highest affinity (specificity) cells are triggered to produce helper cells and factors. The suggestive evidence for oligoclonality is based on a report by Mozes on the ability to make an anti-idiotype antiserum which, while reacting with only 18 -30% of anti-(T,G)-A--L antibody absorbs all HF_{VIVO} and our work (Kontiainen and Feldmann, unpublished) which indicates that a mouse anti-SF_{KLH} can be made which functionally absorbs out the great majority of the SF_{KLH}. Other arguments for this concept are detailed elsewhere (Feldmann, in preparation).

HF_{VIVO} does not bind to anti-Ig immunoadsorbents but has been reported to contain immunoglobulin idiotypic determinants (Mozes 1977). It is not known if HF_{VITRO} also contains idiotypic determinants, although it does bind to a chicken anti-MOPC 104E immunoadsorbent. However, the specificity of this chicken antiserum has

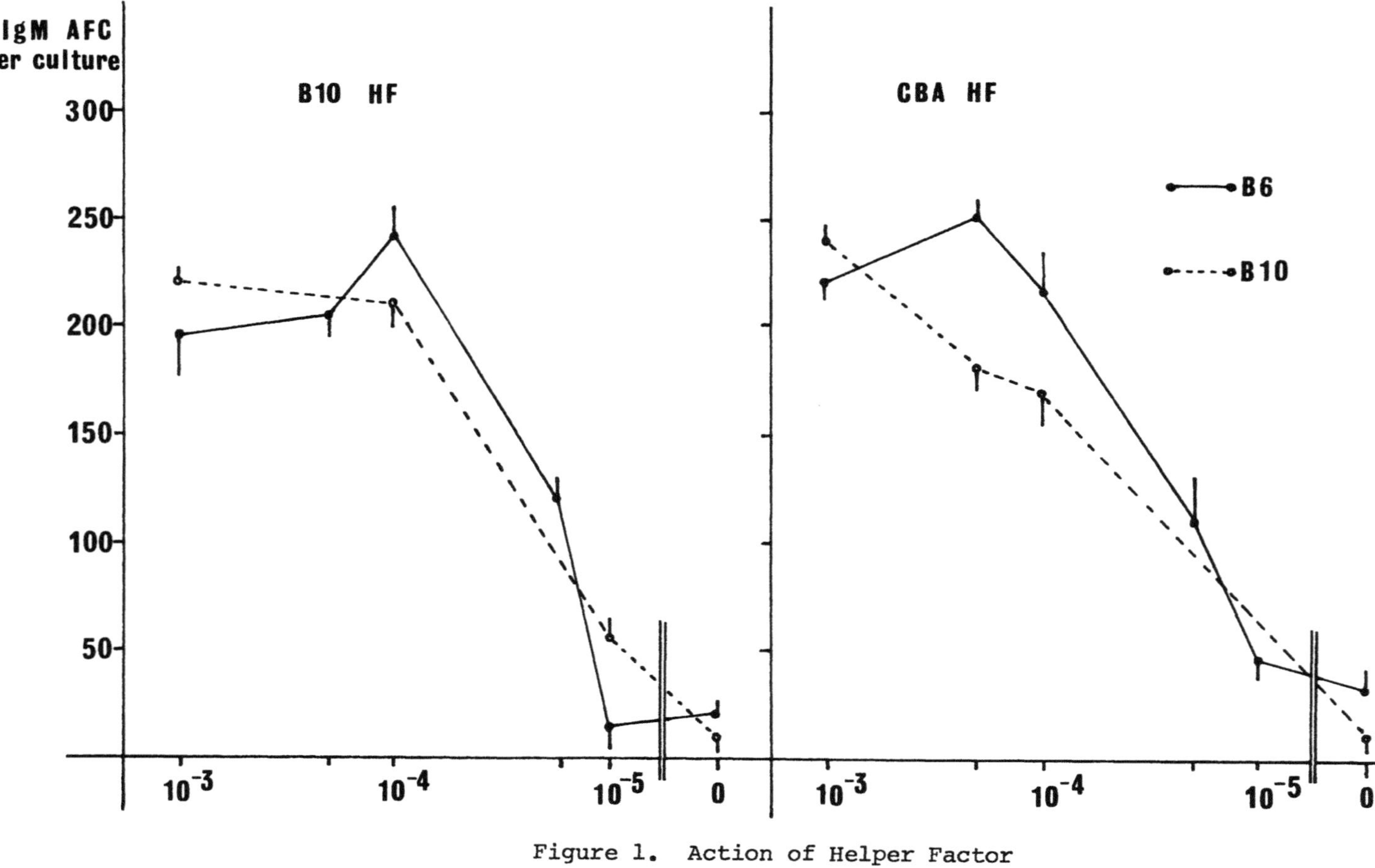

Figure 1. Action of Helper Factor

TABLE 1

SIMILAR SPECIFICITY OF HELPER CELLS AND HELPER FACTOR

Cells	Stimulus (HC/HF)	Response (AFC/Culture) to		
		DNP-TGAL	DNP-PheGAL	DNP-TGProL
B6 spleen	Nil	10 ± 6	7 ± 7	13 ± 3
"	B6 HC_{TGAL}	190 ± 6	13 ± 9	17 ± 7
"	B10 HF_{TGAL}	210 ± 20	30 ± 10	27 ± 9
	CBA HF_{TGAL}	180 ± 6	33 ± 6	30 ± 12
B10 spleen	Nil	-	30 ± 12	13 ± 9
"	B10 HC_{TGProL}	-	-	250 ± 45
"	B10 HC_{PheGAL}	-	223 ± 9	-

Factor used 1:200

not been fully characterised, as it has not been ruled out that carbohydrate and not Ig determinants are recognised; this question is relevant to those determinants recognised on 'IgT' by anti-Ig (Feldmann and Basten 1972).

What Cells Express (T,G)-A--L Ir Genes?

Taussig and Munro classified non-responder mice to (T,G)-A--L as having either a B or a T cell defect, or a defect in both cell types (Munro and Taussig 1975). The basis for the classification was the assumption that the lack of helper factor production implies a T cell defect, and lack of response to helper factor is caused by a B cell defect. Their experiments did not rule out a defect at the level of the macrophages, as this was not examined. There is increasing evidence to suggest that one functional site for Ir gene expression may be at the level of the macrophage (Feldmann 1977, Rosenthal et al. 1977). All T-dependent Ir controlled responses thus far described are macrophage dependent; both helper cell induction and subsequent HF production requires macrophage (Erb and Feldmann 1974, Howie et al. unpublished) and HF action on B cells also requires macrophages (Feldmann 1972, Howie and Feldmann 1977). Thus, an Ir gene defect expressed at the macrophage level could be simply misinterpreted as a T cell or a B cell defect. Using HF_{VITRO} we have classified non-responders as to what appears to be T cell and/or B cell defects. It was of interest that the results of this classification with HF_{VITRO} yielded the same strain distribution (Howie and Feldmann 1977) as previously described with HF_{VIVO} (Munro and Taussig 1975). This is a potent genetic argument that despite some differences (summarised in Feldmann et al. 1977b) the two factors are closely related, if not identical. We are now initiating studies to more closely examine Ir gene defects at the macrophage level.

The effect of macrophage depletion and reconstitution on the ability of (T,G)-A--L HF_{VITRO} to cooperate with F_1 (responder x non-responder) B cells was tested. HF_{VITRO} required macrophages for its action on B cells since F_1 spleen cells depleted of macrophages gave no PFC response to (T,G)-A--L. The responder status of these cells was analysed, by reconstituting with various macrophages. Parental (responder) or F_1 macrophages reconstituted the response whereas non-responder parental macrophages did not. These results suggest the macrophage may be one site for Ir gene expression. However, additional experiments must be done using anti-T cell and complement treated peritoneal exudate cells as a macrophage source to exclude 'suppressive effects' in the non-responder-parental /F_1 combination.

Another indication of Ir genes operating at the macrophage level is the finding that PEC (anti-T cell treated and complement treated) can absorb HF. However, both responder and non-responder macrophages absorb out HF equally, indicating that both have receptors. However, only responder macrophages stimulate B cells for antibody production, and then only if the absorption of HF is performed in the presence of antigen. These results clearly indicate that there is an active macrophage role in the antigen specific induction of B cells.

One observation not yet fully understood regarding the mechanism of action of HF is the following: spleen cells from <u>responder</u> strains or strains with functional B cells challenged in vitro with DNP-(T,G)-A--L and $HF_{(T,G)-A--L}$ produce both anti-DNP and anti-(T,G)-A--L PFC whereas <u>non-responder</u> strains with functional helper factor produce only anti-DNP responses when challenged in a similar manner (Figure 2).

A similar observation has been reported by others (Mozes and Shearer 1971). Thus the simplified concept of non-responsiveness to (T,G)-A--L as being only due to lack of T cell HF production, or of B cells lacking receptors for HF (Munro and Taussig 1975) is regrettably too simple, and needs to be redefined in a more complex manner.

IgM AFC per cult.
300
250
200
150
100
50
B10 HR
B10.A LR
anti-DNP ○·····○ DNP-TGAL
anti-TGAL △- - -△ DNP-TGAL
anti-TGAL ●——● TGAL
10^{-2}
10^{-3}
10^{-4}
10^{-5}
0
concentration of B10 helper factor

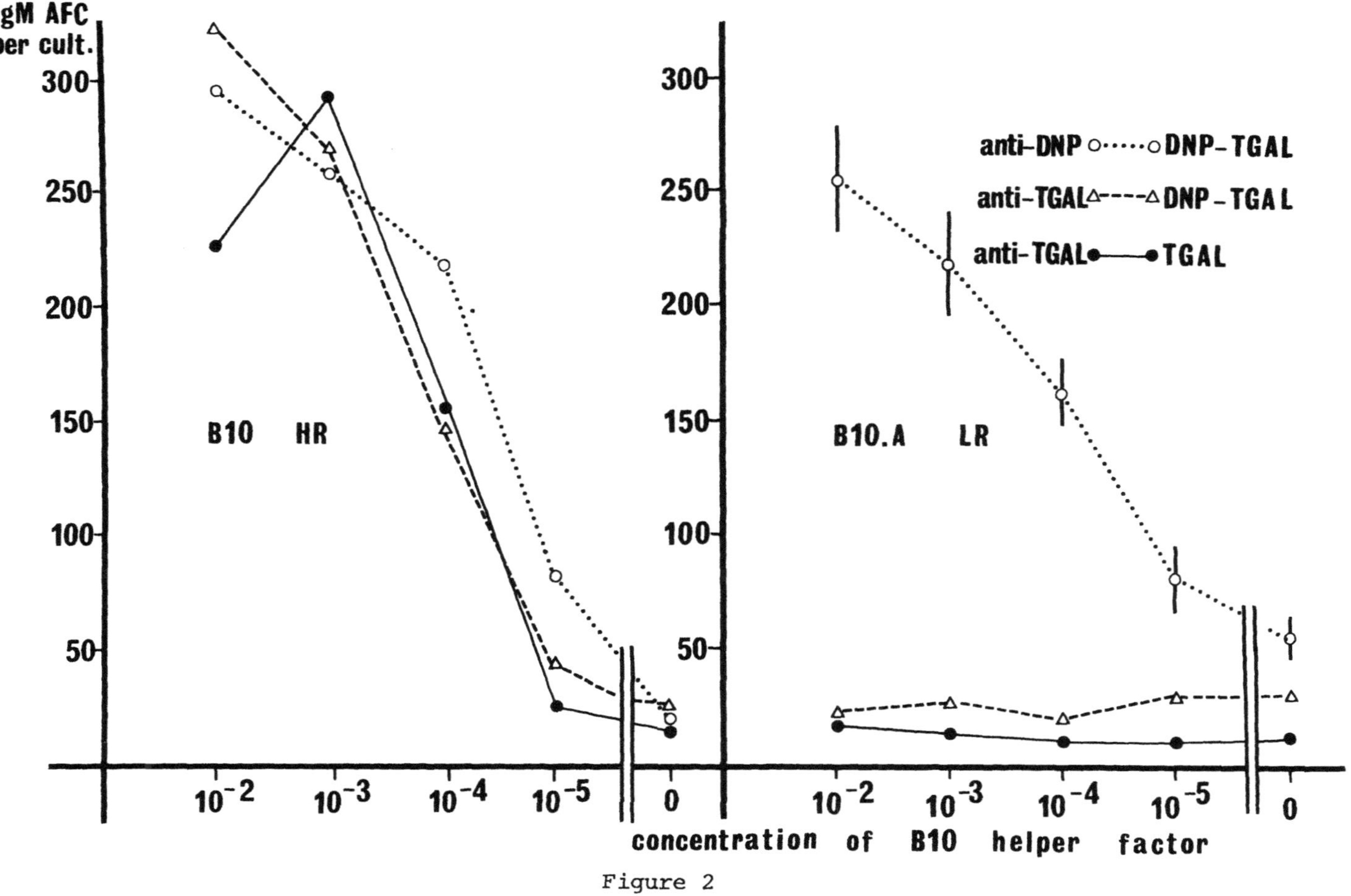

Figure 2

GLPhe Helper Factor

Complementation of at least two Ir gene products from the I-A and I-C subregions are required for antibody responses and T proliferative responses to the synthetic terpolymer, GLPhe (Dorf et al. 1975, Warner et al. 1977). There are data which suggest that both gene products must be expressed on the same cell for response (Schwartz et al. 1976, Katz et al. 1976, Warner et al. 1977). However neither the cellular site(s) of the non-responder defect nor their mechanism of action is fully understood. For this reason, an analysis of the GLPhe response using HF was attempted, since HF_{GLPhe} has not been described previously; responder/non-responder status was based on either T proliferative responses or serum antigen binding capacity. We have succeeded in producing HF_{GLPhe} and are using it to analyse the cellular site(s) of GLPhe-Ir gene products and their mechanism (Baltz et al. submitted).

We used a GLPhe PFC response induced by HF_{GLPhe}. Experiments were done to determine if either I-A or I-C subregion codes for HF_{GLPhe} production or HF_{GLPhe} acceptor site (as has been done using $HF_{(T,G)-A--L}$). The strain distribution patterns of GLPhe responses did not correlate with published data on *in vivo* findings based on serum antigen binding capacity tests or on *in vitro* T cell proliferation responses. $I\text{-}A^k$ allele has been classed as a GLPhe non-responder; however, we found that spleen cells from $I\text{-}A^k$ strains tested (B10.A, B10.BR, CBA) produced HF_{GLPhe^5} and responded to it (Figure 3). *In vivo* data using CBA mice primed and boosted with $GLPhe^5$ produced substantial anti-GLPhe PFC responses. Thus by our criteria, $I\text{-}A^k$ behaves as a responder allele. There are reports that $H\text{-}2^k$ haplotypes exhibit primary responses of 0 to 47% antigen binding capacity (Merryman et al. 1972, Merryman et al. 1975). This is a pertinent point to be clarified since $I\text{-}A^k$ has been used extensively in gene complementation studies; these may need reinterpretation if $I\text{-}A^k$ is a responder to GLPhe. As yet, we have been unable to map to I-A or I-C subregions defects in either the ability to produce HF_{GLPhe} or in the capacity to respond to it.

We have used both $GLPhe^5$ and $GLPhe^9$ in our study. An interesting finding is that B10 mice ($I\text{-}A^b$, $I\text{-}C^b$) neither produce HF_{GLPhe^5} nor respond to it but do produce HF_{GLPhe^9}. Discrimination between $GLPhe^9$ and $GLPhe^5$ has been reported in $H\text{-}2^p$ mice using serum antigen binding capacity tests (Maurer, unpublished). Thus, the GLPhe Ir gene mechanism is by no means clear. It will be of interest to ascertain whether the I-A and I-C gene products determine responses to GPhe or GL determinants on the molecule which could account for the hitherto ambiguous findings. Furthermore, these results emphasise the need to think of Ir genes as regulator genes, rather than absolute determinants of responsiveness.

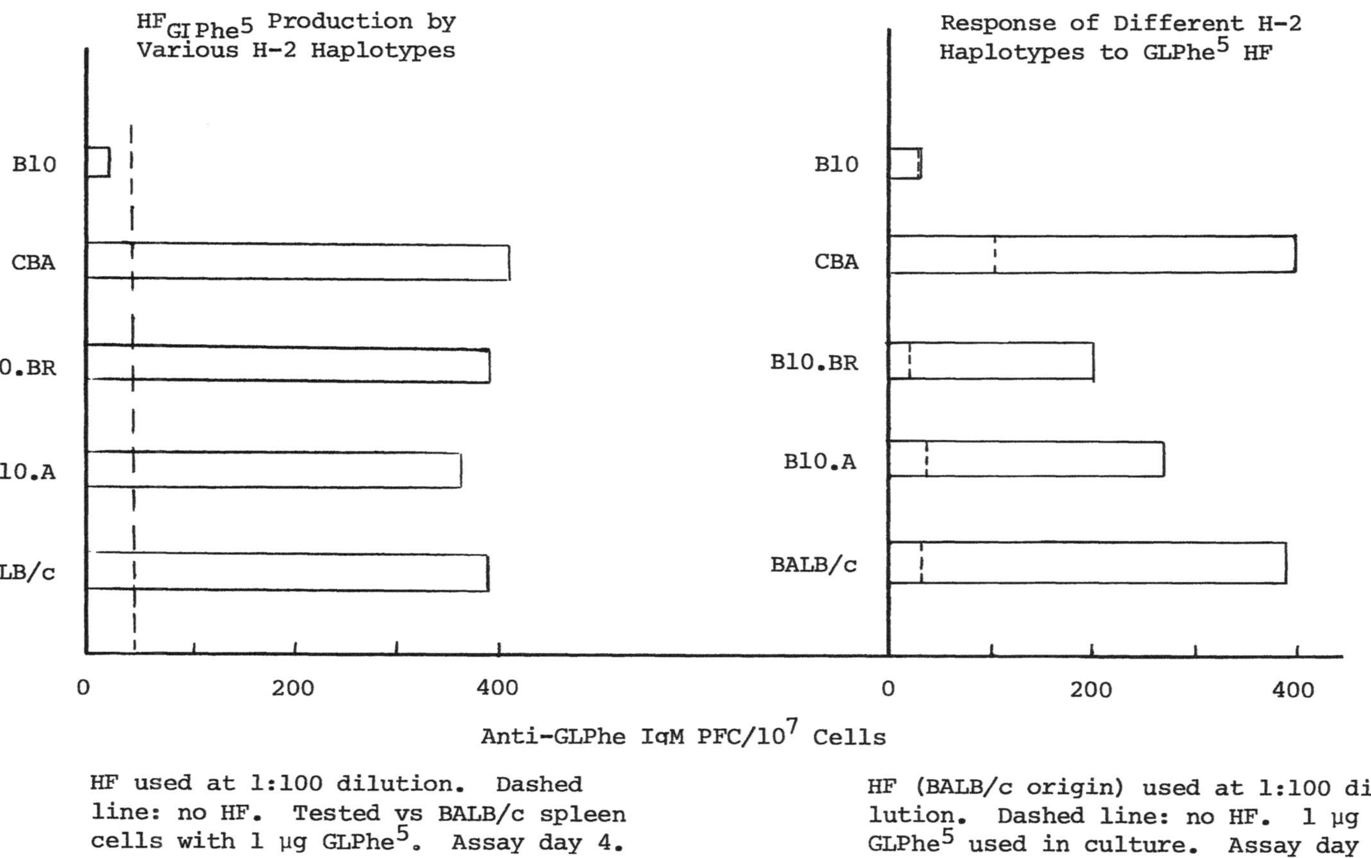

HF used at 1:100 dilution. Dashed line: no HF. Tested vs BALB/c spleen cells with 1 µg $GLPhe^5$. Assay day 4.

HF (BALB/c origin) used at 1:100 dilution. Dashed line: no HF. 1 µg $GLPhe^5$ used in culture. Assay day 4.

Figure 3

Suppressor Factor (SF)

There are numerous reports of suppressive factors or extracts produced by T cells. Factors described by Tada et al. (1976), Taniguchi et al. (1976) and Theze et al. (1977) are extracts of sonicated thymocytes or spleen cells from primed mice. These factors suppress both *in vivo* and *in vitro* IgG, but not IgM responses. The factors are of ∿ 50,000 daltons MW, bear Ia determinants (I-J subregion) and are produced by Ly-2^+3^+ T cells. Their site of action appears to be a T cell, probably of Ly-2^+3^+ phenotype, which interacts with a Ly-$1^+2^+3^+$ to generate more suppressor cells (Tada, personal communication). Some suppressor extracts require I-J homology for action (Tada et al. 1976, Taniguchi et al. 1976) while others do not (Theze et al. 1977).

We have produced SF *in vitro* from metabolically active T cells after challenge with high doses of antigen (Kontiainen and Feldmann 1977). Induction of SC and subsequent SF production requires interaction between two T cells, a SC amplifier (Ly-$1^+2^+3^+$Ia$^-$) and a SC precursor (Ly-$1^-2^+3^+$Ia$^-$) (Feldmann et al. 1977a). SC induction is not dependent on macrophages (or at least needs many fewer macrophages than HC induction) (Feldmann and Kontiainen 1976). SF bears Ia determinants (likely to be of the I-J subregion using KLH as antigen) and is produced by Ly-2^+3^+ T cells (Kontiainen and Feldmann 1977). No H-2 restriction in its action has been found, and unlike suppressor extract, both IgM and IgG responses (*in vivo* and *in vitro*) are suppressed. Its target site is a nylon wool non-adherent, Ly-1^+ T cell, presumably an HC; SF does not act on HF (Table 2) (Kontiainen and Feldmann 1977a). Obviously, the relation of suppressor extracts to SF must be clarified for understanding the role of SF or suppressor extracts in I region control.

Genetically Related Factor (GRF) from Macrophages

The role that macrophages and macrophage derived factors play in genetic control of responses is not well understood. One factor, GRF is produced by macrophages, acts on T_1 lymphocytes (short-lived T cells) and induces them to become helper cells (HC) (Erb et al. 1976). Thus GRF can replace the requirement for intact macrophages in HC induction (2-mercaptoethanol cannot substitute for GRF). GRF is a complex of ∿ 55,000 daltons MW and bears extrinsic antigen and Ia determinants (Erb et al. 1976). The ability to produce GRF is coded for by the I-A subregion, as is the acceptor site for GRF on T_1 cells (Erb et al. 1976a). Thus, at least two gene products within the I-A are required for the production and action of GRF. There is also a requirement for I-A compatibility between macrophages producing GRF and T_1 cells upon which it acts; GRF unlike HF or SF, does not act across allogeneic barriers.

TABLE 2

LACK OF EFFECT OF SF ON HELPER FACTOR (HF) STIMULATED RESPONSES

Stimulus HC/HF	Stimulus Antigen	Suppression	Response anti-DNP-AFC/Culture ± SE
-	TNP-KLH	-	50 ± 25
CBA HC_{KLH}	"	-	677 ± 13
"	"	CBA SF_{KLH} 10%	130 ± 12
CBA HF_{KLH} 0.1%	"	-	257 ± 79
"	"	CBA SF_{KLH} 10%	273 ± 46
"	"	" 1%	363 ± 60

The genetic restriction in GRF-T_1 interaction is not fully understood. Other systems have been described where macrophage-T cell interaction requires genetic compatibility but this occurs only in secondary responses (Pierce et al. 1973). In these systems there is no genetic restriction for primary responses, unlike the GRF-T_1 interaction. This discrepancy cannot be explained at present and needs to be further explored. This question has been reinvestigated recently using a variety of techniques. Using F_1 T cells and parental macrophages it was possible to generate helper cells that cooperated preferentially with B cells and macrophages of the parental haplotype used for initial priming, indicating that genetic restrictions may be induced or selected in vitro. The possibility that suppression may be the mechanism of genetic restrictions was investigated using genetically tolerant chimaeras. In these unprimed mice genetic restrictions still applied, even if suppressor cells were eliminated from our cultures using anti-Ly or anti-Ia antisera (Erb et al. submitted).

The relationship of GRF-Ia to the Ia molecules found on macrophages, T cells and B cells is not known. Furthermore, the relevance of Ia molecules on GRF to its function is not clear. It is known that the Ia antigen portion of GRF is non-covalently bonded and Ia determinants from GRF produced against one antigen (e.g. KLH) will recombine with other antigens (e.g. (T,G)-A--L). This suggests that the Ia molecule may have no, or limited, antigen specificity. If GRF is a reflection of macrophage Ir gene products, this is difficult to reconcile with the evidence for Ir genes demonstrating antigen specificity at the level of macrophage (Feldmann 1977, Rosenthal et al. 1977), unless the nature of these specificities is clearly different from that of Ig molecules. Although only speculative, one site of Ir gene control may be at the level of the macrophage in GRF production and/or at the GRF receptor site on T_1 cells. Experiments are in progress to answer this question.

CONCLUSIONS

We have described our findings of these functionally distinct factors, HF, SF, and GRF, which are associated with the I region and serve as regulatory molecules of the immune system. The biochemical analysis of these factors is just beginning and little is known regarding their structure or their relationship to each other and to other immunoregulatory molecules (such as immunoglobulin). All characterisations done so far are based on using appropriate immunoadsorbent columns followed by testing the absorbed or eluted factor for functional activity. The factors described all bear Ia determinants, but it should be stressed that the relevance of the Ia molecules to the function of the factors and the question as to whether they are Ir gene products is not clear.

The finding that these factors are antigen specific and serve as regulatory molecules in the mouse system both in vivo and in vitro suggests that they are of importance in the immune system. Further knowledge on the structure and function of these I associated factors may help us to understand the nature of I region regulation of the immune response.

ACKNOWLEDGEMENTS

The work described here was supported by the ICRF, MRC, US Public Health Service grant no. IMB RO1 AI 13145-02, the Swiss National Research Foundation, the Finnish Academy of Sciences (S.K.) M.B. is a Fellow of the Leukaemia Society of America, Inc. A.T. is a recipient of an Overseas Fellowship from the Spanish Ministerio de Educacion y Ciencia. SK is a recipient of a Long Term Fellowship from the European Molecular Biology Organisation. S.H. is a recipient of an MRC Postgraduate Fellowship.

REFERENCES

Baltz, M., Maurer, P., Merryman, C. and Feldmann, M. (submitted for publication).
Dorf, M.E., Stimpfling, J.H. and Benacerraf, B. (1975) J. Exp. Med. 141, 1459.
Erb, P. and Feldmann, M. (1974) Nature 254, 352.
Erb, P., Feldmann, M. and Hogg, N. (1976) Eur. J. Immunol. 6, 365.
Erb, P., Meier, B. and Feldmann, M. (1976a) Nature 263, 601.
Erb, P., Meier, B., Kraus, D., von Boehmer, H. and Feldmann, M. (submitted for publication).
Feldmann, M. (1972) J. Exp. Med. 136, 737.
Feldmann, M. and Basten, A. (1972) J. Exp. Med. 136, 49.
Feldmann, M. (1977) Nature, 267, 105.
Feldmann, M. and Kontiainen, S. (1976) Eur. J. Immunol. 6, 302.
Feldmann, M., Beverley, P., Erb, P., Howie, S., Kontiainen, S., Maoz, A., Mathies, M., McKenzie, I. and Woody, J. (1977) Cold Spring Harbor Symp. Quant. Biol. XLI, 113.
Feldmann, M., Beverley, P.C.L., Woody, J. and McKenzie, I.F.C. (1977a) J. Exp. Med. 145, 793.
Feldmann, M., Baltz, M., Erb, P., Howie, S., Kontiainen, S., Woody, J., and Zvaifler, N. (1977b) Progress in Immunol. III (in press).
Howie, S. and Feldmann, M. (1977) Eur. J. Immunol. 7, 417.
Howie, S., Baltz, M. and Feldmann, M. (unpublished data).
Isac, R. and Mozes, E. (1977) J. Immunol. 118, 584.
Katz, D.H., Dorf, M.E. and Benacerraf, B. (1976) J. Exp. Med. 143 906.
Kontiainen, S. and Feldmann, M. (1973) Nature, 245, 285.
Kontiainen, S. and Feldmann, M. (1977) Eur. J. Immunol. 7, 310.
Kontiainen, S. and Feldmann, M. (1977a) J. Exp. Med. (in press).
Merryman, C.F., Maurer, P.H. and Bailey, D.W. (1972) J. Immunol. 108, 937.

Merryman, C.F., Maurer, P.H. and Stimpfling, J. (1975) Immunogenetics 2, 441.
Mozes, E. (1977) Proc. 3rd Ir Gene Conference (in press).
Mozes, E. and Shearer, G.M. (1971) J. Exp. Med. 134, 141.
Mozes, E., Isac, R. and Taussig, M.J. (1975) J. Exp. Med. 141,703.
Munro, A. and Taussig, M.J. (1975) Nature, 256, 103.
Pierce, C.W., Kapp, J.A. and Benacerraf, B. (1973) J. Exp. Med. 137, 405.
Rich, S.S. and Rich, R.R. (1976) J. Exp. Med. 143, 672.
Rosenthal, A.S., Barcinski, M.A. and Blake, I.J. (1977) Nature, 267, 156.
Schimpl, A. and Wecker, E. (1972) Nature New Biol. 237, 15.
Schwartz, R.H., Dorf, M.E., Benacerraf, B. and Paul, W.E. (1976) J. Exp. Med. 143, 897.
Tada, T., Taniguchi, M. and David, C.S. (1976) J. Exp. Med. 144, 713.
Taniguchi, M., Hayakawa, K. and Tada, T. (1976) J. Immunol. 116, 542.
Theze, J., Kapp, J. and Benacerraf, B. (1977) Proc. 3rd Ir Gene Conference (in press).
Warner, C.M., McIvor, J.L., Maurer, P.H. and Merryman, C.F. (1977) Immunogenetics 145, 766.

ACTIVATION OF B CELL SUBSETS BY T-DEPENDENT AND T-INDEPENDENT ANTIGENS

George K. Lewis, Joel W. Goodman, and Raymond Ranken

Department of Microbiology and Immunology
University of California at San Francisco
San Francisco, California 94143

ABSTRACT

The capacity of the trinitrophenyl haptenic group coupled to a series of chemically dissimilar carriers to cross-stimulate putative T-dependent and T-independent B-cell subpopulations was determined by using an *in vitro* limiting dilution technique to generate primary IgM responses. TNP-Ficoll and TNP-dextran, two T-independent antigens with little or no polyclonal mitogenicity, stimulate the same population of anti-TNP precursors, which is distinct from the precursor population activated by TNP-LPS, a T-independent polyclonal mitogen, or by TNP-HRBC, a T-dependent antigen. TNP-LPS and TNP-HRBC activate the same precursor population, indicating that LPS can substitute for the T cell signal in T-dependent B-cell responses, whereas nonmitogenic T-independent antigens cannot. However, the cumulative evidence from this and other laboratories suggests that LPS and T-dependent antigens activate B cells by different mechanisms. TNP conjugates of Ficoll and dextran, which are relatively poor inducers of polyclonal B cell activation, induced larger anti-TNP clones than did TNP-LPS, a strong polyclonal mitogen. Macrophages are required for the anti-TNP-Ficoll/anti-TNP-dextran response, whereas, a similar requirement has not been shown for the anti-TNP-LPS response. Thus, macrophages may function as polyclonal B cell

---

Abbreviations: TNP, trinitrophenyl; LPS, bacterial lipopolysaccharide; HRBC, horse erythrocytes; CR, complement receptor; C3, third component of complement; MHC, major histocompatability complex; DNP, dinitrophenyl; POL, polymenized flagellin; KLH, keyhole limpet hemocyanin; PBA, polyclonal B-cell activator; MØ, macrophage; SRBC, sheep red blood cell; 2-ME, 2-mercaptoethanol; AECM, aminoethyl carbamylmethyl; SD, standard deviation.

activators in T-independent responses. Experiments in which TNP was coupled directly onto the macrophage surface support this hypothesis.

B-cell heterogenity in T-dependent responses is suggested by experiments using the C3 receptor as a marker for functional subpopulations of B cells. Murine T cells cooperate with B cells that carry a receptor for C3 and with at least some B cells which lack the C3 receptor in a primary in vitro antibody response. In vitro culture experiments using populations of B cells fractionated on the basis of the C3 receptor showed that CR+ cells were unable to make T-dependent antibody responses in the presence of anti-C3 antibody, whereas the response of CR- B cells was unaffected. Using irradiated, carrier-primed spleen cells from B10.A mice as a source of helper cells for B cells derived from various congenic strains in an in vitro primary IgM response to TNP-KLH, CR+ B cells cooperated across haplotype differences in the I region of the MHC, whereas CR- B cells did not. Preliminary mapping experiments for the genetic restriction of CR- B cells suggest complementation between the I-A and I-C subregions of the MHC. These findings tenatively suggest the existence of alternative cooperative pathways between T cells and B cell subpopulations.

INTRODUCTION

B lymphocytes are activated to antibody secreting cells by a variety of structurally dissimilar antigens. These B cell responses may be distinguished by their relative dependence upon collaborating T cells. T-dependent antigens are those which show a strict requirement for T cells, in that they are highly sensitive to the standard manipulations which deplete T cells. By contrast, T-independent responses are not affected by routine methods of T depletion. However, the observed differences may be relative and the absolute T independency of any antigen is still in question.

The existence of T-dependent and T-independent responses naturally raises the question whether the same B cell is capable of responding to both types of antigen. In the present communication, we will discuss recent results from our laboratory and others which point to multiple B cell subsets capable of responding to either T-independent or T-dependent antigens. Additionally, we will describe data which suggests the existence of B cell subsets with differing modes of cell-cell collaboration in both T-dependent and T-independent responses.

B CELL HETEROGENEITY IN T-DEPENDENT AND T-INDEPENDENT RESPONSES

Data Based on Cell Separation Procedures

The first successful attempt to separate T-dependent T-independent B cells was reported by Gorczynski and Feldmann (1975), who used velocity sedimentation to separate B cells responding to TNP-KLH from those responding to DNP-POL. For the secondary IgM response, B cells responding to DNP-POL appeared to be larger than B cells responding to TNP-KLH. By contrast, B cells making IgG antibody to TNP-KLH and DNP-POL were of similar size. Such size differences were not as readily apparent when unprimed cells were compared in the same system. However, the B cells responding to T-independent antigens showed a distinct shoulder toward larger sedimentation values when compared with sedimentation profiles for T-dependent B cells.

A different approach to the separation of T-dependent and T-independent B cells involves fractionating cells into subpopulations on the basis of their differential expression of surface markers. Two lines of evidence suggested the C3 receptor as a logical starting point for such a separation. First, Pepys (1974) reported the susceptibility of *in vivo* T-dependent antibody responses to depletion of serum C3 by treatment with cobra venom factor, which did not affect T-independent responses. Secondly, similar results were obtained *in vitro* by Feldmann and Pepys (1974) and by Dukor et al. (1974) using anti-C3 to neutralize the effects of C3 in culture. In these studies, T-independent responses were unaffected by including anti-C3 in cultures of normal or primed spleen cells whereas T-dependent responses were severely depressed. The results suggested that C3 might be involved in T-B collaboration but not in T-independent B cell triggering. Since earlier studies implicated the CR+ B cell as being involved in T-B collaboration, it seemed logical that the CR- B cell might be the principal responder to T-independent antigens. This notion was supported by the resistance of T-independent responses to C3 depletion as well as by the earlier appearance in ontogeny of T-independent responses than of CR+ B cells (unpublished observation).

In order to test the above hypothesis, splenic B cells were separated into CR+ and CR- components by rosetting with C3 coated red cells followed by density gradient centrifugation. On the basis of this procedure, 50-75% of normal adult splenic B cells possess complement receptors. The results from several laboratories are summarized in Table I. The average contribution of CR+ B cells to T-independent responses ranged from a low of 16% (Lewis et al. 1976) to a high of 46% (Parish 1975). The contribution of CR+ B cells was lower for responses to Ficoll and dextran as carriers than responses to POL (Table I). It should be pointed out that POL is a fairly strong polyclonal activator (Coutinho and Moller, 1975) whereas dextran and Ficoll are weak or questionable polyclonal activators. Another potent polyclonal activator, LPS, is capable of activating both CR+ and CR- B cells (Dukor et al. 1974, Lewis et al. 1976, and Hoffman et al. 1976) in keeping with the relationship between polyclonal activation and the ability to stimulate both CR+ and CR- B cells. In the experiments using Ficoll and dextran as carriers, it is not clear whether CR+ B cells are totally unresponsive or are simply less responsive than CR- B cells. This ambiguity results

TABLE I

Responses of CR- B cells to T-Independent Antigens

Antigen	% PFC Response Residing in the CR- B Cell Fraction	Reference
DNP-AE-Dextran	60%, 73%[†]	Dukor et al. (1974)
DNP-POL	54% (97%)[††]	Parish (1975)
DNP-AECM-Ficoll	84%, 72%	Lewis et al. (1976)

† IgM response

†† Numbers in parenthesis represent IgG responses.

from the use of highly manipulated cell populations. Thus, it is possible that CR+ B cells are rendered less responsive consequent to cell separation or, alternatively, that weak CR+ responses reflect the presence of contaminating CR- B cells.

The ability of CR+ and CR- B cells to respond to T-dependent antigens is shown in Table II. Generally, particulate antigens activate both CR+ and CR- B cell subsets; in contrast, monomeric antigens preferentially activate CR+ B cells in the IgM response and both CR+ and CR- B cells in the IgG response. Clearly, if the majority of the precursors for DNP-Ficoll and DNP-dextran lie in the CR- subset while all of the precursors for DNP-MON reside in the CR+ subpopulation, then CR expression serves to delineate T-dependent and T-independent B cell subsets. However, when the response pattern for DNP-POL and HRBC are considered the expression of CR is no longer a useful marker for T-dependency. HRBC and DNP-POL stimulate both CR+ and CR- B cells, raising the question of whether a common hapteni moiety coupled to a T-dependent carrier like HRBC and to a strong PBA will activate the same CR- and CR+ B cells. Additionally, the question remains whether the CR- B cells responding to TNP-Ficoll (T-independent) are the same CR- B cells that respond to TNP-HRBC (T-dependent). These questions are dealt with in the following section.

Data Based on Limiting Dilution Experiments

Recently, with the introduction of appropriate culture methodology by Lefkovits (1972), it has become possible to accurately determine precursor frequencies for a common hapten coupled to a variet

TABLE II

Collaboration of CR+ and CR- B Cells with T Cells

Antigen	Ability of T Cells to Colla-aborate With CR+ B Cells	CR- B Cells	Reference
SRBC	Yes[†]	No	Arnaiz-Villena et al. (1975)
SRBC	Yes	No	Dukor et al. (1974)
HRBC	Yes	Yes	Parish (1975)
DNP-MON	Yes	No	Parish (1975)
DNP-BGG	Yes (Yes)[†††]	No[††] (Yes)	Mason (1976)
TNP-SRBC	Yes	Yes	Hoffman et al. (1976)
SRBC	Yes	Yes	Lewis et al. (1976)
TNP-HRBC	Yes	Yes	Lewis et al. (1977)

[†] Primary IgM response
[††] Secondary IgM response
[†††] Secondary IgG response

of carriers. Using TNP as the hapten, we have prepared conjugates with carriers having broadly different biological activities (Table III). Our experimental approach has been to compare the precursor frequencies for each antigen cultured alone with the precursor frequencies obtained when two antigens are cocultured. In the case of a single B-cell subset at limiting dilution, the fraction of non-responding cultures will be: (1) $P(0) = e^{-n\lambda}$ where P(0) is the fraction of non-responding cultures, n is the number of cells per culture well, and λ is the number of cells containing one precursor. Generally, for m subsets, the fraction of non-responding cultures is given by the following equation: (2) $P(0) = 1 - (1-e^{-n\lambda})^m$. Since we can only compare two carriers at a time, we have m = 2 for the case where the two antigens activate distinct B cell subsets. In this instance equation (2) becomes:

$$(3) \quad P(0) = 1 - (1-e^{-n\lambda_1})\ (1-e^{-n\lambda_2})$$

where λ_1 and λ_2 represent the number of cells containing one precursor for TNP on carrier 1 or carrier 2. If the two antigens activate the same subset then m = 1 and we obtain equation (1). In practice, strict additivity of the precursor frequencies is only compatible with the case where m = 2 and both antigens activate

TABLE III

Immunological Properties of Antigens

Antigen	Requires T Cells	Requires A Cells	Stimulates Polyclonal Ig Synthesis	Stimulates Polyclonal DNA Synthesis
TNP-Ficoll	-	++++	±	±
TNP-dextran	-	++++	+	+
TNP-LPS	-	±	++++	++++
TNP-HRBC	++++	++++	-	-

different subsets. If the precursor frequencies are not additive, then m = 1 and the two antigens activate the same subset. In equation (3) λ_1 must approximate λ_2 in order to make a valid comparison between the two antigens. If $\lambda_1 >> \lambda_2$ then the term $(1-e^{-n\lambda_2})$ becomes neglible and we obtain $m \doteq 1$, in which case the test is invalid. This has not occurred in our studies to date.

To compare the precursor frequencies of TNP Ficoll and TNP-dextran, .05 ng of each antigen was added separately or in combination into cultures containing $1x\ 10^4 - 8 \times 10^4$ normal spleen cells from C57Bl/6S mice. Precursor frequencies, determined after four days of culture, were 13.2 ± 1.2 for TNP-Ficoll, 14.0 ± 1.3 for TNP-dextran, and 13.7 ± 1.3 for the two antigens in the same cultures (Table IV). Since the precursor frequency was the same whether cells were cultured with the antigens individually or together, the data clearly suggest that the same B cells respond to TNP-Ficoll and TNP-dextran.

TABLE IV

Splenic Precursor Frequencies from Limiting Dilution Experiments Comparing TNP-Ficoll and TNP-Dextran

Antigen	Precursors Per 10^6 Spleen Cells ± SD
TNP-Ficoll	13.2 ± 1.2
TNP-Dextran	14.0 ± 1.3
TNP-Ficoll + TNP-Dextran	13.7 ± 1.3

For a similar comparison of cells responsive to TNP-Ficoll and to TNP-LPS, cultures were established containing .05 ng TNP-Ficoll, 5 ng TNP-LPS, or both, and the precursor frequency was determined in the usual manner. In this set of experiments, the frequencies per 10^6 spleen cells were 16.1 ± 1.5, 31.3 ± 2.5, and 45.5 ± 3.6 for TNP-Ficoll, TNP-LPS, and the combination, respectively (Table V). The strict additivity of these responses suggests that different B cell subsets are activated by TNP-Ficoll and TNP-LPS. Since TNP-Ficoll and TNP-dextran stimulate the same subpopulation of B cells, it follows that TNP-LPS and TNP-dextran also trigger independent subsets of cells.

To determine if the ability to respond to TNP-Ficoll, a T-independent antigen, and to TNP-HRBC, a strictly T-dependent antigen, is shared by a common pool of B cells, varying number of spleen cells serving as a source of B cells were cultured with an excess of mitomycin-C treated carrier primed cells in the presence of one or both antigens. T-helper cell excess in these cultures was established by the ability to obtain responses in 100% of the cultures when 10^5 normal spleen cells were cultured with the carrier-primed cells.

The precursor frequency for TNP-Ficoll in this series of experiments was 8.3 ± .8 per 10^6 spleen cells, that for TNP-HRBC was 14.7 ± 1.3, and 26.3 ± 2.1 precursors were found for TNP-Ficoll plus TNP-HRBC (Table VI). The additivity of these frequencies indicates that different B cells respond to the two antigens. Since TNP-Ficoll (or TNP-dextran) appears to activate a subset of anti-TNP precursors distinct from those reactive to either TNP-LPS or TNP-HRBC, it was clearly of interest to determine if the latter two antigens, one T-independent and the other T-dependent, activated the same or different subsets. To address this question, cultures were established with a constant number of nylon-wool passed spleen cells from mice primed with HRBC plus from 1 x 10^4 to 8 x 10^4 normal spleen cells as a source of B cells. The cultures contained 5 ng of TNP-LPS, 3 x 10^4 TNP-HRBC, or both antigens. In this series of experiments TNP-LPS stimulated 83.3 ± 7.4 precursors per 10^6 spleen cells, TNP-HRBC generated a response of 31.3 ± 2.4 cells per 10^6 spleen cells, and the two antigens together triggered 71.4 ± 6.4 precursors per 10^6 spleen cells. These figures provide strong evidence that the subset of B cells responsive to TNP-HRBC resides within the population activated by TNP-LPS.

Clearly, these studies suggest marked B cell heterogeneity in T-independent and T-dependent responses. Similar studies were reported recently by Quintans and Cosenza (1976) for the anti-phosphoryl-choline response in Balb/c mice and by Jennings and Rittenberg (1976) for DNP. Our studies agree with Quintans and Cosenza in that T-dependent and T-independent precursors segregated from one another at limiting dilution. Additionally, our studies demonstrate that

TABLE V

Splenic Precursor Frequencies from Limiting Dilution Experiments Comparing TNP-Ficoll and TNP-LPS

Antigen	Precursors Per 10^6 Spleen Cells ± SD
TNP-Ficoll	16.1 ± 1.5
TNP-LPS	31.3 ± 2.5
TNP-Ficoll + TNP-LPS	45.5 ± 3.6

TABLE VI

Splenic Precursor Frequencies from Limiting Dilution Experiments Comparing TNP-Ficoll and TNP-HRBC

Antigen	Precursors Per 10^6 Spleen Cells ± SD
TNP-Ficoll	8.3 ± .8
TNP-HRBC	14.7 ± 1.3
TNP-Ficoll + TNP-HRBC	26.3 ± 2.1

although TNP-LPS and TNP-HRBC activate the same B cell subset, they do so by different mechanisms, since the anti-TNP-HRBC response is partially inhibited by anti-mouse C3 (Lewis et al. 1977) whereas the anti-TNP-LPS response is not.

CELLULAR COLLABORATION BETWEEN B CELL SUBSETS, T-CELLS, AND MACROPHAGES IN T-INDEPENDENT AND T-DEPENDENT RESPONSES

Collaboration Between T-Independent B Cells and Macrophages

Several years ago, Mosier et al. (1974) reported that the *in vitro* response to DNP-Ficoll was independent of macorphages. Shortly thereafter, we noted that the *in vivo* response to TNP-Ficoll was highly susceptible to carageenan treatment, suggesting that T-independent responses could be abrogated by more exhaustive procedures for MØ depletion. The macrophage dependence of the in vitro anti-hapten-Ficoll response has been substantiated by Chused et al. (1976) and by Lee et al. (1976). These workers used Sephadex-G10 filtration and phagocytosis of carbonyl iron to remove macrophages in their respective investigations. In this section, data will be presented which demonstrates an absolute requirement for macrophages in T-independent responses, and a possible mode of action for macrophages in these responses will be formulated.

In their original studies, Mosier et al. (1974) used adherence to plastic for depletion macrophages in the anti-DNP-Ficoll and anti-SRBC responses. This technique markedly reduced the anti-SRBC response while leaving the anti-DNP-Ficoll response intact. Recent studies in our laboratory using a modified plastic adherence procedure have shown a macrophage dependence for both anti-TNP-Ficoll and anti-TNP-dextran responses. Since it was previously shown that these two antigens stimulate the same B cell subset, 21 individual responses were normalized and plotted versus the fraction of macrophages remaining

$$(\text{\% macrophages remaining} = \frac{\text{\% phagocytic cells after depletion}}{\text{\% phagocytic cells before depletion}})$$

after depletion on plastic. As shown in Figure 1, variable degrees of macrophage depletion were obtained; consequently, the anti-TNP responses were also variably depleted. The slope of the response curve was 0.91 in the absence of 2-mercaptoethanol suggesting a single hit phenomenon for the interaction between macrophages and T-independent B cells. Interestingly, inclusion of 2-ME completely rescued the response even in those cultures with the most exhaustive macrophage depletion, thus raising the question whether 2-ME replaces MØ entirely or merely amplifies the activity of residual MØ. In order to determine if T-independent B cells can be activated directly by antigen in the presence of 2-ME, the carbonyl iron procedure of Lee et al. (1975) was used to exhaustively deplete normal spleen cells of macrophages. These cells were then cultured for 4 days in the presence of antigen, 2-ME, and, in some cultures, highly purified peritoneal exudate macrophages. In this experiment (Figure 2) cultures containing MØ depleted spleen cells, antigen, and 2-ME gave background PFC responses (2 ± 3 IgM anti-TNPFC/culture). When enriched MØ were titrated into the cultures, a linear relationship between MØ number and PFC response was obtained in the range from 3.12×10^3 to 6.3×10^4 MØ per culture. The slope in this region was 1.13, again suggesting a single hit phenomenon for the interaction between T-independent B cells and macrophages. Thus, TNP-Ficoll responsive B cells only recognize antigen in the presence of macrophages. 2-ME apparently amplifies the macrophage-dependent function, but fails to substitute for the cells.

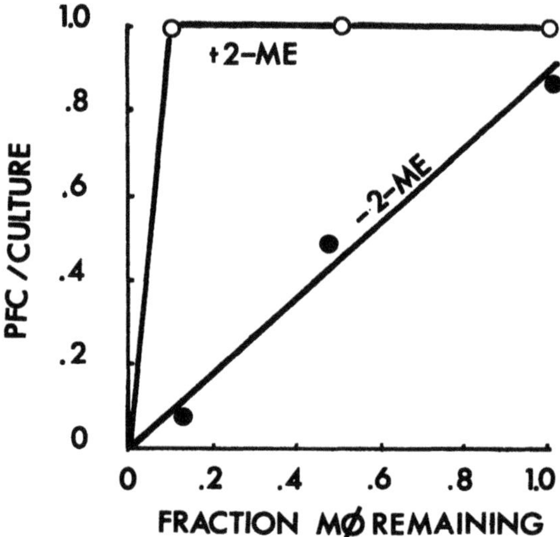

FIGURE 1. Effect of MØ depletion on T-independent responses. Normal BDF, spleen cells were depleted of MØ by a modified plastic plate adherence technique and cultured for 4 days in the presence of 5 ng ml^{-1} TNP-Ficoll or 5 ng ml^{-1} TNP-dextran. Each point represents the normalized values for 21 individual responses. SD ≤ .15 x sample mean.

The above data are especially relevant when considered in the context of the current controversy about the mechanisms of B cell activation. According to the Coutinho and Möller hypothesis (1975), all T-independent antigens are polyclonal B cell activators (PBA), immunoglobulin receptors serving only to focus the PBA onto the appropriate receptor, thereby triggering an antigen specific response. Higher concentrations of PBA would obviate the need for antigen focusing, thus resulting in the activation of many more clones of B cells. The model is opposed by a number of others which propose an active role for immunoglobulin receptors in B-cell activation (for review, see Transplant. Rev. vol. 23). Thus, the existence of a potent T-independent antigen with little or no polyclonal mitogenicity would constitute a strong agrument against the Coutinho-Möller hypothesis. During the course of the above limiting dilution studies, it was noted that TNP-Ficoll and TNP-dextran induced clonal burst sizes which were always comparable to or larger than the burst size for TNP-LPS (Table VII). The clonal burst size is given by

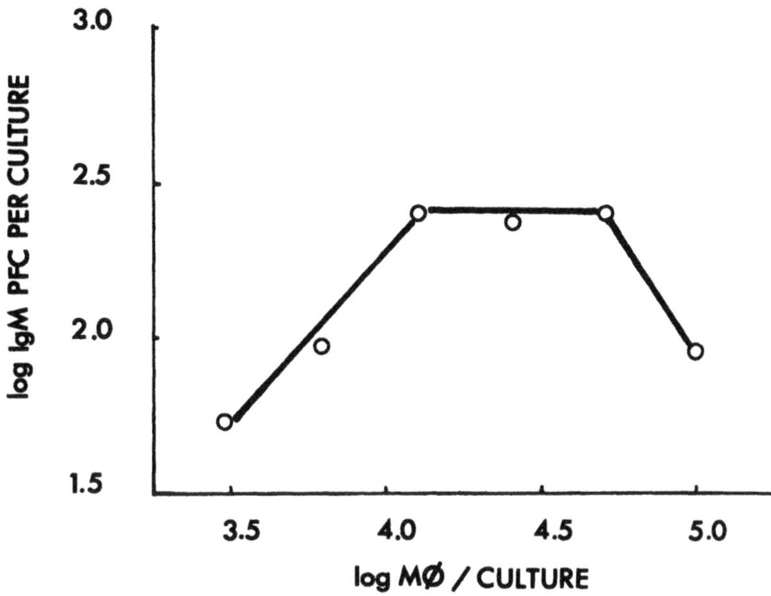

FIGURE 2. Absolute requirement for macrophages in the anti-TNP-Ficoll response. Normal BDF, spleen cells were depleted of MØ using carbonyl iron and cultured for 4 days in microcultures in the presence of 5 ng ml TNP-Ficoll and 5 x 10^{-5} M 2-ME. Mitomycin-C treated peritoneal macrophages (≥ 98% phagocytic cells after overnight adherence to plastic) were pulsed into MØ depleted cultures at the time of culturing. SD ≤ .12 x sample mean.

the following relationship: (4) $B(n) = \frac{\text{PFC/culture}}{\text{Precursors/culture}}$

and is dependent on the PFC generation time. According to Coutinho-Möller, the clonal burst size might reflect the size of the B cell population activated by the PBA as well as the generative potential of the carrier. The assumption is made that V region markers would be spread randomly among the population of B cells possessing mitogen receptors. As shown in Table VII, TNP-Ficoll and TNP-dextran activate smaller subsets than TNP-LPS, but with a greater generative potential (larger burst size). This is difficult to reconcile with the known PBA activities of these antigens (Table III) and appears to argue against the "single non-specific signal" theory. However, Table III and the data presented above suggest an alternative interpretation. The TNP-Ficoll and TNP-dextran responses are absolutely dependent on the presence of MØ, whereas it has been difficult to consistently deplete the TNP-LPS response under identical conditions. Therefore, it is possible that MØ themselves act as PBA, and that

TABLE VII

Burst Size of Clones Responding to T-Dependent and T-Independent Antigens

Experiment	Antigen	Burst Size ± SD
1	TF[†]	26.8 ± 3.1 (19.7 ± 5.8)
	TH	34.8 ± 5.8 (42.4 ± 10.7)
2	TF	14.5 ± 2.0
	TD	14.4 ± 2.0 (14.6 ± 0.5)
3	TF	15.4 ± 1.7
	TL	11.1 ± 1.0 (8.9 ± 5.4)
4	TL	13.1 ± 1.7
	TH	50.9 ± 14.0

† TF, TNP-Ficoll; TH, TNP-HRBC; TD, TNP-dextran; TL, TNP-LPS. ( ) = mean ± SD for all experiments.

for weakly mitogenic antigens like Ficoll, the MØ serves as the prime proliferative signal. Akin to soluble antigens, MØ associated PBA activity could be focused onto the relevant B cell consequent to interaction between the hapten (TNP) and Ig receptors. This concept is supported by the recent observation of Opitz et al. (1976) demonstrating MØ associated PBA activity.

In order to test the above hypothesis, TNP was directly coupled onto highly purified populations of peritoneal exudate macrophages. Using these TNP-MØ as the sole source of antigen, significant in vitro PFC responses were obtained. As shown in Figure 3, titration of TNP-MØ into normal spleen cells yields a linear plot when $\log_{10}$ PFC is plotted versus $\log_{10}$ TNP-MØ/culture. Interestingly, the slope of this plot is 0.57 which suggests that one TNP-MØ activates more than one B cell. This type of response is seen only with hapten-modified MØ since normal MØ only marginally increased PFC responses. Normal spleen cells and normal macrophages did not give rise to significant polyclonal responses. These results are not at variance with Opitz et al. (1976) since they observed PBA activity only when MØ were cocultured with normal spleen cells for a period of 18 hours. After this incubation period, MØ were removed by carbonyl iron adherence and the non-adherent cells cultured for the remainder of a 4 day culture period. If the MØ were not removed, then there was a marked reduction in the response. Generally, later experiments have shown that MØ-depleted spleen cell populations give increased

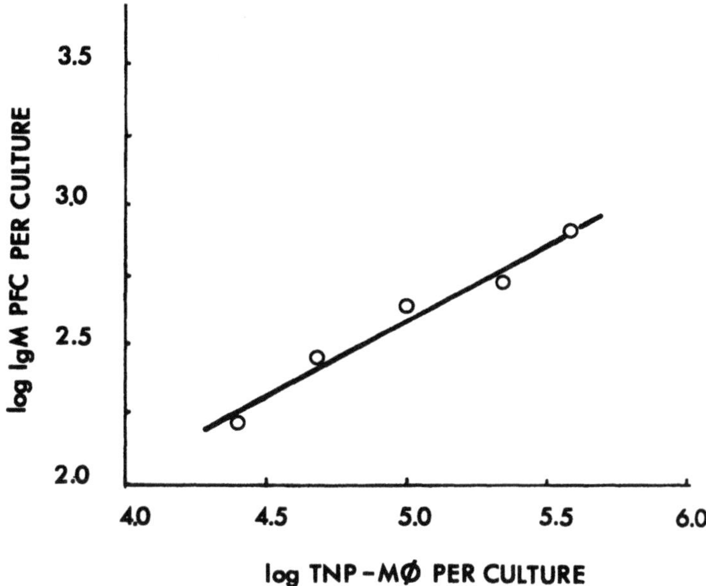

FIGURE 3. Immunogenicity of TNP-MØ. Highly enriched peritoneal MØ (> 99% phagocytic) were coupled with TNP and added to .5 ml cultures of normal BDF_1 spleen cells containing 5 x 10^{-5}M 2-ME. Day 4 response SD ≤ .12 sample mean.

anti-TNP responses to TNP-MØ. Preliminary experiments using anti-Thy-1 serum suggest the T-independence of the anti-TNP-MØ response; however, these results require confirmation by more rigorous methods for removing T cells. Assuming that this response is T-independent, a strong argument can be made for the aforesaid proposition that the macrophage acts as a PBA in the recognition of antigen by T-independent B cells. Clearly, it is of interest to determine the exact nature of this interaction at both the genetic and molecular levels. Preliminary experiments suggest the importance of Ia-bearing macrophages in the TNP-Ficoll response, implicating the cell interaction genes in T-independent responses.

Collaboration between T-Dependent B-Cell Subsets and T-Cells

As shown in Table II, the B cell response to T-dependent antigens is heterogeneous with respect to CR- and CR+ B cell participation. In light of this, the possibility that CR- and CR+ B cells collaborate differently with T cells was investigated. A precedent for this idea is the evidence that Cr- B cells require activated macrophages to collaborate with T-cells, whereas CR+ B cells cooperate readily with T cells in the presence of normal macrophages (Hoffmann et al. 1976).

Since CR+ and CR- B cells are distinguished from one another by the complement receptor, the requirement for C3 by these two B cell subsets in T-B collaboration was investigated. Feldmann and Pepys (1974) and Dukor et al. (1974) first reported the selective inhibition of T-dependent responses by anti-C3 cultures of mouse spleen cells, which did not affect T-independent responses. Therefore, a rabbit anti-mouse C3 antiserum was prepared and its effects on collaboration of CR+ and CR- B cells with T cells was investigated.

The ability of anti-C3 to interfere with cooperation between T cell and B cell subpopulations in the response to TNP-HRBC was determined by culturing whole spleen cell preparations or spleen cell preparations depleted of CR+ cells with and without anti-C3 serum or purified antibody. In order to maximize cooperation between T cells and CR- B cells, donor mice were carrier primed 7 days earlier with 4×10^8 horse erythrocytes. As shown in Table VIII, anti-C3 serum reduced the anti-TNP-PFC response of unfractionated spleen cells by 78%. This figure is reasonably consistent with the expected values of 56 to 76%, based on the proportion of CR+ B cells found experimentally. In addition, the CR- B cell compartment appears to be functionally heterogeneous (Lewis et al. 1976), which may contribute to the extent of reduction of the PFC response by anti-C3 serum. In contrast, the response of CR- spleen cells was unaffected by the inclusion of anti-C3 in the culture medium (585 ± 68 PFC/culture vs. 620 ± 55 PFC/culture). Equivalent results have been obtained with purified anti-C3 antibody in place of absorbed antiserum (data not shown). Since the whole spleen cell preparation differed from the CR- spleen cell population by only the CR+ cells, we conclude that the CR+ cells comprise the population which is affected by anti-C3. The anti-C3 preparations have been shown to be noncytoxic for unfractionated spleen cells, CR+ cells, and CR- cells. These data suggest that the anti-C3 effect is not due to a general depletion of CR+ B cells resulting from the reaction between anti-C3 and C3 remaining on the surface of CR+ B cells consequent to the separation procedure.

These results differ from those of Feldmann and Pepys (1974) and Dukor et al. (1974) in that complete inhibition of the primary IgM response by anti-C3 was not obtained . Recently, this antiserum was shown to possess substantially more activity against C3d than C3b, and since fetal calf serum, which is a good source of C3b inactivator was used in the rosetting procedure, these results may have been obtained with C3d rosettes only. Therefore, it is possible that the CR- B cells have receptors for C3b and that this population was not inhibited because of the preferential activity of the antiserum for C3d. Resolution of this point is presently in progress.

TABLE VIII

Effect of Anti-C3 on the Cooperation between T-Cell and B-Cell Subpopulations in the In Vitro Response to TNP-HRBC

Cell Population†	Anti-C3††	Anti-TNP IgM PFC††† Culture ± S.D.	% Inhibition
Whole spleen	-	790 ± 60	
Whole spleen	+	170 ± 29	78
CR- spleen cells	-	585 ± 68	
CR- spleen cells	+	620 ± 55	0

† HRBC primed spleen cells

†† 1:40 dilution of rabbit anti-mouse C3 serum

††† Indicator cells were TNP-SRBC

While the ability to inhibit at least one pathway of T-B collaboration with an antiserum against a component of C3 is suggestive of differing modes of collaboration of T cells with CR+ and CR- B cells, independent evidence was sought to strengthen this conclusion. For this purpose, the ability of CR+ and CR- B cells to collaborate across haptotype barriers in the primary in vitro IgM response was determined. B10.A mice were primed with 50 μg of KLH in CFA to provide a syngeneic MØ-T cell interacting population. Seven days after priming, spleen cell suspensions were irradiated with 1200r and cultured with CR+ or CR- B cells in the presence of TNP-KLH. The B cell subsets were derived from either syngeneic B10.A mice or B10 congenic mice differing from B10.A predominantly in the K or D end of the MHC. Culturing B10.A CR+ or CR- B cells with syngeneic carrier primed B10.A T cells gave 378 ± 31 and 342 ± 60 IgM PFC per culture, respectively (Table IX). When B10.A T cells were cultured with CR+ B cells from B10.BR mice (I-C,S,G,D difference) or B10.D2 mice (K,I-A,I-B,I-J,I-E difference) the respective responses were 791 ± 48 IgM PFC per culture and 302 ± 27 IgM PFC per culture. In contrast, culturing carrier primed T cells from B10.A mice with CR- B cells from B10.BR or B10.D2 mice gave no detectable responses. These data confirm the ability of at least some B cells to collaborate across MHC barriers in the primary IgM response and suggest that genetic restriction may occur in B cell subsets. It is possible to tentatively map the genes responsible for the restriction of the CR- B cell subset to the I region of the MHC. Identity at the K or D ends is insufficient to permit collaboration, as is identity at I-A

TABLE IX

Cooperation Between B-Cell Subsets and Congenic T Cells

MØ + T Cells	B Cells		PFC/Culture	MHC DIFF.	Genotype T/B						
					K	IA	IB	IJ	IC	S	D
		CR+	342 ± 60	NONE	k	k	k	k	d	d	d
B10.A	B10.A				k	k	k	k	d	d	d
		CR-	378 ± 71	NONE							
		CR+	791 ± 48		k	k	k	k	d	d	d
B10.A	B10.BR			IC,S,D	k	k	k	k	k	k	k
		CR-	0								
		CR+	302 ± 27		k	k	k	k	d	d	d
B10.A	B10.D2			K,IA,IB,IJ	d	d	d	d	d	d	d
		CR-	0								

through I-E. Thus there must be either a complementing gene system between a region from I-A to I-E and I-C or, alternatively, there must be a new I region gene between I-E and I-C. Additionally, it must be emphasized that positive and negative allogeneic effects have not been formally excluded as explanations for these data. This problem is being approached by attempting to use helper factors to replace T cells, thereby avoiding allogeneic responses.

CONCLUSIONS

The results described in this communication prompt the following conclusions:

1. T-dependent and T-independent antigens activate different B cell subsets.
2. T-independent antigens with different properties activate different B cell subsets.
3. Some T-independent responses have an absolute requirement for macrophages.
4. Macrophages may function in T-independent responses as polyclonal B activators.
5. An individual B cell may be activated by more than one mechanism.
6. Tentatively, CR+ and CR- B cells collaborate with T cells via different pathways.

ACKNOWLEDGMENTS

This work was supported by National Institutes of Health grants AI-05664 and AI-11983. George Lewis is the recipient of a U.S. Public Health Service Postdoctoral Fellowship.

REFERENCES

Chused, T.M., Kassan, S., and Mosier, D.E. (1976) J. Immunol. 116: 1579.
Coutinho, A., and Möller, O. (1975) Adv. Immunol. 21:113.
Dukor, P., Dierich, F.M., Gisler, R.H., Schumann, G., and Bitter-Suermann, P. (1974) Prog. Immunol. 3:111.
Feldmann, M., and Pepys, M.B. (1974) Nature 249:159.
Gorczynski, R.M., and Feldmann, M. (1975) Cell. Immunol. 18:88.
Hoffmann, M.K., Hämmerling, V., Simon, M., and Oettgen, H. (1976) J. Immunol. 116:1447.
Jennings, J., and Rittenberg, M.B. (1976) J. Immunol. 117:1749.
Lee, K.C., Shiozawa, C., Shaw, A., and Diener, E. (1976) Eur. J. Immunol. 6:63.

Lefkovits, I. (1972) Eur. J. Immunol. 2:360.

Lewis, G.K., Ranken, R., Nitecki, D.E., and Goodman, J.W. (1976) J. Exp. Med. 144:382.

Lewis, G.K., Ranken, R., and Goodman, J.W. (1977) J. Immunol. 118 1744.

Mosier, D.E., Johnson, B.M., Paul, W.E., McMaster, P.R.B. (1974) J. Exp. Med. 139:1354.

Opitz, H.G., Opitz, V., Lemke, H., Huget, R., and Flad, H.D. (1976) Eur. J. Immunol. 6:457.

Parish, C.R. (1975) Transplant. Rev. 25:98.

REGULATION OF ANTI-HAPTEN ANTIBODY SECRETION BY CARRIER-SPECIFIC SUPPRESSOR T CELLS

R.W. Warren, R.C. Griffith and J.M. Davie

Washington University School of Medicine

St. Louis, MO 63110

ABSTRACT

Carrier-primed T lymphocytes can suppress high avidity IgG anti-hapten antibody secretion within 90 min. *in vitro* if the suppressor and target cells are primed with the same carrier determinants. Suppression seems to be directed to the antibody secreting cell since the effect is rapid and does not depend on macrophages or T cells in the target cell population. Suppression can be blocked by inclusion of soluble carrier in the cell mixture or by treatment of the target cells with anti-carrier antibody or pronase. Moreover, suppression can be augmented by PFC exposure to the soluble hapten-carrier conjugate.

Finally, carrier specificity may be altered by preincubation of the target population with a hapten-heterologous carrier before addition of suppressor cells specific for the heterologous carrier. Thus, it is likely that high avidity suppression depends upon immunogen bound to the surfaces of antibody secreting cells which serves as a target for suppressor cells or molecules.

INTRODUCTION

The ability of T lymphocytes to suppress specifically an antibody response is a well-recognized phenomenon which has been implicated in idiotypic (Eichmann, 1974; Owen *et al.*, 1977) and allotypic (Herzenberg *et al.*, 1976) suppression, and several forms of antigen-induced suppression, such as an avidity modification (Tada *et al.*, 1975) and some forms of tolerance (Elson and Taylor, 1974;

Sanfilippo and Scott, 1974). In these various systems, several targets for suppression have been identified including macrophages, B cells and helper T cells.

In this paper, we will summarize work from our laboratory (Warren _et al._, 1976; Warren and Davie, 1977a,b) which demonstrates that suppressor T cells can inhibit antibody formation directly most likely following recognition of immunogen on the surface of antibody secreting cells. Thus, exposure of immune splenocytes to suppressor cell population _in vitro_ or injection of suppressor cells into hyperimmune animals results in rapid inhibition of high avidity IgG antibody secretion.

AVIDITY MODIFICATION _IN VIVO_

Tada and Takemori (1974) demonstrated that spleen or thymus cells from hyperimmunized animals suppressed the primary and secondary IgG plaque forming cell (PFC) response and showed that this T cell dependent effect preferentially inhibited high avidity PFC (Takemori and Tada, 1974). Our own interest in this system has centered on the nature of the target cell and the mechanism by which avidity dependence is mediated. The experimental system we have employed uses activated thymocytes (ATC) as a source of suppressor cells. ATC were prepared by the injection of 10^8 AKR thymocytes into lethally irradiated syngeneic recipients along with 100 μg antigen in saline. Six to 8 days later, cell suspensions of their spleens, which served as a source of ATC, were injected into DNP-KLH immunized recipients. The effects of the ATC on the avidity of the anti-DNP secondary response was measured by a technique based on hapten inhibition of plaque formation where high avidity PFC are more easily inhibited by free hapten than low avidity PFC. Fig. 1 demonstrates that injection of varied numbers of DNP-KLH ATC 4 weeks after primary immunization markedly alters the avidity distribution of the secondary anti-DNP response to DNP-KLH when measured 12 days later. Selective suppression of high avidity IgG and augmentation of middle avidity PFC are seen, effects which resulted in no change in total PFC. In this and all other experiments reported here, ATC had no reproducible effect on IgM PFC.

The suppressive cell in ATC is most likely a T cell as shown in Table I: Anti-θ treatment of ATC removes suppression capacity and the suppressor cell does not adsorb to nylon columns. In addition, the suppressive cell seems specific for carrier determinants (Table II). Both DNP-KLH and KLH ATC can suppress high avidity IgG PFC responses of DNP-KLH primed mice, while DNP-BGG ATC are without effect.

While the carrier specificity and T cell dependence argue against the role of antibody itself on the observed suppression,

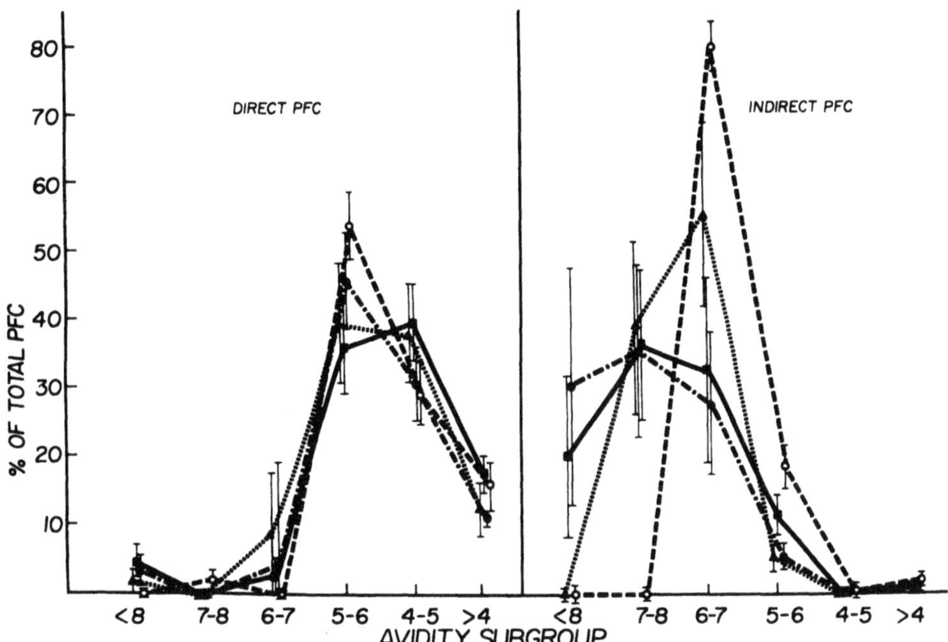

Fig. 1: ATC dose effect of secondary response PFC. Direct PFC (left panel) and indirect PFC (right panel) of mice given 100 μg DNP-KLH in CFA in the thighs, followed 4 weeks later by 0 (■), 2.8 x 10^6 (●), 9.2 x 10^6 (▲), or 28 x 10^6 (o) ATC directed against DNP-KLH. The secondary immunization, 100 μg DNP-KLH in saline i.p. was given 8 days after ATC. All groups were assayed at 12 days. (From Warren et al., 1976).

the kinetics of antibody-mediated suppression are clearly different from ATC-mediated suppression (Fig. 2). For an antibody-mediated suppression model, we chose a thymus independent antigen, DNP-dextran known to induce both IgM and IgG anti-DNP antibodies (Rude et al., 1976). Suppression was achieved by the injection of 200 μg of mouse anti-α(→3) dextran antibody (Hansburg et al., 1976) at various times before and after immunization with 100 μg of DNP-dextran in saline, and measuring the anti-DNP PFC response 4 days after immunization. It can be seen in the left panel of Fig. 2 that anti-carrier antibody suppresses both IgM and IgG anti-hapten responses if given as late, but no later than 1-2 days after immunization. On the other hand, carrier-specific ATC are suppressive not only when given 1 week before second antigen administration as shown in previous experiments, but also when given even 4 days after antigen administration (Fig. 2, right panel), which is the day of PFC assay. In addition, IgM PFC are never affected by ATC. From kinetic considerations alone, it is probable that anti-carrier

Table I: Suppression is T cell mediated*

Recipient	DNP-KLH ATC	INDIRECT PFC/10^6 VIABLE CELLS total	<7
DNP-KLH primed	None	359 (1.2)	116 (2.1)
	$4x10^6$	447 (1.2)	20 (1.5)
	$4x10^6$+anti-θ	379 (1.1)	138 (3.3)
	$2.2x10^6$ after nylon	441 (1.3)	3 (1.5)

*Recipients were immunized with 100 μg DNP-KLH in CFA and 1-2 months later were given a) 0, $4x10^6$ or $4x10^6$ anti-θ pretreated DNP-KLH ATC or $18.4x10^6$ ATC passed over nylon wool, producing $2.2x10^6$ effluent cells. Five or six days later, 100 μg DNP-KLH in saline was given i.p., plaque assay followed 4 days after boost. Shown are the geometric means and standard errors of the total indirect PFC response and the highest avidity subgroups (<7); underlined numbers are different from control (p<0.01). (Modified from Warren _et al_., 1976).

Table II: Suppression is carrier specific*

Recipient	ATC specificity	INDIRECT PFC/10^6 VIABLE CELLS total	<7
DNP-KLH	None	568 (1.4)	194 (1.4)
primed	DNP-KLH	599 (1.5)	10 (3.0)
	KLH	1867 (1.4)	6 (7.4)
	DNP-BGG	115 (1.6)	185 (1.4)

*Recipients were immunized with 100 μg DNP-KLH in CFA and 1 month later were given 0 or 9-10 x 10^6 ATC primed with 100 μg of the antigens listed. One week later, all animals were given 100 μg DNP-KLH in saline i.p.; plaque assay followed 4 days later. Shown are the geometric means and standard errors of the total indirect PFC response and the highest avidity subgroups (<7); underlined numbers are different from control (p<0.01). (Modified from Warren _et al_., 1976).

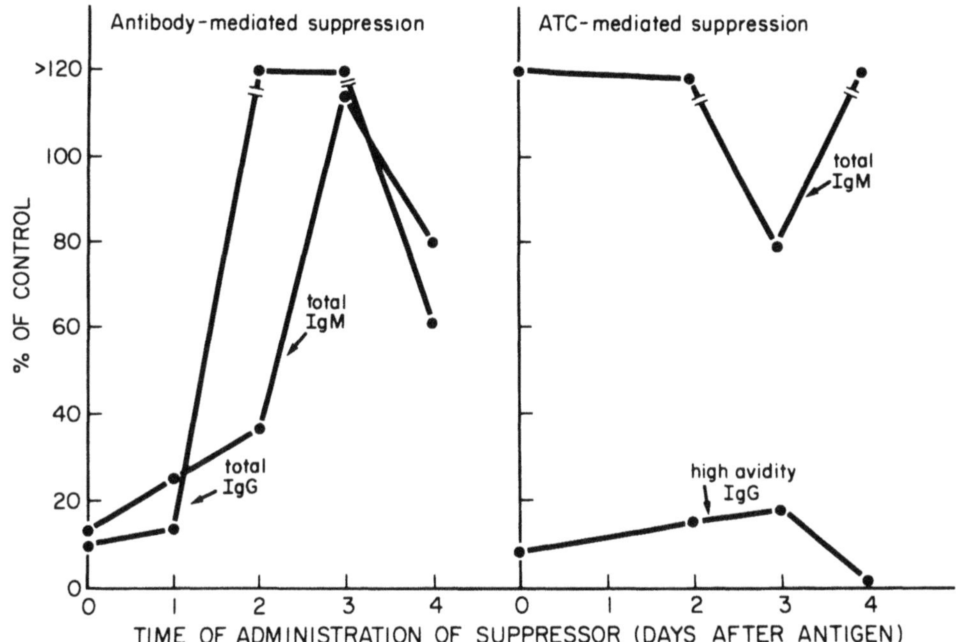

Fig. 2: Kinetics of antibody-mediated and ATC-mediated suppression.

Left panel: Mice were immunized with 100 μg DNP-dextran and anti-DNP PFC were measured 4 days later. At 0, 1, 2, 3 and 4 days after immunization, groups of 4 mice were given 200 μg of anti-dextran antibodies. Right panel: Mice were immunized with 100 μg DNP-KLH in CFA; 6 weeks later, they received 100 μg of DNP-KLH in saline and their spleens were assayed 4 days later for PFC. On 0, 2, 3 and 4 days after secondary immunization, animals received about 10×10^6 DNP-KLH ATC i.v.

antibody suppresses an early event in the response to antigen, whereas ATC suppression likely suppresses a late event.

T CELL SUPPRESSION IS RAPID

Since ATC were suppressive at all times tested, it was possible that suppression would be detectable with *in vitro* incubation of ATC and splenocytes. This was indeed shown to be the case. When ATC were mixed in equal numbers with hyperimmune splenocytes for 90 min. at 37°C under tissue culture conditions, preferential suppression of high avidity IgG PFC was seen.

Fig. 3 demonstrates the specificity of the effect.

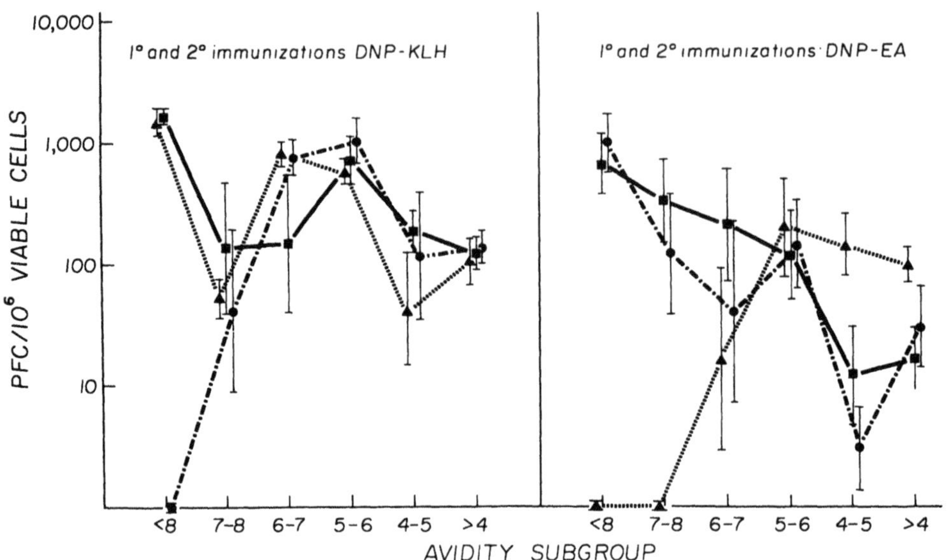

Fig. 3: Carrier specificity of late-acting suppressor activity.

Mice were primed with 100 μg of DNP-KLH or DNP-EA in CFA and 8 weeks later boosted i.p. with 100 μg of the homologous antigen in saline. Assay followed 4 days later, and no ATC (■), 10×10^6 DNP-KLH ATC (●), or 10×10^6 DNP-EA ATC (▲) were mixed with 20×10^6 DNP-KLH immune (left panel) or DNP-EA immune (right panel) splenocytes. Only homologous carrier ATC produced significant total PFC suppression ($p < 0.01$ for both DNP-KLH and DNP-EA hyperimmune cells). Indirect PFC are shown: direct PFC showed no effect. (From Warren and Davie, 1977a.)

If the anti-DNP PFC comes from animals immune to DNP-KLH, then DNP-KLH ATC, but not DNP-EA (egg albumin) ATC, are suppressive for high avidity PFC. Conversely, DNP-EA primed PFC are sensitive to only DNP-EA ATC. Just as in the *in vivo* suppression, the *in vitro* effect depended on Thy 1.1-bearing, nylon nonadherent cells; carrier specific ATC were equally suppressive as hapten-carrier primed ATC.

Since helper T cells are not thought to influence the immune response so late, the possibility of suppressor cells decreasing helper cell activity is unlikely. Nonetheless, we have not yet separated suppressor from helper function, both known to exist in ATC populations. We have, however, demonstrated that T depleted splenocyte populations remain susceptible to ATC populations. In addition, we have been able to remove the bulk of macrophages from both the target and suppressor cell populations by repeated plastic dish adsorption, again without affecting the suppressive function.

For these several reasons we feel it most likely that the PFC itself is the target for ATC suppression.

ROLE OF ANTIGEN IN SUPPRESSION

If this is so, the carrier-specific T cell or its factor must have the ability to distinguish between anti-hapten PFC which presumably differ only in the avidity of the immunoglobulin they secrete. The most likely means by which this difference could be expressed at the level of the B cell would be by the varying capacities of B cells to bind antigen to their surfaces. These antigen molecules in turn could be specific targets for T cells or their products.

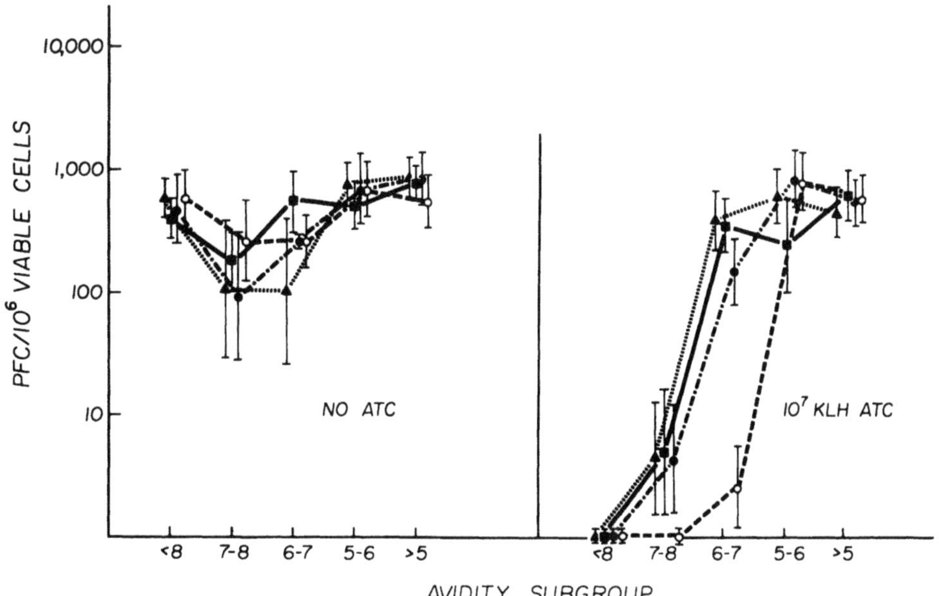

Fig. 4: Modification of suppression by preincubation of hyperimmune cells with antigen.

Mice were given 100 µg DNP-KLH in CFA, in the thighs, followed 10 weeks later by 100 µg DNP-KLH in saline i.p. Just before PFC assay 4 days later, immune spleen subfractions (about 8×10^6 cells) were preincubated with no antigen (■), 10 µg/ml KLH (●), 10 µg/ml DNP-EA (▲), or 10 µg/ml DNP-KLH (o). After washing, these cells were (right panel) or were not (left panel) incubated for 90 min. at 37°C with 10^7 KLH ATC. Total indirect PFC/10^6 were significantly reduced for all groups receiving ATC ($p<0.01$) and of these, preincubation of hyperimmune cells with DNP-KLH further reduced total PFC/10^6 ($p<0.05$). (From Warren and Davie, 1977b).

Evidence to support this hypothesis is reasonably strong. The *in vitro* exposure of DNP-KLH hyperimmune cells to DNP-KLH but not KLH or DNP-EA sensitizes the population to KLH ATC, producing an avidity dependent increase in the observed suppression (Fig. 4).

In a related experiment, DNP-KLH hyperimmune cells become sensitive to EA ATC (contrary to the normal carrier specificity) if hyperimmune cells are preincubated with DNP-EA but not EA alone nor EA mixed with DNP-KLH (Table III).

Thus, we propose that high avidity B cells recognize and bind specific haptenic determinants of the hapten-carrier conjugate, and thereupon gain surface carrier determinants which then serve as targets for carrier specific suppressor T cells and/or their soluble

Table III: Antigen mediated shift in the carrier specificity of suppression of DNP-KLH primed splenocytes*

Antigen Pulse	EA ATC	INDIRECT PFC/10^6 VIABLE CELLS total	<8
0	0	3108	705
EA	0	2931	675
DNP-KLH	0	3360	852
EA+DNP-KLH	0	2940	124
0	10^7	2800	819
EA	10^7	2869	1189
DNP-EA	10^7	2178	13
EA+DNP-KLH	10^7	3003	558

*1° immunization, 100 μg DNP-KLH in CFA; 2°, 100 μg DNP-KLH in saline, 6 weeks later; just prior to assay 4 days later, 8×10^6 immune spleen cells were preincubated with 10 μg/ml EA, DNP-EA, or 10 μg/ml EA and DNP-KLH for 1 hour at 37° C. The cells were washed twice, then incubated with 10^7 EA ATC for 90 min at 37°C. Underlined number is significantly different ($p<0.001$) from its control groups. (Modified from Warren and Davie, 1977b).

products, resulting in depression of antibody secretion. This concept is illustrated in Fig. 5.

As further support of this idea, DNP-KLH hyperimmune cells are protected from KLH ATC by prior incubation with anti-KLH but not normal guinea pig immunoglobulin (Table IV). Moreover, KLH ATC activity is specifically blocked by incubation with KLH (but not DNP-KLH) before mixture with target cells. This result favors a theory of physical blockade of suppressor molecules by KLH (presumably, DNP-KLH bound to suppressor would be an active complex). In addition, KLH produces a dose-dependent emergence of high avidity PFC when added to the ATC-hyperimmune cell mixture, and lower avidity suppressible PFC are first protected. This finding is consistent with the concept that lower avidity PFC, possessing fewer targets for suppressor binding, would first escape a suppression threshold in a suppressor limited system.

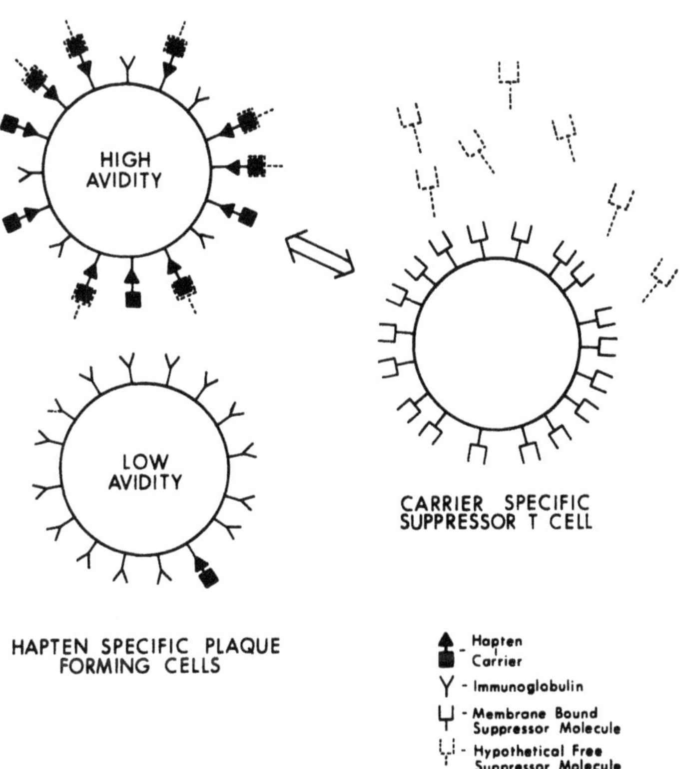

Fig. 5: Proposed mechanism for late acting suppression

Table IV: Protection against suppression by anti-carrier antibody; preincubation with hyperimmune cells*

Immunoglobulin Pulse	KLH ATC	INDIRECT PFC/10^6 VIABLE CELLS total	<8
-----	0	4476	656
anti-KLH	0	5290	798
normal Ig	0	4745	879
-----	10^7	3332	<u>0</u>
anti-KLH	10^7	5013	1267
normal Ig	10^7	3886	<u>0</u>

*1° immunization, 100 μg DNP-KLH in CFA; 2°, 100 μg DNP-KLH in saline, 8 weeks later; just prior to assay 4 days later, 10^7 hyperimmune splenocytes were incubated for 1 hr, 0°C with 0.13 mg/ml anti-KLH Ig or 0.17 mg/ml normal guinea pig Ig, then washed; KLH ATC were added, and incubated 90 min. at 37°C. Underlined numbers are significantly different ($p<0.001$) from control groups. (From Warren and Davie, 1977b).

Finally, and most impressive, is the loss of sensitivity of hyperimmune cells to ATC by prior treatment with pronase, suggesting the importance of membrane bound proteins. Even after regrowth of surface proteins, DNP-KLH hyperimmune cells remain insensitive to KLH ATC, unless the cells are first incubated with DNP-KLH (Table V).

COMMENTS

It seems clear that hapten-carrier conjugates remain on the surface of high avidity antibody secreting cells for at least 4 days after antigen administration and that this antigen provides the focus for carrier-specific, T cell-mediated suppression. Preliminary experiments to examine PFC directly for carrier determinants by radiolabelled anti-carrier antibody support this notion.

Table V: Loss and recovery of suppressibility following pronase treatment of hyperimmune cells*

Immune Splenocyte Pretreatment				INDIRECT PFC/10^6 VIABLE CELLS	
Pronase	Culture for Ig regrowth	DNP-KLH Pulse	KLH-ATC	total	<8
0	0	0	0	3359	482
0	0	0	10^7	2767	10
+	0	0	0	2266	209
+	0	0	10^7	2156	226
+	+	0	0	72277	15662
+	+	0	10^7	52949	13607
+	+	10 μg/ml	0	59889	10934
+	+	10 μg/ml	10^7	45958	164

*1° immunization, 100 μg DNP-KLH in CFA; 2° 100 μg DNP-KLH in saline, 6 weeks later; immediately before assay 4 days later, hyperimmune spleen cells were pronase treated, then incubated for 90 min. at 37°C with 10^7 KLH ATC. One set of pronase-treated hyperimmune cells, before incubation with ATC, were placed in culture for 20 hrs at 37°C in 5% CO_2; the population was rosetted with TNP-SRBC, then incubated for 1 hr on ice with 10 μg/ml DNP-KLH; after washing the hyperimmune cells twice, 10^7 KLH ATC/ml were added, and incubation continued for 90 min. at 37°C. Approximately 8×10^6 hyperimmune cells comprised each group. Total PFC recovery from group 3 to group 5 approximately 30%. Underlined numbers are significantly different ($p<0.001$) from control groups. (From Warren and Davie, 1977b).

What remains unclear is the relationship of this mechanism of suppression to others which clearly point to other cellular targets. Of particular importance are the extensive studies of Tada and his coworkers (1975) of suppressor T cells which also preferentially suppress high avidity IgG anti-hapten antibody production, but which are thought to act by inhibiting helper T cell activity. How, in fact, suppressed helper activity is translated into an avidity dependent antibody suppression remains problematic, particularly in view of Sanfilippo and Scotts' (1976) demonstration that helper cell unresponsiveness does not seem to alter the avidity of antibody. Nonetheless, direct effects of suppressor T cells on helper function have been described in the allotype suppression system of Herzenberg (1976). However, even in this system, Bosma and Bosma (1977) showed that suppressor cells acted directly on plasmacytoma cells bearing the appropriate allotypic determinants.

Whether, in fact, these disparate results of suppressor cell targets reflect multiple suppressor cell populations each specific for a different target cell, or whether a single suppressor population can act on several types of target cells is not clear. The results of our studies would indicate that if suppressor T cells act on several different target cells antigen will likely be found on each.

ACKNOWLEDGEMENTS

This research was supported by USPHS grants AI-11635, GM-02016, and CA-09118 and by grant SPF-13 from the American Cancer Society.

REFERENCES

Bosma, M.J. and Bosma, G.C. (1977) J. Exp. Med. 145, 743.

Eichmann, K. (1974) Eur. J. Immunol. 5, 511.

Elson, C.J. and Taylor, R.B. (1974) Eur. J. Immunol. 4, 682.

Hansburg, D., Briles, D.E. and Davie, J.M. (1976) J. Immunol. 117, 569.

Herzenberg, L.A., Okumura, K., Cantor, H., Sato, V.L., Shen, F.W., Boyse, E.A. and Herzenberg, L.A. (1976) J. Exp. Med. 144, 330.

Owen, F.L., Ju, S. and Nisonoff, A. (1977) J. Exp. Med. 145, 1559.

Rude, E., Wrede, J. and Gundelach, M.L. (1976) J. Immunol. 116, 527.

Sanfilippo, F. and Scott, D.W. (1974) J. Immunol. 113, 1661.

Sanfilippo, F. and Scott, D.W. (1976) Cell. Immunol. 21, 112.

Tada, T. and Takemori, T. (1974) J. Exp. Med. 140, 239.

Tada, T., Taniguchi, M. and Takemori, T. (1975) Transplant. Rev. 26, 106.

Takemori, T. and Tada, T. (1974) J. Exp. Med. 140, 253.

Warren, R.W. and Davie, J.M. (1977a) J. Immunol., in press.

Warren, R.W. and Davie, J.M. (1977b) J. Exp. Med., in press.

Warren, R.W., Murphy, S. and Davie, J.M. (1976) J. Immunol. 116, 1385.

GENETIC CONTROL OF THE T-LYMPHOCYTE PROLIFERATIVE RESPONSE TO CYTOCHROME _C_

Ronald H. Schwartz, Alan M. Solinger, Michiel Ultee and Emanuel Margoliash

The Laboratory of Immunology, NIAID, NIH, Bethesda, Md. and the Department of Biochemistry and Molecular Biology, Northwestern University, Evanston, Ill.

Abstract

Cytochromes _c_ have been used as antigens in a murine T-lymphocyte proliferation assay in order to characterize the nature of determinants whose recognition is under immune response (Ir) gene control. The cytochromes are advantagous as antigens because 1) they have well-characterized primary and tertiary structures, 2) they are antigenically simple, differing from mouse cytochrome _c_ at only a small number of amino acid residues, and 3) there exist a large number of evolutionary variants which can be used to locate antigenic sites by cross-stimulation. In the present studies, the T-lymphocyte proliferative response to pigeon cytochrome _c_ was shown to be under the control of two complementing major histocompatibility (MHC)-linked Ir genes in mice of the $H\text{-}2^a$ and $H\text{-}2^k$ haplotypes. Mice of the $H\text{-}2^b$, $H\text{-}2^d$, $H\text{-}2^p$, $H\text{-}2^q$, $H\text{-}2^s$, and $H\text{-}2^u$ haplotypes were low or nonresponders. Complementation was demonstrated by showing that an F_1 hybrid between two nonresponder recombinant strains, B10.A(4R) and B10.A(5R), could respond to pigeon cytochrome _c_. The determinant on the cytochrome recognized in this immune response was located to the C-terminal portion of the molecule around residues 89 and/or 100. This was shown by the failure of closely related cytochromes from the Pekin duck and chicken to cross-stimulate T lymphocytes immune to pigeon cytochrome; positions 89 and 100 carry the only residues different from those in mouse cytochrome _c_ that are unique to pigeon cytochrome among the three bird cytochromes tested. This localization was further substantiated by demonstrating that the cyanogen bromide cleavage-fragment (residues 81-104) from pigeon cytochrome, but not the same fragment from Pekin duck cytochrome, was as good a stimulant of T cells immune to the whole molecule as the intact cytochrome. These results identify the immunogenic site on the molecule as one which differs from mouse cytochrome c by only one or two amino-acid residues. Thus, T-cell immune responses, which are under MHC-linked Ir gene control, are as capable as antibody responses of recognizing subtle differences in protein structure. However, the ability of T cells to respond equally well to stimulation with polypeptide fragments or with the whole molecule suggests either that T-cell recognition involves certain differences from B cell recognition or that in some cases the fragments possess a similar spatial structure to that of the corresponding segment in the native protein.

* * * *

The importance of the study of globular proteins as model antigens for dissecting the immune response has only recently begun to be reappreciated. Proteins were eclipsed for many years by the seemingly simpler synthetic poly-amino acids. Although the latter antigens offer simplicity in composition, they are heterogeneous in molecular weight and spatial conformation and often differ in antigenic properties from one preparation to the next. In contrast, biochemical studies of many globular proteins have now given us a thorough understanding of the amino acid sequence of the molecules and in many cases precise knowledge of their three-dimensional structure. Furthermore, enzymic and chemical cleavage of these molecules into fragments sometimes makes it possible to localize antigenic determinants (Reichlin, M., 1975).

Cytochrome c, a heme protein of the mitochondrial respiratory chain, has proved to be an extremely useful antigen for the study of the immune response (Reichlin 1975, Urbanski and Margoliash 1977 a,b). It is a globular protein, composed of a single polypeptide chain of a little over 100 amino acids (Figure 1). The amino acid sequences of over 85 examples of this protein from different eukaryotic sources are known (Dayhoff and Eck, 1972; Borden and Margoliash, 1976) and the three-dimensional structure of three of them has been determined at high resolution (Figure 1). The spatial conformation of these three cytochromes, horse, tuna and bonito, were found to be identical, implying a uniformity of conformation for all eukaryotic cytochromes c (Dickerson and Timkovich, 1975). Thus, this group of proteins represents an excellent system with which to study the effects of amino-acid sequence variations on the antigenicity of a globular protein, independent of changes in conformation. The existence of well caracterized, closely related evolutionary variants has provided the major means for localizing antigenic determinants on the molecule without fragmentation through the study of immune cross-reactions (Urbanski and Margoliash, 1977 a,b).

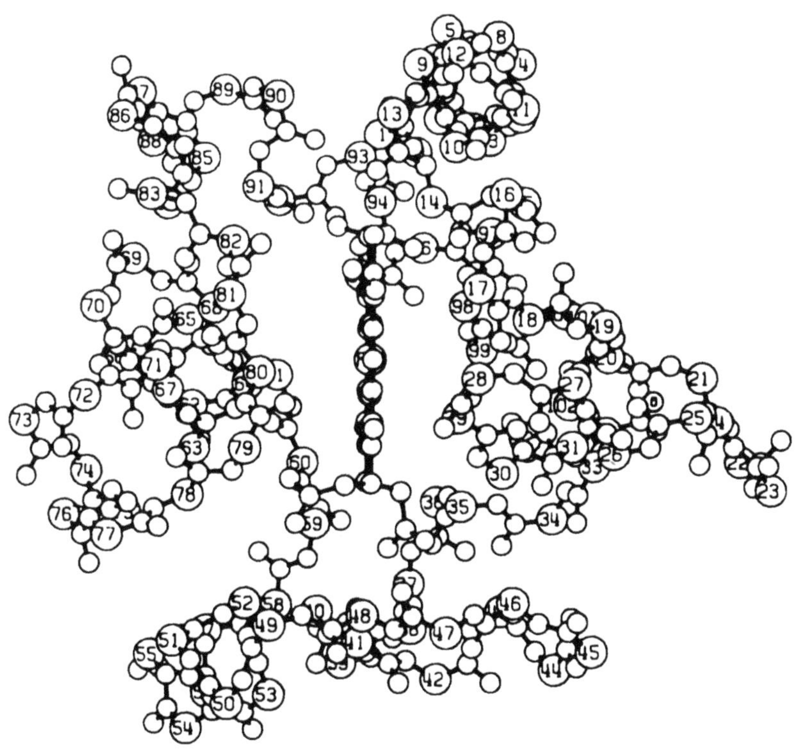

Figure 1. A representation of the spatial structure of the backbone peptide chain of cytochrome c, as derived from the x-ray crystallographic analysis of the tuna protein (Swanson *et al.*, 1977; and Takano *et al.*, 1977). The view is of the front of the molecule, namely the surface containing the exposed edge of the heme along pyrrole rings II and IV. The larger circles represent the α-amino nitrogen atoms with the residue numbers displayed in them. The heme is a square structure in the center of the figure, seen edge on.

The mouse has been an ideal animal for the study of the genetic control of the immune response because of the existence of a large number of inbred strains as well as recombinant and congenic-resistant lines (Klein, 1975). The recent development of a T-lymphocyte proliferation assay for the mouse, has allowed our laboratory to study the genetic control of the immune response at the T-cell level (Schwartz _et al._, 1975,1977; Schwartz and Paul, 1976). In particular, synthetic polypeptides and protein antigens have been used to demonstrate that immune response (Ir) genes exert control over the T-lymphocyte proliferative response (Schwartz and Paul, 1976). In the present studies we have carried out an analysis of the T-lymphocyte proliferative response to cytochrome _c_ in an attempt to locate the antigenic determinants whose recognition is under Ir gene control.

All cytochromes _c_ were prepared by the procedure of Margoliash and Walasek (1967) as modified by Brautigen _et al._ (1977). This procedure insured the strict absence of any of the polymeric and deamidated artifactual forms of the protein that commonly contaminate the preparations. Mice of the C57BL/10 Sn (B10) H-2 congenic series were immunized in the hind foot pads with 0.016, 0.16, 1.6 or 8 nmol. (0.2, 2, 20 or 100μg, respectively), of various cytochromes _c_ emulsified in Freund's complete adjuvant. Two to three weeks later, thioglycollate-induced peritoneal exudate cells were harvested and passed over nylon wool columns. The nonadherent peritoneal exudate, T-lymphocyte-enriched cells (PETLES) were cultured in microculture wells at 2×10^5 cells per well, for 5 days in the presence or absence of antigen. Stimulation was assessed by measuring the incorporation of a 1μCi pulse of ^{3}H-methyl-thymidine 16-18 hr prior to terminating the cultures (Schwartz _et al._, 1975, 1977 and Schwartz and Paul, 1976). The data are mainly expressed as the difference between the mean of the antigen-stimulated and control cultures (ΔCPM).

The dose-response curve of PETLES from B10.A mice immunized with 8 nmol of human cytochrome _c_ is shown in figure 2. A T-cell proliferative response of substantial magnitude was observed. Beginning at a concentration of 0.016μM the response rose to a peak of 37,900 (ΔCPM) at a concentration of 1.6μM and then decreased slightly thereafter. The concentration required to achieve a half-maximal stimulation was approximately 0.1μM. Human cytochrome _c_ was a very potent immunogen. Immunization with 1.6 nmol (20μg) or as little as 0.16 nmol per mouse resulted in a significant PETLES proliferative response. Only immunization with 0.016 nmol failed to elicit a response.

In an attempt to analyze the antigenic determinants present on human cytochrome _c_ responsible for eliciting the T-cell proliferative response, PETLES from mice immunized to human cytochrome _c_ were challenged _in vitro_ with cytochromes _c_ obtained from other

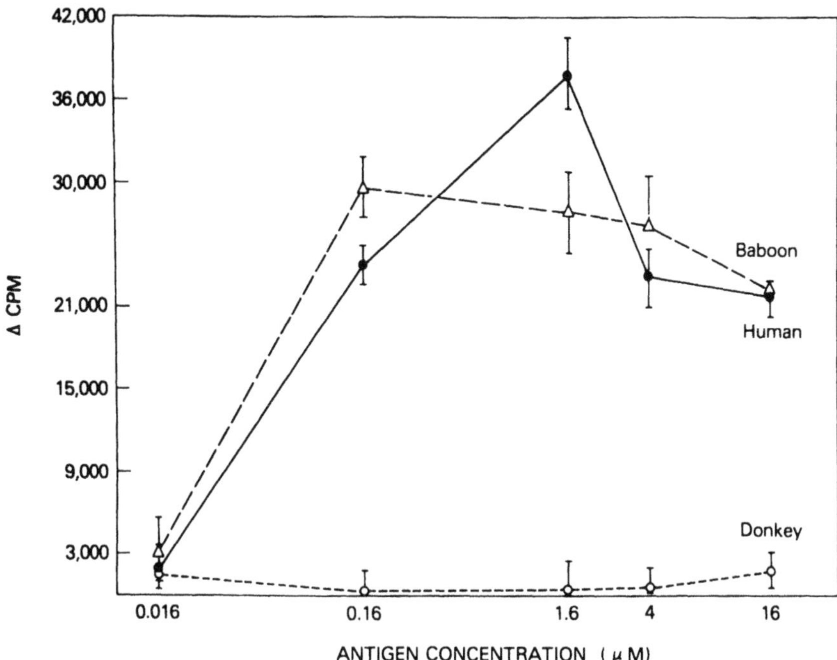

Figure 2. The T-lymphocyte proliferative response to human cytochrome c (●) baboon cytochrome c (Δ) or donkey cytochrome c (0) by PETLES from B10.A mice primed with 8 nmol of human cytochrome c. The ordinate denotes the difference in cpm of ^{3}H-thymidine incorporated between cultures stimulated with the cytochromes and control cultures stimulated with medium alone (ΔCPM).

species. The assumption we made was that cross-stimulations would be observed in those cases in which the variant cytochromes shared antigenic determinants with the immunizing cytochrome. The results with human cytochrome c as the immunogen were not very fruitful. Of all the cytochromes examined, only baboon cytochrome c showed any cross-stimulation. The human cytochrome sequence differs from the mouse cytochrome sequence in 9 amino-acid positions. Thus, there exist 9 potential antigenic sites on human cytochrome c if each amino acid difference constitutes a site. Of these 9 differences baboon protein shares 8 in common with human cytochrome. Therefore, it is not surprising that baboon cytochrome c gives essentially an identical dose response curve (Figure 2) to that of human cytochrome c. In fact, PETLES from B10.A mice immunized to baboon cytochrome c were also stimulated identically by human and baboon cytochromes. The same was true in the B10 strain. In contrast to these complete cross-reactions, cytochromes which share only one potential antigenic site with human cytochrome did not cross-stimulate. For example, donkey cytochrome, which carries a proline at position 44 similar to the human protein (as compared to an alanine in mouse cytochrome *c*) did not stimulate PETLES from B10.A mice immunized to human cytochrome *c* (Figure 2). In all, 4 of the 9 variant residues in human cytochrome *c* were examined in this manner and none showed any cross-reactions. These results may mean that the T-cell antigenic sites lie among the other 5 positions, or that several amino-acid substitutions taken together are needed to constitute an antigenic site. In the latter case, our approach would not fully eliminate any regions of the molecule as possible T-cell stimulating determinants.

To simplify our approach we turned to the study of cytochromes which differed only minimally in composition from mouse cytochrome *c*. An example of an antigen of this type is rabbit cytochrome *c* which differs from mouse at two sites, a valine for alanine substitution at position 44 and an aspartic acid for glycine substitution at position 89. Rabbit cytochrome *c* was not as immunogenic as human cytochrome *c*. Immunization of several strains with 1.6 nmol of rabbit cytochrome did not result in a significant PETLES proliferative response. Only the 8 nmol (100μg) immunization dose elicited sufficient priming to be seen in the secondary T-cell assay (Table 1). Unfortunately, it also revealed a surprising finding, namely, that mouse cytochrome *c* could cross-stimulate PETLES immunized to high doses of rabbit cytochrome (Table 1). This had never been observed in PETLES from mice immunized with human cytochrome *c*, although it was readily reproducible when rabbit cytochrome *c* was the immunogen. Therefore, several strains were immunized with mouse cytochrome *c* to determine if this cytochrome was immunogenic. As shown in Figure 3 mouse cytochrome *c*

TABLE I

T-LYMPHOCYTE PROLIFERATIVE RESPONSE TO RABBIT CYTOCHROME *c*[a]

Mouse Strain	Proliferative Response (CPM ± SEM)		
	Medium	Rabbit Cytochrome	Mouse Cytochrome
B10	1,600 ± 300	19,400 ± 1,000	7,100 ± 2,800
B10.A	700 ± 200	11,500 ± 400	8,500 ± 1,000

[a] 2×10^5 PETLES from B10 or B10.A mice immunized with 8 nmol of rabbit cytochrome *c* were stimulated *in vitro* with various concentrations of rabbit or mouse cytochrome *c*. Only the maximum responses are shown.

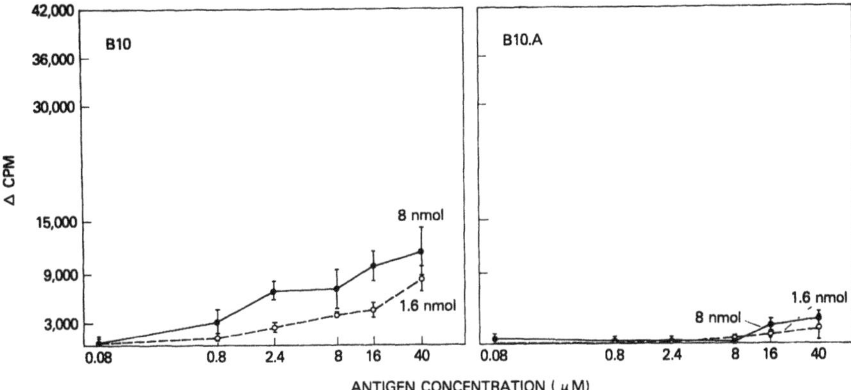

Figure 3. The T-lymphocyte proliferative response to various concentrations of mouse cytochrome c by PETLES from B10 (left panel) or B10.A (right panel) mice primed with 8 nmol (●) or 1.6 nmol (0) of mouse cytochrome c.

was immunogenic to some degree. The magnitude of the PETLES response was greater the higher the immunization dose (compare 8 with 1.6 nmol) and varied consistently from strain to strain (compare B10 with B10.A). However, at no time was it as potent an immunogen as human cytochrome. It would thus appear that the mouse is not completely tolerant to its own cytochrome c, possibly because this protein is mainly sequestered in the mitochondria, which have an intracellular localization. In any event this "autoimmune" response made analysis of the immune response to rabbit cytochrome c difficult to carry out. Although one might suspect that the clones of T cells which respond to the rabbit specific determinants are independent of the clones of T cells which respond to the shared mouse and rabbit determinants and that the rabbit specific response could be calculated by subtracting the response to the mouse cytochrome, one can not prove this assumption for the T cell assay because the end point in the assay, thymidine incorporation, gives no measure of specificity. We, therefore, concluded that the clearest results would come from analysis of those cytochromes which did not show significant cross-stimulation with mouse cytochrome.

Pigeon cytochrome c was one antigen which met our requirements for a potent but specific immunogen. It was highly immunogenic in B10.A mice when administered at 1.6 nmol per mouse (Figure 4). The half maximal response occurred at a concentration of approximately 0.3μM. Furthermore, the PETLES could not be stimulated by any dose of mouse cytochrome c from 0.08μM to 40μM (Figure 4). Even PETLES from B10.A mice immunized with 8 nmol of pigeon cytochrome showed only a negligible cross-reaction with mouse cytochrome (≤ 10% of the pigeon response at an equivalent dose) (Figure 5). Finally, unlike the case with human cytochrome, two closely related bird cytochromes, chicken and Pekin duck, failed to give any cross-stimulation (Figure 5). Pigeon cytochrome c differs from mouse cytochrome c at 7 amino acid positions. Of these 7, Pekin duck and chicken cytochrome each share 4 of the residue changes of pigeon cytochrome and together they share 5 of the 7 sites. Thus, their failures to cross-stimulate suggest that none of those 5 sites alone, nor two different combinations of 4 sites together, represent the antigenic determinants. By this process of elimination the amino acid substitutions at positions 89 and 100 represent the best candidates for the immunogenic determinants on the molecule. On the other hand, one should be cautioned that this analysis is based entirely on negative data i.e. the failure of related cytochromes to cross-stimulate. It is possible that the chicken and Pekin duck cytochromes fail to stimulate because the immunogen in pigeon cytochrome c is a non-cytochrome trace contaminant. We consider this possibility highly unlikely because of the very high degree of purity of the preparation, that is certainly greater than 99%.

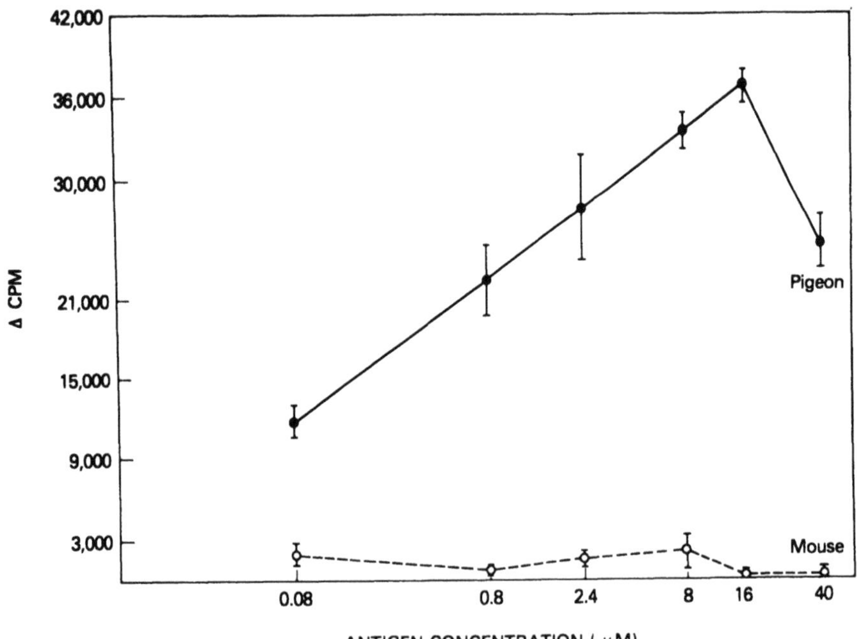

Figure 4. The T-lymphocyte proliferative response to pigeon (●) or mouse (O) cytochrome c by PETLES from B10.A mice primed with 1.6 nmol of pigeon cytochrome c.

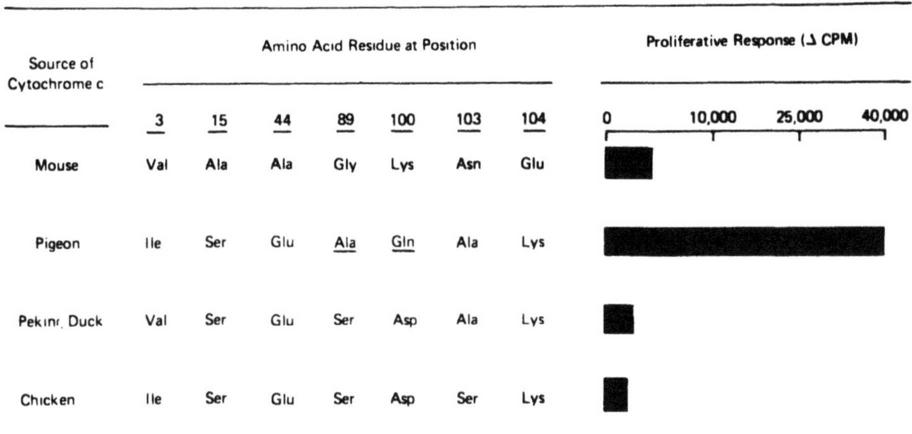

Source of Cytochrome c	Amino Acid Residue at Position						
	3	15	44	89	100	103	104
Mouse	Val	Ala	Ala	Gly	Lys	Asn	Glu
Pigeon	Ile	Ser	Glu	Ala	Gln	Ala	Lys
Pekin Duck	Val	Ser	Glu	Ser	Asp	Ala	Lys
Chicken	Ile	Ser	Glu	Ser	Asp	Ser	Lys

Figure 5. A list of the 7 positions at which pigeon cytochrome c differs from mouse cytochrome c and the amino acids at each of these positions in mouse, pigeon, Pekin duck and chicken cytochromes c. The bar graph at the right shows the T-lymphocyte proliferative response to each of the four cytochromes by PETLES from B10.A mice primed with 8 nmol of pigeon cytochrome c.

Furthermore, even if as high as a 1% contaminant existed, it would probably not be present in sufficient amounts to be immunogenic (1.6 picomoles in 0.16nmol, the lowest immunization dose which gave a significant response). However, one would ideally like to demonstrate that cytochromes having an alanine residue at position 89 or a glutamine residue at position 100 could cross-stimulate PETLES from B10.A mice primed to pigeon cytochrome. Thus, we turned to a different approach, cross-stimulation with antigen fragments, in order to confirm the localization of the antigenic site(s).

Cross-Stimulation of PETLES Immune to Pigeon Cytochrome c with Cyanogen Bromide Cleavage-Fragments of the Cytochrome.

Earlier studies on the genetic control of the T-lymphocyte proliferative response to staphylococcal nuclease demonstrated that PETLES from mice immunized to the whole molecule could be stimulated to proliferate *in vitro* by peptide fragments of the protein (Berzofsky *et al*. In Press; and this book). Only some of the fragments stimulated, and which ones stimulated changed according to the mouse strain examined. It thus appeared that T-lymphocytes could recognize some antigenic determinants whether they were present in the native structure or in polypeptide fragments of the protein.

Similar experiments with cytochrome c led to clear cut results. Pigeon cytochrome c was cleaved with cyanogen bromide and the three fragments (residues 1-65, 66-80, and 81-104), as well as some uncleaved whole molecules, were separated by Sephadex G-50 chromatography in 7% formic acid (Corradin and Harbury, 1970). Similar fragments of the noncross-reacting Pekin duck cytochrome c were also prepared for controls. B10.A mice were immunized with intact pigeon cytochrome and their PETLES challenged *in vitro* with equal molar concentrations of the whole molecule or the various fragments. As shown in Table 2 the C-terminal fragment (residues 81-104) was the only one of the three pigeon peptides that elicited a response. In fact it stimulated better than the intact molecule, whether or not the latter had been exposed to the cleaving conditions. The other two fragments did not give significant stimulation and neither did the C-terminal fragment isolated from Pekin duck cytochrome. Thus, the stimulation with fragment (81-104) from pigeon cytochrome c was highly specific.

These results lead to two important conclusions. One is the localization of the antigenic site in pigeon cytochrome c to the portion of the molecule between residues 81 and 104, the same region identified by the cross-stimulation results obtained with the evolutionary variants. Thus, we seem to be on firm ground in assigning the antigenic site(s) of pigeon cytochrome recognized by B10.A T-lymphocytes to the region of the molecule around the positions 89 and/or 100. The second and possibly more provocative conclusion, is that T-lymphocytes would appear to recognize antigenic determinants in the fragmented molecule at least as well, if not better, than they recognize these determinants in the intact protein. This is in striking contrast to the specificities of most antibody molecules reactive against soluble protein antigens. Such antibodies are exquisitely sensitive to the tertiary structure of the antigen (Sela, 1969 and Benjamini *et al.*, 1972). It is possible that the particular determinants recognized by the present T cells tend to maintain their native conformation even in polypeptide fragments. For example, the stimulatory fragment (residues 81-104) of pigeon cytochrome c contains all 17 residues which make up the largest α helix in the protein (residues 87-103). Thus, the fragment may still retain the α helical conformation which may be required for stimulation. On the other hand, the ability of T-cell receptors to recognize equally well the same determinants in either the native or fragmented form of the protein may turn out to be a fundamental difference between B cell and T cell antigen recognition. In addition, it should not be over-looked that the T-cell responses thus far detected appear to be much more restricted than the responses of B-cells. In the above example only 2 of the 7 variant residues in pigeon cytochrome c seem to be involved in the T-cell proliferative response, and a similar phenomenon was noted with human cytochrome *c*. In contrast, at the B cell level, in every case so far studied, all variant residues on the cytochrome molecules elicited an antibody response (Reichlin, 1975; Urbanski and Margoliash, 1977 a,b). The reasons for this difference remain to be determined.

Genetic Control of the T-lymphocyte Proliferative Response to Pigeon Cytochrome *c*.

Having localized a T-cell antigenic determinant on pigeon cytochrome *c* to the regions around residues 89 and 100, we next

TABLE 2

CROSS-STIMULATION OF PETLES FROM B10.A MICE IMMUNIZED TO PIGEON CYTOCHROME WITH CYANOGEN BROMIDE CLEAVAGE-FRAGMENTS OF CYTOCHROME *C*

Cytochrome Source	Stimulating Fragment (residues)[a]	Proliferative Response (ΔCPM)
Pigeon	Intact (1-104)	19,000
Pigeon	Intact (CnBr-treated)	22,200
Pigeon	1-65	4,700
Pigeon	66-80	300
Pigeon	81-104	31,600
Duck	1-65	< 0
Duck	66-80	1,300
Duck	81-104	6,600

[a] 2×10^5 PETLES from B10.A mice primed with 1.6 nmol of pigeon cytochrome *c* were stimulated *in vitro* with 8μM of pigeon cytochrome (Intact), pigeon cytochrome exposed to the cleavage conditions but recovered intact (CnBr-treated) or the three cyanogen bromide cleavage-fragments, residues 1 to 65, 66 to 80 and 81 to 104 from either pigeon or Pekin duck cytochrome *c*.

attempted to determine whether MHC-linked immune response (Ir) genes were involved in the recognition of these determinants. Mice of the B10-H2 congenic series were immunized with 1.6 nmol of pigeon cytochrome c and their PETLES assayed for responsiveness to pigeon cytochrome, mouse cytochrome and purified protein derivative of tuberculin (PPD) (Table 3). This series of strains includes different MHC-haplotypes on the same C57BL/10Sn non-H-2 background (Klein, 1975). Thus, differences in responsiveness can be directly attributed to differences in MHC genes. As shown in Table 3, only 2 of the 8 B10 congenic strains tested responded well to pigeon cytochrome i.e. mice of the $H\text{-}2^a$ and $H\text{-}2^k$ haplotypes. In both cases the response was specific for pigeon cytochrome in that no significant stimulation was observed with mouse cytochrome. The nonresponder and low responder strains, $H\text{-}2^b$, $H\text{-}2^d$, $H\text{-}2^p$, $H\text{-}2^q$, $H\text{-}2^s$, and $H\text{-}2^u$ were clearly selective poor responders since in all cases their PETLES responded to PPD. Because the $H\text{-}2^a$ haplotype (kkkkkdddd)* is felt to be a natural recombinant between the high responder $h\text{-}2^k$ and the nonresponder $H\text{-}2^d$ haplotypes, it would appear that only B10 congenic strains possessing k alleles in the K and I regions of the MHC can respond to pigeon cytochrome. Thus, the Ir gene control of the response to pigeon cytochrome is as restricted as the Ir gene control for any of the synthetic polypeptides (Shreffler and David, 1975).

An even more interesting complexity of the Ir gene control of the response to pigeon cytochrome was revealed when genetic mapping studies were attempted. Several recombinant strains exist between the B10.A and B10 strains in which the cross-over event occurred within the I region (Klein, 1975 and Shreffler and David, 1975). Because B10.A is a responder to pigeon cytochrome and B10 a nonresponder the recombinants could be used to localize the immune response genes more precisely. As shown in Table 4 PETLES from both the B10.A (4R) and B10.A (5R) recombinant strains did not respond to pigeon cytochrome i.e. they behaved like the nonresponder B10 strain. The failure of the recombinants to respond could not be attributed to the acquisition of a suppressive gene product from the B10 parent, since responsiveness was dominant over nonresponsiveness as shown by the good proliferative response to pigeon cytochrome of PETLES from $(B10.A \times B10)F_1$ mice (Table 4). Thus, the failure of the B10.A (4R) (kkbbbbbbb) to respond must be the result of a loss of $H\text{-}2^k$ genetic material to the right of the I-A subregion and the failure of the B10.A (5R) (bbbkkdddd) to respond must be the result of a loss of $H\text{-}2^k$ genetic material to the left of the I-J subregion. These observations suggest either that a single Ir

*Letters refer to the haplotype source of origin of the K, I-A, I-B, I-J, I-E, I-C, S, G and D alleles of the major histocompatibility complex. See Klein, 1975.

TABLE 3

MHC-LINKED Ir GENES CONTROL THE T-LYMPHOCYTE

PROLIFERATIVE RESPONSE TO PIGEON CYTOCHROME C

Mouse Strain	H-2 Haplotype	T-Lymphocyte Proliferation (ΔCPM) to Pigeon Cytochrome	Mouse Cytochrome	PPD
B10.A	a	36,900[a]	1,900	77,300
B10	b	1,200	300	73,400
B10.D2	d	1,600	1,200	39,400
B10.BR	k	39,200	2,600	55,800
B10.P	p	2,900	800	100,300
B10.Q	q	1,200	1,700	28,700
B10.S	s	3,600	3,000	10,900
B10.PL	u	1,000	100	93,000

[a] Underlined responses to pigeon cytochrome are those which were statistically significantly different from the response to mouse cytochrome by a Student's t test.

gene controlling the proliferative response to pigeon cytochrome is located in the I-B subregion or that more than one Ir gene controls the response. To distinguish between these two alternatives [B10.A (4R) x B10.A (5R)]F_1 hybrids were bred and examined for their response to pigeon cytochrome. A failure to respond would indicate a single gene in I-B, as the (4R x 5R)F_1 is still homozygous for the low responder b allele at I-B. On the other hand, a response by this strain would indicate gene complementation and suggest that at least two genes control the response (Dorf and Benacerraf, 1975 and Schwartz *et al.*, 1976). The results in Table 4 demonstrate quite clearly that the latter explanation is correct. The cross between the two nonresponders produced a responder strain. Therefore, the T-lymphocyte proliferative response to pigeon cytochrome is controlled by two MHC-linked Ir genes, one mapping to the left of the I-B subregion in K or I-A and the other to the right of the I-B subregion in I-J, I-E, or I-C.

TABLE 4

GENETIC MAPPING OF THE Ir GENES CONTROLLING THE T-LYMPHOCYTE PROLIFERATIVE RESPONSE TO PIGEON CYTOCHROME *C*

Mouse Strain	MHC Alleles[a] K A B J E C S G D	Proliferative Response (ΔCPM)[b] to Pigeon Cytochrome c
B10.A	k k k k k d d d d	18,500
B10	b b b b b b b b b	800
(B10.A x B10) F_1	k k k k k d d d d / b b b b b b b b b	19,700
B10.A (4R)	k k b b b b b b b	100
B10.A (5R)	b b b k k d d d d	2,300
(4R x 5R) F_1	k k b b b b b b b / b b b k k d d d d	18,800

[a] Capital letters refer to the genetic regions of the major histocompatibility complex (MHC). A B J E and C are the subregions of the I region. Small letters refer to the haplotype source of the genes in each region or subregion.

[b] 2×10^5 PETLES from mice immunized with 1.6 nmoles of pigeon cytochrome *c* were stimulated *in vitro* with 8μM of pigeon cytochrome.

In conclusion, these studies have demonstrated the potential usefulness of cytochrome c as an antigen for analyzing the genetic control of the immune response at the T-cell level. On the one hand the structural features of a well characterized globular protein with an array of evolutionary variants provides a powerful means of localizing antigenic determinants. On the other hand, the limited sequence differences between the antigen and the cytochrome of the responding species ensures a relatively restricted immune response which will be under easily discernible MHC-linked Ir gene control. As a result it should be possible to delineate at the structural level what type of antigenic determinants are under Ir gene control and whether these determinants are identical to those recognized by antibody molecules. In the case of pigeon cytochrome discussed in this paper it was demonstrated that the ability to respond to a region of the molecule located near positions 89 and/or 100 is controlled by two separate MHC-linked Ir genes of the k haplotype. Thus, even such complexities as two gene complementation would appear to be amenable to this approach and one may indeed hope that the use of cytochrome c as an antigen in the proliferation assay will lead to a better understanding of this aspect of the T-cell response.

Acknowledgments

We wish to thank Dr. William E. Paul for many helpful and stimulating discussions. The authors are also grateful to Dr. R.E. Dickerson for providing the stereo diagram of the structure of cytochrome c from which Figure 1 was made.

References

Benjamini, E., Scibienski, R.J., and Thompson, K. (1972). Contemp. Top. Immunochem. 1, 1.

Berzofsky, J.A., Schwartz, R.H., Schechter, A.N., and Sachs, D.H. Proc. Third Ir Workshop. H.O. McDevitt, Ed. Academic Press, New York. In press.

Borden, D. and Margoliash, E. (1976). Handbook of Biochemistry and Molecular Biology, Vol. 3. G.D. Fasman (Ed.) The Chemical Rubber Co., Cleveland, pp. C-156-161.

Brautigan, D.L., Ferguson-Miller, S., and Margoliash, E. (1977) Methods in Enzymology. In press.

Corradin, G. and Harbury, H.A. (1970). Biochem. Biophys. Acta. 221, 489.

Dayhoff, M.O. and Eck, R.V. (1972). Atlas of Protein Sequence and Structure, Nat. Biomed. Res. Found., Washington.

Dickerson, R.E. and Timkovich, R. (1975). The Enzymes, Third Edition, Vol. XI, P.D. Boyer (Ed.) Academic Press, New York, p. 397.

Dorf, M.E. and Benacerraf, B. (1975) Proc. Natl. Acad. Sci. U.S.A. 72, 3671.

Klein, J. (1975). Biology of the Mouse Histocompatibility-2 Complex. Springer-Verlag, New York, pp. 16-39.

Margoliash, E. and Walasek, O.F. (1967). Methods in Enzymology Vol. X, R.W. Estabrook and M.E. Pullman (Eds.) Academic Press, New York, p. 339.

Reichlin, M. (1975). Adv. Immunol. 20, 71.

Schwartz, R.H., Jackson, L., and Paul, W.E. (1975). J. Immunol. 115, 1330.

Schwartz, R.H., Dorf, M.E., Benacerraf, B., and Paul, W.E. (1976). J. Exp. Med. 143, 897.

Schwartz, R.H. and Paul, W.E. (1976). J. Exp. Med. 143, 529.

Schwartz, R.H., Horton, C.L., and Paul, W.E. (1977). J. Exp. Med. 145, 327.

Sela, M. (1969). Science 166, 1365.

Shreffler, D.C. and David, C.S. (1975). Adv. Immunol. 20, 125.

Swanson, R., Trus, B.L., Mandel, N., Mandel, G., Kallai, O.B. and Dickerson, R.E. (1977). J. Biol. Chem. 252, 759.

Takano, T., Trus, B.L., Mandel, N., Mandel, G., Kallai, O.B., Swanson, R. and Dickerson, R.E. (1977). J. Biol. Chem. 252, 776.

Urbanski, G.J. and Margoliash, E. (1977a). Immunochemistry of Enzymes and their Antibodies, M.R.H. Solton, Ed. John Wiley & Sons, New York, p. 204.

Urbanski, G.J. and Margoliash, E. (1977b). J. Immunol. 118, 1170.

INDEPENDENT PRECURSORS FOR THYMUS DEPENDENT AND THYMUS INDEPENDENT IgG MEMORY B CELLS

Marvin B. Rittenberg and Thomas V. Tittle

Department of Microbiology and Immunology
University of Oregon Health Sciences Center
Portland, Oregon 97201

ABSTRACT

Spleen cells from mice primed with the thymus dependent antigen trinitrophenyl keyhole limpet hemocyanin several months earlier can be cultured *in vitro* to give vigorous IgG antihapten PFC responses to thymus dependent and thymus independent forms of the hapten. The IgG memory precursors responding to these two forms of the hapten constitute functionally distinct subpopulations which we have designated as $B_{1\gamma}$ and $B_{2\gamma}$ to represent the precursor cells responding to the thymus independent and thymus dependent antigens respectively. Four types of evidence for these subpopulations are presented 1) the responses to the two types of antigen are additive when both forms are added to the same culture; 2) the precursor frequency for the thymus dependent and thymus independent populations is different although expansion over primary IgM precursor frequencies was not detectable; 3) the avidities of the PFC elicited by each antigen are distinct; the thymus independent antigens elicit lower avidity PFC; 4) selective killing of one population can be accomplished by BUdR and light treatment without affecting the other population.

INTRODUCTION

Several laboratories including our own have reported that IgM precursor B lymphocytes responding to thymus dependent (TD) and thymus independent (TI) forms of the same hapten may represent functionally distinct subpopulations of B lymphocytes (3,11,15,18,19). The relationship between these subpopulations is still the subject of speculation, but it has been argued that TI and TD responding B lymphocytes represent immature and mature forms respectively of the same cell lineage (3); however, the evidence for this is circumstantial, and it is also possible that they represent distinct subpopulations with origins at the stem cell stage. Delineation of the ontogenetic relationship between TD and TI responding B lymphocytes is clearly of importance to understanding the developmental patterns of the humoral immune network.

Recently we described in vitro IgG secondary responses of large magnitude to TD and TI forms of the trinitrophenyl (TNP) or dinitrophenyl (DNP) haptens in spleen cells from mice primed to the TD antigen trinitrophenyl hemocyanin (TNP-KLH)(27). These results provided in vitro confirmation of an in vivo study by Braley-Mullen using TD and TI forms of pneumococcal polysaccharide-SIII (1) and emphasized the ability of TI antigens to trigger IgG memory B cells. Here we present evidence to indicate that, like IgM precursors, the precursors of IgG memory also appear to be divisible into functionally distinct subpopulations of TI and TD responding cells. Based on avidity differences in the PFC populations elicited, this functional differentiation may be marked by differences in V region gene expression.

MATERIALS AND METHODS

Mice

Adult female Balb/c mice were obtained from Charles River Breeding Labs., Willmington, Mass. and were caged in groups of 6 with free access to water and food.

Antigens

Trinitrophenylated-keyhole limpet hemocyanin (TNP-KLH) was prepared as described previously(21) and had a mole ratio of TNP_{1067}-KLH. TNP-T4 bacteriophage was prepared as described previously (10). Dinitrophenylated-dextran (DNP-dextran) was a gift from Dr. M. Feldmann.

Immunization

Mice were primed at 2-3 months of age with 3 injections of TNP-KLH-bentonite as previously described (2).

Cell Culture

Spleen cells from at least 3 mice primed 2-4 months previously were pooled and cultured using microtiter plates (12). Culture medium was supplemented with 5 x 10^{-5}M 2-mercaptoethanol (12) and nucleosides (4). The antigen dose is indicated in the results.

Plaque Assays

Anti-TNP plaque-forming-cells (PFC) were detected using TNP-haptenated sheep red blood cells (TNP-SRBC) as prepared previously (22). Cells from 8 replicate microcultures were pooled and plated as one culture for PFC (5). Three such pooled cultures were assayed per experimental point. Cells producing IgM anti-TNP antibody were detected by direct plating. Cells producing IgG anti-TNP antibody were detected by adding goat anti-mouse IgG antiserum (6) and antimouse μ chain antiserum to suppress IgM PFC (17).

Avidity Determinations

IgG PFC were assessed as above with TNP-ε-aminocaproic acid incorporated into the plaque assay at various molar concentrations (7). Diluent was added in place of free hapten for controls. Cells at each concentration of inhibitor and controls were plated in quadruplicate with cultured cells diluted so that control slides had 250-300 PFC per slide.

Selective Suicide

5 bromouridine deoxyribose (10^{-6} M final concentration, BUdR) was added to cultures 48 hrs after initiation (20). The cultures were illuminated either for 3 hours on day 3 or for 2 hours on days 3 and 4; the latter had a more pronounced effect. After the final illumination the cultures were washed and reincubated with fresh culture medium either with or without additional antigen.

Limiting Dilution Analysis

Precursor frequencies for TD and TI antigens were obtained by culturing cells under conditions where B cells were limiting (19). Sufficient helper function was assured by adding helper primed Mitomycin C treated spleen cells (25). Sixty wells were cultured per experimental point. The number of positive wells was determined by plaque assay of individual wells. The precursor frequency was calculated by the Poisson statistic as in (19).

RESULTS

Previously we have shown that spleen cells from mice primed by three weekly injections of the TD antigen TNP-KLH developed a vigorous anti-TNP IgG response when placed *in vitro* for 7-9 days with either TD or TI antigens and that the responses to these two forms of the hapten were equal in magnitude(27). At the same time we noted that there was a difference in the relative requirement for 2-mercaptoethanol between the TD and TI initiated responses and that the kinetics of these responses differed. These distinctions led us to ask whether the IgG memory cells responding to TD and TI antigens were different B lymphocytes as has been shown for the primary IgM response (3,11,15,18,19).

A simple first experiment was the addition of TD and TI antigens either alone or simultaneously to the same culture. If these antigens were stimulating different B cell subpopulations, the response of the culture challenged simultaneously with both antigens would be expected to equal the sum of the individual responses. Table I shows the results of one of 4 such addition experiments. Spleen cells from TNP primed mice were challenged with optimum doses of either TNP-T4 or TNP-KLH or both antigens simultaneously. The cells were cultured for 5 or 7 days, harvested and assayed for anti-TNP IgG PFC. On day 5 we observed 8000 PFC/10^6 for both TNP-T4 and TNP-KLH stimulated cultures. If the TD and TI responses

TABLE I

ADDITION OF IgG RESPONSES ON DOUBLE CHALLENGE WITH TD AND TI ANTIGENS

Antigen	Anti-TNP PFC/10^6 Days in Culture 5	7
TNP-T4[a] (TI)	8519 ± 606[b]	22771 ± 2097
TNP-KLH (TD)	8504 ± 1407	12298 ± 291
TNP-T4 + TNP-KLH	20691 ± 96	37264 ± 6537
Expected if Additive	17023	35069

[a] Antigen doses were optimal: TNP-T4 (6 x 10^6 PFU/ml), TNP-KLH (0.02 μg/ml).

[b] IgG PFC enumerated in the presence of a suppressive amount of anti-IgM antiserum. Mean ± standard error.

were additive as has been shown for primary IgM responses, we would have expected 17,000 PFC/10^6, and we observed 20,000 in the simultaneously challenged culture; as predicted the results were additive. Likewise, on day 7 we observed 22,000 and 12,000 PFC/10^6 cells for TNP-T4 and TNP-KLH stimulated cultures respectively; we expected 35,000 PFC/10^6 based on simple addition, and we observed 37,000 PFC/10^6 in cultures challenged simultaneously with both antigens. Thus addition experiments support the notion that separate subpopulations of IgG memory cell precursors are responding to TD and TI antigens.

Having observed addition by simultaneous challenge with TD and TI antigens, we have carried out preliminary analysis of the frequencies of TD and TI IgG memory precursors. To date we have only evaluated frequencies based on day 5 of culture. Typical results are shown in Table II where the TI precursor frequency is nearly 5 times greater than that of the TD precursors. We have encountered technical difficulties in getting cultures to persist beyond day 5 in the micro system used for precursor analysis. The total number of precursors in each category may ultimately be shown to be greater as later days of culture are evaluated. The important point, however, is that the number of TI IgG precursors has consistently been larger.

As a third approach we have examined the avidity distribution of the PFC stimulated by TD and TI antigens using hapten inhibition as described by Goidl and Siskind (7). Results typical of a large number of such experiments are shown in Fig. 1. They indicate that, whereas the TI antigen elicits only a narrow range of low avidity PFC (10^{-5} M TNP-ε-amino caproic acid (EACA) was the lowest concentration which inhibited the TI response), The TD antigen elicited a more heterogeneous range of PFC of higher avidity. Furthermore, we can exclude the possibility that the TI antigen selectively blocks the expression of high avidity PFC since

TABLE II

FREQUENCY OF TD AND TI IgG PRECURSORS

Antigen	IgG Precursors/10^5 Spleen Cells[a]
TNP-T4[b] (TI)	1.2[c]
TNP-KLH (TD)	0.26

[a] Assayed on day 5 of culture.
[b] Optimum doses: TNP-T4 (1.5 x 10^6 PFU/ml), TNP-KLH (0.002 μg/ml).
[c] Calculated from Poisson statistic as in (4) using 60 cultures per dilution point in limiting dilution analysis.

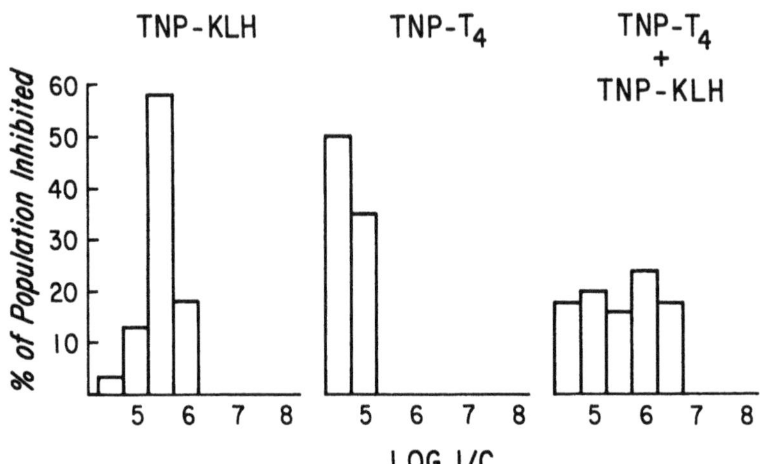

Figure 1. Avidity of IgG PFC generated by TD or TI antigens *in vitro*. The inhibitor TNP-EACA in varying molar concentrations was added to the plaque assay and compared to controls in which diluent was added in place of inhibitor. The assay contained anti-IgM antiserum to suppress IgM PFC as well as anti-IgG antiserum and complement. Cells were harvested on day 5 of culture.

The abscissa represents $\log_{10}$ of the inverse of the free hapten concentration used as inhibitor. The ordinate represents the percentage of the total population of PFC which were inhibited. Avidity increases to the right. The antigen used to stimulate the *in vitro* response is shown at the top. Optimal concentrations of antigen were used: TNP-T4 (6×10^6 PFU/ml), TNP-KLH (0.002 μg/ml).

when both TD and TI antigens were added to the same culture, both high and low avidity PFC were detected.

Finally, we designed suicide experiments using BUdR and light to eliminate specifically one antigen-responding population prior to stimulation by a second antigen. In these experiments TNP primed spleen cells were cultured with an optimum dose of TNP-T4 or without antigen. BUdR was added to antigen stimulated cultures on day 2 followed by either 3 hours of illumination on day 3 or 2 hours of illumination on days 3 and 4. After the final illumination, the cells were washed, and antigen, either TI or TD, was added and the cells recultured. Typical results are shown in Table III. As can be seen the presence of the TI antigen prior to BUdR and light treatment greatly reduced the subsequent response to rechallenge with the TI antigen but did not affect the response to the TD antigen TNP-KLH. We have done the reciprocal experiment (*i.e.* TNP-KLH added first), and have obtained similar results. However, in these

TABLE III

SELECTIVE KILLING OF TI IgG PRECURSORS BY BUdR + LIGHT[a]

Challenged with TNP-T4	% of Control Response			
Rechallenged with[b]	Exp 1[c]	Exp 2	Exp 3	Exp 4
TNP-T4 (TI)	37	21	8	4
DNP-Dextran (TI)	nd	nd	13	1
TNP-KLH (TD)	249	186	192	380

[a] Cells were challenged with TNP-T4 on day 0 of culture. BUdR (1×10^{-6} M final concentration) was added on day 2. In Exp 1 and 2 the cells were illuminated 24 hrs later for 3 hrs. In Exp 3 and 4 the cells were illuminated 24 and 48 hrs later for 2 hrs on each day. Immediately after illumination the cells were centrifuged, washed and rechallenged with the TD or TI antigens as indicated.

[b] Antigen doses were optimal: TNP-T4 (1.5×10^6 PFU/ml), DNP-dextran (0.01 μg/ml), TNP-KLH (0.002 μg/ml).

[c] Assayed 5 days (Exp 1,2,3) or 7 days (Exp 4) after rechallenge. The control cultures were treated with diluent in place of BUdR and illuminated, washed and challenged with antigen as the experimental groups.

latter experiments we have not yet ruled out the possible effect of BUdR on activated helper T cells. The experiments using the TI antigen first, however, clearly indicate that it is possible to abolish the response to the TI antigen without affecting the response to the TD antigen. We have observed in all BUdR experiments that elimination of one responding population increases the response to the unaffected population dramatically. It is possible that this reflects removal of a B cell crowding effect (24) or more likely an elimination of suppressor cells or their precursors which may also be cycling (26) in these cultures and, therefore susceptible to BUdR treatment. However, we have not yet investigated this aspect.

DISCUSSION

The results reported here for IgG memory precursors are in keeping with those reported previously for IgM precursors (3,11,15,

18,19) and thus lend themselves to the interpretation that B cell precursors responding to thymus dependent and thymus independent antigens represent functionally distinct subpopulations.

Simultaneous addition of TD and TI antigens to the same culture resulted in addition with the response equalling the sum of the responses to each antigen alone. Although not shown the secondary IgM responses were also additive. In some experiments synergistic responses greater than those expected from simple addition were obtained. Such synergy has also been observed in primary addition experiments of this type (11,19). Quintans and Cosenza (19) observed synergy in the IgM response only if the TD response was initiated 24 hours before adding the TI antigen and suggested that some TD responsive B cells may have been driven to TI along a common differentiation pathway. On the other hand since we found that synergy could result from simultaneous addition of both TD and TI antigens, we, therefore, suggested that nonspecific T cell factors might be able to affect TI B cells after initial triggering (11). This has remained true in those instances where we have observed synergy in IgG responses. However, the explanation for synergy remains unanswered.

We have found consistently that the TI IgG memory precursors were more numerous than TD precursors. We were surprised, however, to find that the number of precursors was not larger since they are within the range reported previously for IgM precursors (19). We cannot, for the present, state whether these numbers reflect the actual numbers of precursors and that memory has developed in these mice through an unequal division mechanism in which the total memory pool has not expanded or whether it reflects a technical problem. We have succeeded in measuring precursor frequencies only on day 5 in the micro cultures used for limiting dilution analysis (19) and these cultures have not generated the PFC expansion we observe on days 7 and 9 in conventional micro Mishell-Dutton cultures (27). Thus it is possible that IgG precursors which would not be triggered until later stages of _in vitro_ culture escape detection. The important point here, however, is that the number of precursors differs for the two populations.

Two aspects of the secondary IgG memory response to TD and TI antigens shown here differ from those previously reported for IgM responses. The first is that there are apparent differences in the avidity distribution of PFC stimulated by the TD and TI antigens (Figure 1). We have observed this consistently for IgG memory populations; PFC stimulated by either TNP-T4 or DNP-dextran are of low avidity; whereas a broad spectrum of higher avidity PFC are generated by TNP-KLH. On the contrary no differences in avidity were detected in primary IgM PFC stimulated by TD and TI forms of either TNP (11) or phosphoryl choline (19). Whether this reflects the technical difficulty of measuring relative avidity of IgM responses or a fundamental difference in IgM and IgG precursors cannot be determined at present. However, the results among IgG precursors may be taken as evidence that functional differentiation to TD and TI responsiveness reflects differences in V region gene expression.

The narrow spectrum of avidities found among TI IgG PFC suggests that the TI antigens are not serving here as polyclonal activators since we would expect all of the available avidity classes to be expressed in the latter case. The results are in keeping with the view that expression of high avidity PFC reflects a thymus dependent element in avidity maturation (16).

The second way in which this study of TD and TI responding IgG precursors differs from IgM studies is that we were able to achieve substantial elimination of the TI response with BUdR and light treatment without affecting the TD response upon subsequent addition of antigen. Similar types of experiments utilizing the hot thymidine pulse technique were attempted with the phosphoryl choline IgM system but were inconclusive due to technical problems (19). In this regard we have observed in all of our BUdR experiments that secondary IgM precursors are considerably less sensitive to this treatment than IgG precursors although selective killing is still observed (not shown). The results of these suicide experiments constitute a powerful argument for functionally distinct subopulations but do not allow us to draw a conclusion concerning their developmental relationship.

It appears from several types of evidence then that there are functionally differentiated subpopulations of B lymphocytes which differ in their ability to read the hapten carrier complex and to distinguish those which are thymus independent from those which are thymus dependent. These subpopulations were originally termed B_1 and B_2, respectively, by Playfair and Purves (18). Two hypotheses for their ontogenetic development are shown in Fig. 2 which is based on the model of Cambier _et al._ (3) who suggested a common pathway of development from stem cell $\rightarrow B_1 \rightarrow B_2$ based on properties which B_1 cells in the adult have in common with immature neonatal B cells. The alternative view proposed by Quintans and Cosenza (19) is that B_2 cells may be precursors of B_1. Obviously it is also possible that B_1 and B_2 are "separate categories" of cells as suggested recently by Kincade (14) who found CBA/N mice to be devoid of colony-forming B cells (immature, B_1?). Since CBA/N mice do have adequate numbers of B_2 cells, they respond to TD antigens but poorly, if at all, to TI antigens (9,23), they do not fit readily into the $B_1 \rightarrow B_2$ model. Our demonstration of $B_{1\gamma}$ and $B_{2\gamma}$ memory populations further complicates this picture; they could arise from $B_{1\mu}$ and $B_{2\mu}$, respectively, if the separate lineage

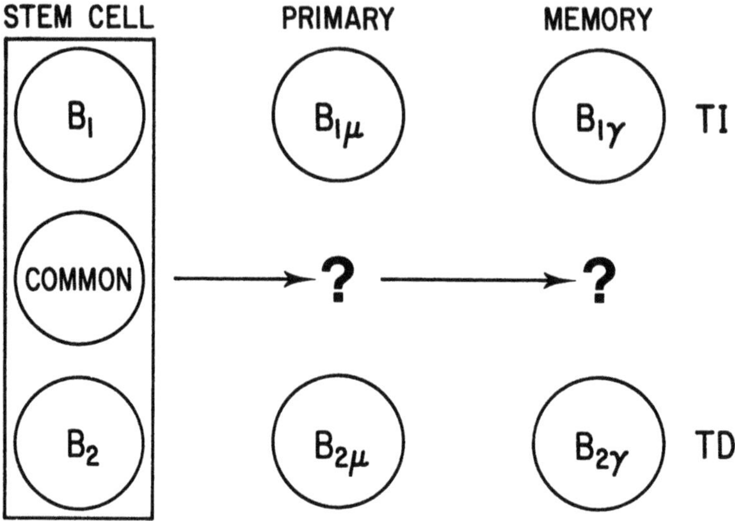

Figure 2. Functional differentiation among primary and memory B lymphocyte precursors.

hypothesis is correct or from a common precursor. If the latter were true, we would favor $B_{2\mu}$ as the immediate precursor since it was the TD antigen which primed for the subsequent TI IgG response. Clearly it is too early to predict which of these ontogenetic schemes is correct. Furthermore, Kimoto et al. (13) recently reported obtaining secondary IgE responses to both DNP-ovalbumin and DNP-ficoll. Although they did no analysis for independent TD and TI subpopulations, we can expect that similar subpopulations probably exist for all Ig classes.

Presumably the development of these functionally distinct subpopulations during the course of evolution was subjected to a selective pressure which ensured their survival. Perhaps the selective rationale will become apparent once the developmental relationships between TD and TI responding populations of B cells from virgin precursor to memory population is delineated. Thus delineation of these relationships should remain an important topic for the foreseeable future.

ACKNOWLEDGEMENTS

This work was supported by a grant from the Medical Research Foundation of Oregon and Grant Number CA 17228 from the National Institutes of Health.

We wish to thank K. Pratt for excellent technical assistance. We also thank Dr. M. Feldmann for DNP-dextran and Dr. A. Malley for anti-IgM antiserum.

REFERENCES

1. Braley-Mullen, H. (1975) J. Immunol. 115, 1194.
2. Bullock, W.W. and Rittenberg, M.B. (1970) J. Exp. Med. 132, 926.
3. Cambier, J.C., Vitetta, E.S., Uhr, J.W. and Kettman, J.R. (1977) J. Exp. Med. 145, 778.
4. Click, R.E., Benck, L. and Alter, J.B. (1972) Cell. Immunol. 3, 264.
5. Cunningham, A. and Szenberg, A. (1968) Immunology 14, 599.
6. Dresser, D.W. and Wortis, H.H. (1965) Nature 208, 859.
7. Goidl, E.A. and Siskind, G.W. (1974) J. Exp. Med. 140, 1285.
8. Gorczynski, R. and Feldmann, M. (1975) Cell. Immunol. 18, 88.
9. Janeway, C.A., Jr. and Barthold, D.R. (1975) J. Immunol. 115, 898.
10. Jennings, J.J., Baltz, M.L. and Rittenberg, M.B. (1975) J. Immunol. 115, 1432.
11. Jennings, J. and Rittenberg, M.B. (1976) J. Immunol. 117, 1749.
12. Kappler, J.W. (1974) J. Immunol. 112, 1271.
13. Kimoto, M., Kishimoto, T., Noguchi, S., Watanabe, T. and Yamamura, Y. (1977) J. Immunol. 118, 840.
14. Kincade, P.J. (1977) J. Exp. Med. 145, 249.
15. Lewis, G.K., Ranken, R., Nitecki, D.E. and Goodman, J.W. (1976) J. Exp. Med. 144, 382.
16. Okomura, K., Metzler, C.M., Tsu, T.T., Herzenberg, L.A. and Herzenberg, L.A. (1976) J. Exp. Med. 144. 345.
17. Pierce, C.W., Johnson, B.M., Gershon, H.E. and Asofsky, R. (1971) J. Exp. Med. 134, 395.
18. Playfair, J.H.L. and Purves, E.C. (1971) Nature (New Biol.) 231, 149.
19. Quintans, J. and Cosenza, H. (1976) Eur. J. Immunol. 6, 399.
20. Raidt, D.J., Mishell, R.I. and Dutton, R.W. (1968) J. Exp. Med. 128, 681.
21. Rittenberg, M.B. and Amkraut, A.A. (1966) J. Immunol. 97, 421.
22. Rittenberg, M.B. and Pratt, K.L. (1969) Proc. Soc. Exp. Biol. Med. 132, 575.
23. Sher, I., Ahmed, A., Strong, D.M., Steinberg, A.D. and Paul, W.E. (1975) J. Exp. Med. 141, 788.
24. Stocker, J.W. (1976) Immunology 30, 181.
25. Swain, S.L. Trefts, P.E., Tse, H.Y-S. and Dutton, R.W. (1977) Cold Spring Harbor Symposia on Quant. Biol. XLI part 2, 597.
26. Sy, M-S., Miller, S.D. and Claman, H.N. (1977) J. Immunol. 119, 240.
27. Tittle, T.V. and Rittenberg, M.B. Cellular Immunol., In press.

Immune Responses to Synthetic Polymers and to Proteins

INTRODUCTION

David H. Katz

Department of Cellular and Developmental Immunology
Scripps Clinic and Research Foundation
LaJolla, California 92037

Before we begin this afternoon's session which is entitled "Immune Responses to Synthetic Polymers" I would like to spend about five minutes to make a few points which are perhaps along more philosophical lines. One of the things that has impressed me and I am sure would impress particularly anybody, particularly those entering our field as newcomers, is the seemingly enormous complexity of the cellular aspects of the immune system. I'm not referring solely to the various regulatory mechanisms and interactions that go on in the system, but the seemingly endless number of lymphocyte subpopulations and sub-subpopulations. Complicating matters further are, of course, the multiple factors that are specific, non-specific, global and so forth that appear to play intimate roles and selective roles for each of these various sub-subpopulations of cells. I emphasize the word <u>appear</u> because I think that it's not unwise to view what has happened during the logarithmic growth phase of the field of Cellular Immunology in the past seven or eight years with some degree of caution at this point. I say this because it's not totally unlikely that we've let these complexities run away with us in a certain sense. For example, despite the fact that we now recognize the existence of clearly defined lymphocyte subpopulations of both classes, very few of us openly discuss the possibility that each of these subpopulations could very well be capable of performing multiple functions. A very good example of this, from a historical point of view, is the fact that not too many years ago B cell precursors of different heavy chain isotypes were thought to be all separate in their lineage; today, of course, we know that this is not true, that there are very sophisticated and as yet undefined genetic mechanisms which allow a single progenitor cell to switch its isotype expression. This is, therefore, an example of what appeared to be the existence of many different cells of the same specificity which actually turned out not to be the case once we learned more about B cell ontogeny. Another point in this regard is the fact that there are very well-known, and probably many other yet to be defined, molecular feedback mechanisms which exist in the immune system (as in other systems, of course, with the endocrine system being perhaps the best example to keep in mind) that allow amplification (or contraction) of regulatory effects that could give the appearance of unique and selective cell functions associated with each different regulatory mechanism.

My point is that biological systems have evolved in such a way as to use such molecular feedback mechanisms to bring very complex interaction systems, in terms of final effector activities, into a much simpler functional framework. In this way, fewer cells can perform rather complex regulatory functions, although it might appear that such regulatory functions involve relatively large numbers of cells. I only point this out because it would not be surprising, at least to me, if five years from now we find ourselves viewing some of the ever-branching pathways and models that we have all been proposing and debating during the preceding years as retrospectively somewhat humorous in terms of what we might know at that time. With that I would like to turn the floor over to Stu Schlossman who will talk to us about T cell regulation of restricted B cell responses.

T-CELL REGULATION OF RESTRICTED B-CELL RESPONSES

A. Campos-Neto, H. Levine, and S. F. Schlossman

Division of Tumor Immunology, Sidney Farber Cancer Institute and the Department of Medicine, Harvard Medical School, Boston, Massachusetts 02115

INTRODUCTION

In earlier studies it was shown that synthetic and chemically well-defined Dnp-oligolysines did induce both cellular and humoral immunity in guinea pigs, and that this response was under immune response gene control (1,2). Sera of guinea pigs of genetic responder strain immunized with synthetic Dnp-oligolysine peptides have been shown to contain highly specific antibodies of restricted heterogeneity which could discriminate Dnp-oligolysines with minimal changes in hapten position, chain length, D-lysine-alanine substituents (3-7). Like specificity has been shown in T-cell responses of responder guinea pigs to these simple antigens since they could also discriminate equally well the homologous immunizing antigen from closely related ones in assays measuring antigen-induced delayed hypersensitivity, tritiated thymidine incorporation, and mediator production (8-9). Non-responder animals, in contrast, lack a T-cell response to these antigens and the antibody produced in the absence of T-cells, while Dnp-specific, could not discriminate one Dnp-oligopeptide from another (6). Exquisite specificity of antibody in animals with highly specific T-cell responses and the lack of it in non-responder guinea pigs immunized to the same antigen suggested that T-cells could select specific B-cell clones to proliferate (10). To test this possibility, studies were undertaken to explore antigen-induced B-cell responses in both strain 2 and 13 guinea pigs in the presence and absence of Dnp-oligolysine-specific T-cells. These experiments will emphasize the role of specific T-cells in the selection and amplification of unique B-cell clones.

MATERIALS AND METHODS

Peptides. Synthetic Dnp-oligolysine peptide antigens were prepared as described previously (2,3). For this study the following peptides were used: α,Dnp-Lys_3, α,Dnp-Lys_8, α,Dnp-Lys_9, α,Dnp-Lys_{10}, α,Dnp-Lys_{15}, ε,Dnp-Lys_3, ε,Dnp-Lys_8, ε,Dnp-Lys_9 and ε,Dnp-Lys_{12}. The octapeptides Lys-Ala_6-Lys(Dnp), Lys_2-Ala_5-Lys(Dnp), Lys_3-Ala_4-Lys(Dnp) and Lys_4-Ala_3-Lys(Dnp) were synthesized according to the method of Kalir et al. (11), using insoluble polimeric active esters of lysine and alanine for stepwise prolongation of the peptide chain.

Animals and immunizations. Inbred strain 2 and 13 guinea pigs of both sexes weighing 400-600 g were used in all studies. Each animal was injected with 150 μg of a given peptide in saline emulsified with an equal volume of Complete Freund's Adjuvant (CFA) containing 1 mg/ml of *Mycobacterium tuberculosis* H_{37}Ra (Difco Laboratories, Detroit, Michigan). Each guinea pig received a total of 0.8 ml of the emulsion CFA-antigen among the four footpads.

Skin tests. Two to three weeks after immunization, the guinea pig's flanks were shaved and injected intradermally with 0.1 ml of a PBS solution containing 10 μg of the immunizing antigen. As a control, 0.1 ml of PBS without antigen was also injected. The test sites were observed at 24 hrs. and the extent of induration and erythema was measured. Delayed reactions with induration equal or larger than 5 mm in diameter were considered positive (12).

In vitro antigen-induced incorporation of ^{3}H-thymidine. Immunized guinea pigs were killed by bulbar dislocation between 2-3 weeks after immunization. Inguinal and axillary lymph nodes were aseptically removed and teased in RPMI (Gibco, Grand Island, New York), supplemented with 1% L-glutamine (200 mM), 1% penicillin-streptomycin (5000 units penicillin and 5000 mcg streptomycin/ml) and 10% normal guinea pig serum (Rockland, Gilbertsville, PA). The cells were counted and the viability was assessed by trypan blue exclusion. Dead cells were removed as described previously (13). Viability greater than 95% was invariably obtained.

For antigen-induced proliferation, 10^6 cells in a volume of 0.2 ml were cultured in flat-bottomed Microtest II plates (Falcon Plastics, Oxnard, CA). Cultures were done in triplicate, in the presence of various concentrations of the homologous (immunizing) and heterologous antigens. After 24 hours of incubation at 37°C in a humidified atmosphere of 95% air and 5% CO_2, the cultures were pulsed with 20 μl of RPMI solution containing 0.2 μCi of ^{3}H-thymidine (specific activity 0.9 Ci/mM, Schwartz-Mann, Orangeburg, NY). After an additional 24 hr incubation, the cultures were harvested on a MASH II apparatus. (Microbiological Associates, Bethesda, MD). The incorporation of ^{3}H-thymidine was measured by scintillation spectroscopy. Results are expressed as mean c.p.m. ± standard error of the mean. Stimulation index is the ratio of ^{3}H-thymidine incorporation by 10^{6} cells in the presence of antigen to c.p.m. incorporation by unstimulated cultures.

Antibody response. The anti-Dnp antibody response was assayed by isoelectric focusing as reported previously (14). Briefly, thin layer polyacrylamide gels containing 2% (w/v) ampholine carrier ampholytes (pH range 5 to 8 and 7 to 10 (LKB, Stockholm, Sweden) were prefocused to remove persulfate. The antisera were then electrofocused for 14 hrs. at 4°C, after which time the antibody isoelectric spectra were developed by overlay with ^{131}I-α,N(4-hydroxyphenylacetyl)-ε-N-Dnp-L-Lysine. The plates were processed as previously described and autoradiographs made by 4-21 hr. exposure to Agfa-Gevaert Osray M3 X-ray films.

The purification and characterization of guinea pig anti-Dnp antibody was previously described in detail (6,15). Fluorescence quenching of immunoabsorbant purified anti-Dnp antibody was carried out as previously described (6,16,17).

Immunoelectrophoresis. Immunoelectrophoresis was performed through agarose gel plates (Immunotec II, Behring Diagnostics, Somerville, NJ) using barbital buffer pH 8.2, 0.04 ionic strength. Rabbit antisera reacting specifically with guinea pig IgG2 was a gift of Dr. R. Asofsky (N.I.H., Bethesda, MD).

"B" guinea pigs. "B" guinea pigs were prepared by thymectomy of normal adult strain 2 guinea pigs and lethal irradiation (1000 r) on day 15. Immediately following irradiation the animals were reconstituted with 100 - 150 X 10^{6} syngeneic bone marrow cells. Thirty days later the guinea pigs were immunized as described above.

"E" Rosettes. E rosette test was performed using fresh rabbit erythrocytes according to the method of Stadecker *et al.* (18).

RESULTS

In vitro responses to Dnp-oligolysines and related compounds. Both strain 2 and 13 guinea pigs were immunized with α,Dnp-Lys_9 and skin tested with 10 μg of antigen 21 days following immunization. All strain 2 and no 13 guinea pigs developed delayed skin hypersensitivity. Both lymph node cells and serum were obtained from each of the animals immunized with α,Dnp-Lys_9. The anti-hapten antibody was purified from both strain 2 and 13 animals and the yield was similar to that previously described (6,14).

The binding energies of α,Dnp-Lys_3, α,Dnp-Lys_5, α,Dnp-Lys_8, α,Dnp-Lys_9, α,Dnp,Lys_{15}, ε,Dnp-Lys_9, Lys_4-Ala_3-Lys(Dnp) and dinitrophenol with purified strain 2 anti α,Dnp-Lys_9 antibody was obtained by fluorescence quenching (Fig. 1). As shown, the maximal $-\Delta F^o$ is obtained with α,Dnp-Lys_9, the homologous immunizing antigen. Peptides containing fewer lysyl residues, such as α,Dnp-$Lys_{3,5,8}$ and those containing more α,Dnp-Lys_{15} resulted in a decrease in binding energy when compared to α,Dnp-Lys_9. Similarly, either placing the dinitrophenol group on the carboxyl terminal end of the nonapeptide, or substitution of lysines with alanine residues also resulted in a marked decrease in binding energy. Dinitrophenol had a $-\Delta F^o$ of approximately 2000 cal/M less than α,Dnp-Lys_9.

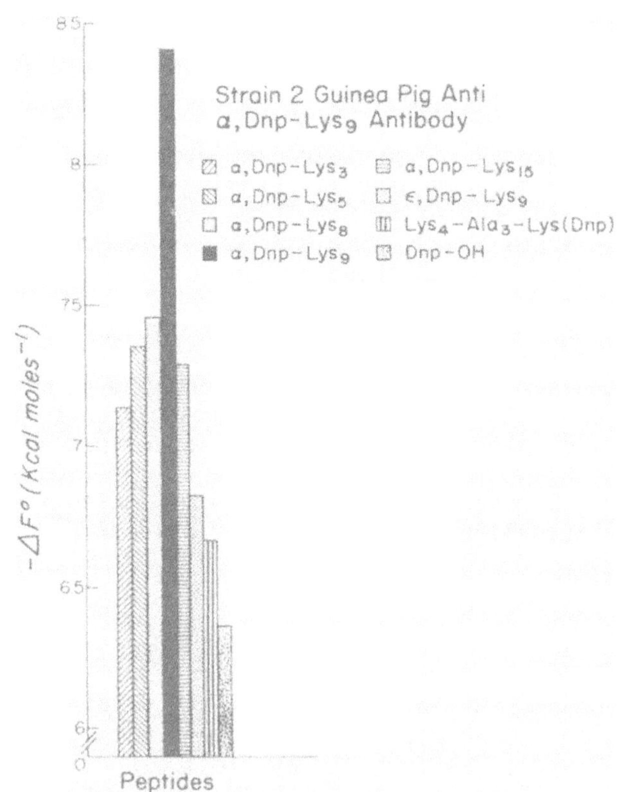

Fig. 1. Binding energies ($-\Delta F^o$) of Dnp-oligolysines and dinitrophenol obtained with strain 2 anti α,Dnp-Lys_9 antibody.

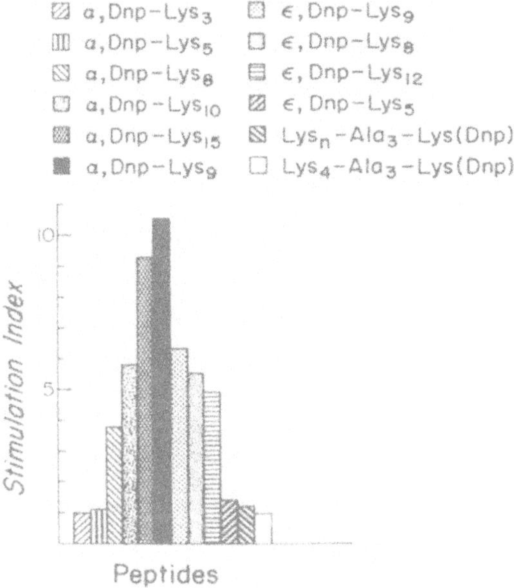

Fig. 2. In vitro proliferative response of lymph node cells from strain 2 guinea pigs immunized with α,*Dnp-Lys*$_9$.

Lymph node cells were obtained from these animals, and the effect of the homologous immunizing antigen and closely related peptides in stimulating thymidine incorporation in cell culture is shown in Figure 2. It is apparent that α,Dnp-Lys$_9$ produced maximal stimulation. All peptides were compared at 20 nanamoles/ml; stimulation indices obtained at different antigen concentrations gave similar results. As indicated, α,Dnp-Lys$_3$, α,Dnp-Lys$_5$ were non-stimulatory, whereas cross-reactions were seen with α,Dnp-Lys$_8$, α,Dnp-Lys$_{10}$, α,Dnp-Lys$_{15}$, and ε,Dnp-Lys$_{8,9}$, and $_{12}$. No stimulation was seen with Lys$_n$-Ala$_3$-Lys(Dnp) peptides or non-immunogenic ε,Dnp-Lys$_3$ and $_5$. These studies (representing the mean of 3 strain 2 guinea pigs sensitized with α,Dnp-Lys$_9$) indicate that the homologous immunizing antigen could be discriminated from a series of closely related antigens. Previous studies have shown that this in vitro response was mediated by T-cells and that while macrophages were necessary, the specificity could not be attributed to either B-cells or macrophages (19). Thus, both in vitro T-cell responses as well as antibody produced in responder animals were exquisitely specific for the homologous immunizing antigen.

TABLE I

Incorporation of ^3H Thymidine by Lymph Node Cells from Guinea Pigs Immunized with α,Dnp-Lys_9 in CFA[a]

Strain	Experiment	Antigen		
		Medium	α,Dnp-Lys_9	PPD
2	1	473 ± 46	6668 ± 325	31586 ± 2372
	2	692 ± 12	7423 ± 196	35246 ± 865
	3	726 ± 53	5381 ± 277	35631 ± 1823
13	1	1021 ± 64	1122 ± 119	25127 ± 1609
	2	837 ± 74	844 ± 5	26119 ± 1467
	3	1187 ±191	1187 ± 33	31082 ± 518

(a) All experiments were done in triplicate and results are expressed in CPM of the mean ± standard error.

In contrast, strain 13 guinea pigs immunized with α,Dnp-Lys_9 despite producing normal levels of anti-Dnp antibody, neither developed delayed skin reactions nor were their lymph node cells stimulated in culture to incorporate thymidine by either α,Dnp-Lys_9 or related peptides. Nevertheless, strain 13 guinea pig cells could be shown to respond well to PPD (Table I).

Antibody from strain 13 animals was purified and as shown in Figure 3, could not disciminate α,Dnp-Lys_9 from related peptides. The binding energy for α,Dnp-Lys_9 was comparable to that obtained with α,Dnp-Lys_3, α,Dnp-Lys_5, α,Dnp-Lys_8, α,Dnp-Lys_9, α,Dnp-Lys_{15}, α,Dnp compounds and dinitrophenol. Thus, in strain 13 animals, there is an absence of both specific T and B-cell responses to α,Dnp-Lys_9. It should also be emphasized that the purified antibodies from both strain 2 and 13 were predominantly IgG2 as measured by immunoelectrophoresis and showed lines of identity by gel diffusion (results not shown). In addition, both sets of antibody were highly restricted in heterogeneity comprised of 1-2 clones when measured by isoelectric focusing and hot hapten overlay (not shown).

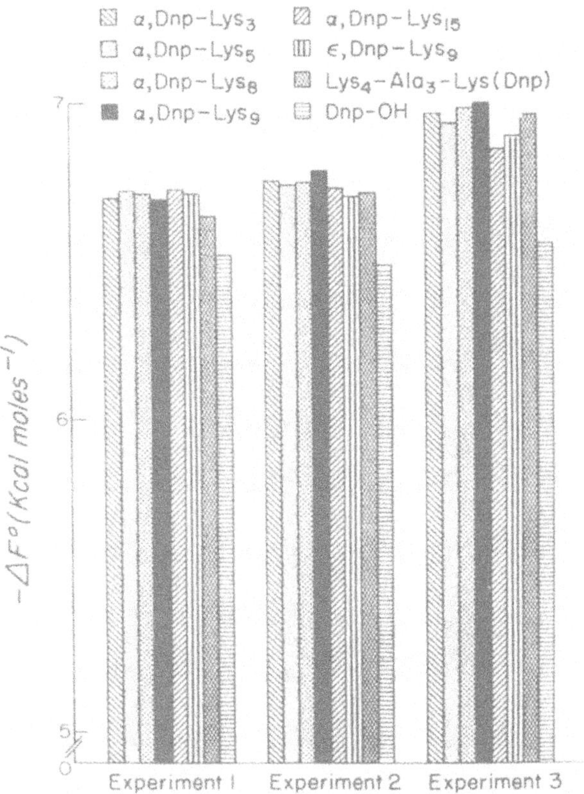

Fig. 3. Binding energies (-ΔF°) of Dnp-oligolysines and dinitrophenol obtained with strain 13 anti α,Dnp-Lys$_9$ antibody.

<u>Response of strain 2 and 13 guinea pigs to Dnp-Oligopeptides not under immune response gene control</u>. As shown above, there was a distinct difference between the response of strain 2 and 13 guinea pigs to peptides under Ir gene control. One could generate in strain 2 animals T-cells and antibody with comparable, if not identical specificity; strain 13 guinea pigs lacking the Ir gene could not develop a specific T-cell response and the synthesized antibody had not specificity. To test whether or not these differences were related to the Ir gene or were the property of other factors in these animals, both strain 2 and 13 guinea pigs were immunized with Lys-Ala$_6$-Lys(Dnp). Neither strain 2 nor 13 guinea pigs developed delayed skin reactivity to this peptide, whereas both strains developed significant quantities of circulating antibodies. In this case, strain 2 guinea pigs behaved like strain 13

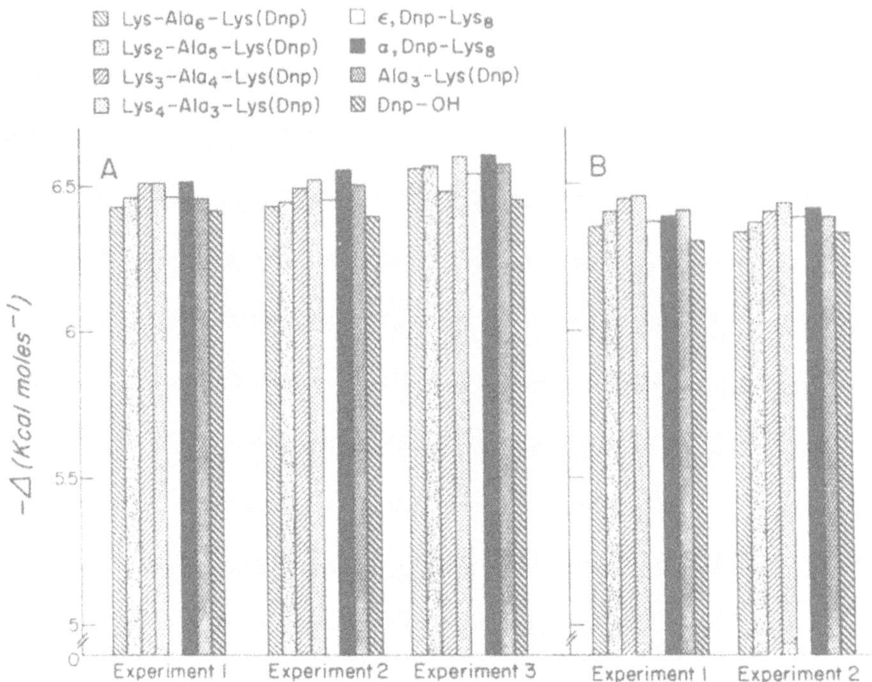

Fig. 4. *Binding energies ($-\Delta F^{o}$) of Dnp-oligopeptides and dinitrophenol to: (A) strain 2 anti-Lys-Ala_6-Lys(Dnp) andtibody, (B) strain 13 anti-Lys-Ala_6-Lys(Dnp) antibody.*

guinea pigs sensitized to α,Dnp-Lys_9. As shown in Figure 4A, purified antibody from 4 strain 2 guinea pigs immunized with Lys-Ala_6-Lys(Dnp) could not discriminate Lys-Ala_6-Lys(Dnp) from any closely related peptides including Lys_2-Ala_5-Lys(Dnp), Lys_4-Ala_3-Lys(Dnp), Lys_3-Ala_4-Lys(Dnp), α,Dnp-Lysines or dinitrophenol. These antibodies, like those produced above in strain 13 guinea pigs to α,Dnp-Lys_9, were hapten-specific since dinitrophenol had a binding energy similar to that obtained with the immunizing peptide. Similarly, as shown in Figure 4B, the antibody from strain 13 guinea pigs immunized with Lys-Ala_6-Lys(Dnp) were not specific for the homologous antigen. Again, these antibodies were hapten specific. Lymph node cells from both strain 2 and 13 animals were harvested and set up in culture with these peptides and could not be triggered to proliferate in response to the immunizing and related antigens (Table II). Purified antibody from these animals was predominantly IgG2 antibody and highly restricted by IEF.

TABLE II

Incorporation of ^3H Thymidine by Lymph Node Cells from Guinea Pigs Immunized with Lys-Ala_6-Lys(Dnp) in CFA[a]

Strain	Experiment	Antigen		
		Medium	Lys-Ala_6-Lys(Dnp)	PPD
2	1	793 ± 62	847 ± 93	28463 ± 1685
	2	1169 ± 101	1247 ± 112	27532 ± 3484
	3	1337 ± 109	1428 ± 130	32403 ± 788
13	1	1170 ± 93	1188 ± 68	25723 ± 134
	2	738 ± 69	751 ± 47	25240 ± 432
	3	455 ± 35	497 ± 56	21700 ± 796

(a) All experiments were done in triplicate and results are expressed in CPM of the mean ± standard error.

Response of strain 2 "B" guinea pigs to α,Dnp-Lys_9. One could argue that the specific antibody response in strain 2 guinea pigs to α,Dnp-Lys_9 was regulated by a specific T-cell response. In the absence of specific T-cells, the antibody produced was incapable of discriminating the homologous immunizing antigen from closely related ones.

To test the hypothesis that specific T-cells were required to select a unique B cell response, strain 2 guinea pigs were deprived of T-cells. Normal strain 2 guinea pigs were thymectomized, irradiated, and reconstituted with bone marrow cells from syngeneic donors and challenged with α,Dnp-Lys_9 in Complete Freund's Adjuvant. Three weeks following challenge these "B" guinea pigs were skin tested and bled. All animals were skin test negative for α,Dnp-Lys_9 and PPD. In these T-deprived animals, there was a marked deficiency of lymph node T-cells since only 5% of their cells formed rabbit E rosettes compared to 40-50% of cells obtained from intact guinea pigs.

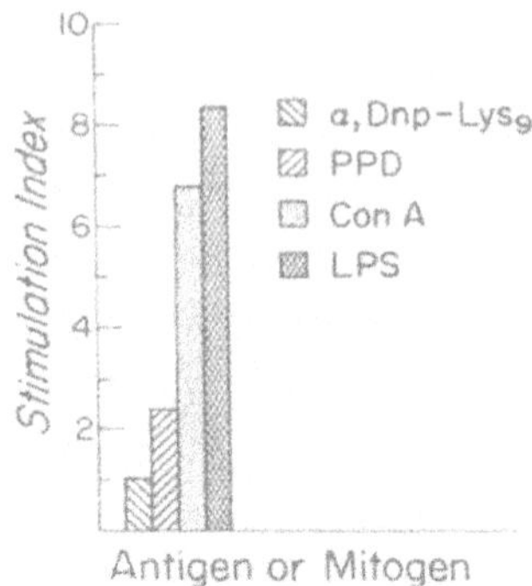

Fig. 5. In vitro proliferative response of lymph node cells from strain 2 "B" guinea pigs immunized with α,Dnp-Lys$_9$ in CFA.

As shown in Figure 5, lymph node cells from B guinea pigs immunized with α,Dnp-Lys$_9$ in Complete Freund's Adjuvant did not respond _in vitro_ to α,Dnp-Lys$_9$ and at best minimally to PPD. The response to ConA was also minimal compared to normal animals, and whereas the response to LPS was within normal limits. These results are consistent with the fact that the majority of the cells are B-cells. A more striking difference is seen in the antibody formed in these animals. B guinea pigs immunized to α,Dnp-Lys$_9$ developed a significant antibody response which was comparable to that found in the intact strain 2 guinea pig immunized to α,Dnp-Lys$_9$ (~150 μg Ab/ml of serum). As shown in experiments 1, 2, and 3 of Figure 6A, the antibody formed could not discriminate α,Dnp-Lys$_9$ from dinitrophenol or any of the other related Dnp-oligopeptides tested. These results are in marked contrast to other strain 2 guinea pigs possessing T-cell responses which were immunized with the same antigen (Figure 6B). It should also be emphasized that not only was the title of antibody similar to the intact animal in these strain 2 "B" guinea pigs, but that the antibody was predominantly IgG2 as measured by immunoelectrophoresis and Ouchterlony and restricted in heterogeneity as measured by isoelectric focusing.

DISCUSSION

The present studies indicate that B-cells in guinea pigs having specific T-cells have the capacity to elaborate molecules which are specifically reactive with the immunizing antigen. Thus, the

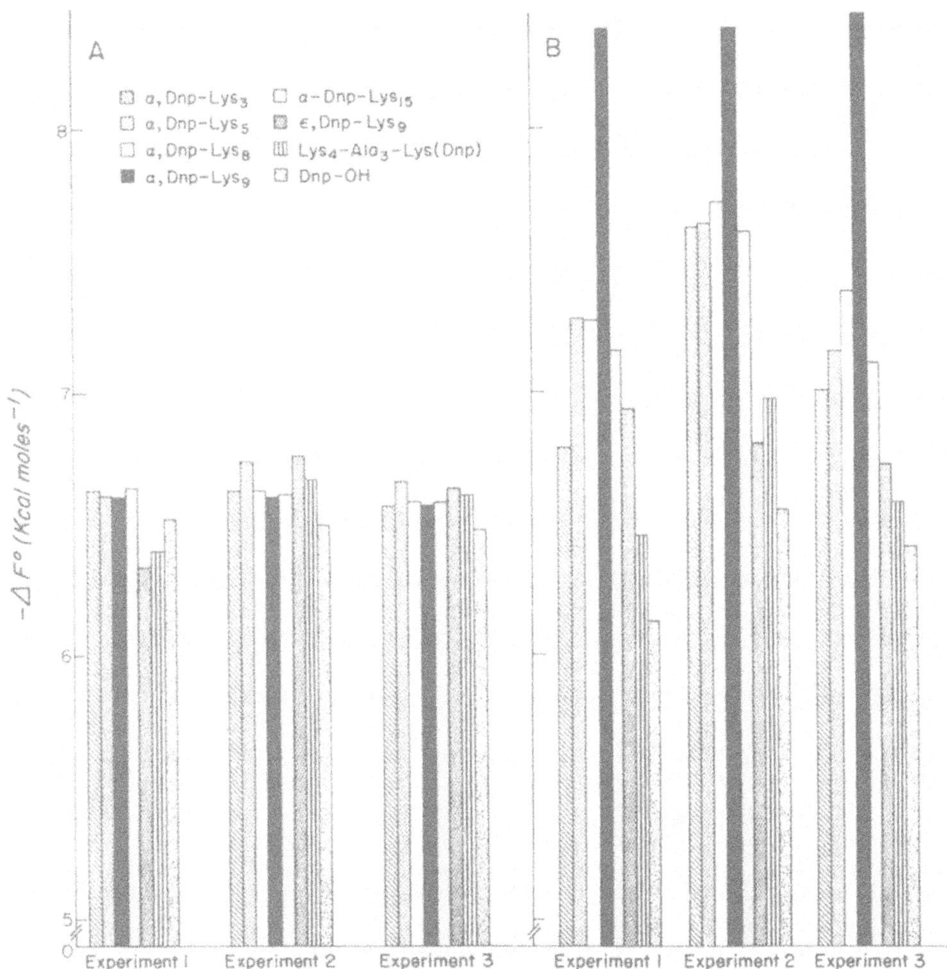

Fig. 6. Binding Energies ($-\Delta F^{O}$) of Dnp-oligolysines and dinitrophenol to: (A) strain 2 "B" guinea pigs anti-α,Dnp-Lys_9 antibody and (B) conventional strain 2 guinea pigs anti-α,Dnp-Lys_9 antibody.

antibody formed to α,Dnp-Lys_9 in genetic responder animals is restricted in heterogeneity, of the IgG class and can specifically distinguish α,Dnp-Lys_9 from a series of closely related antigens which include α,Dnp-$Lys_{3,5,8,15}$, ε,Dnp-Lys_9, Lys_4-Ala_3-Lys(Dnp) and dinitrophenol. In such animals, like specificity is shown for T-cells in vitro as measured by antigen induced thymidine incorporation; the homologous immunizing antigen can be discriminated from a variety of closely related antigens and maximal antigen-induced triggering obtained with α,Dnp-Lys_9. Both sets of observations clearly illustrate the specificity of T and B-cells to antigens regulated by Ir genes. Antigens which do not induce specific T-cell responses such as Lys-Ala_6-Lys(Dnp) in strain 2 and 13 guinea pigs, and α,Dnp-Lys_9 in strain 13 guinea pigs can also induce IgG antibody of restricted clonality. In contrast, both anti-Lys-Ala_6-Lys(Dnp) from strain 2 and 13 guinea pigs, and anti-α,Dnp-Lys_9 from strain 13 guinea pigs are only Dnp-specific and are incapable of distinguishing the dinitrophenol group from any of the Dnp-oligolysines used to induce the immune response. Thus, one could argue that in the absence of specific immune response genes and associated T-cell responses, specific antibody cannot be generated. To emphasize this point, strain 2 "B" guinea pigs were prepared by thymectomy, lethal irradiation, and reconstitution with bone marrow cells and immunization with α,Dnp-Lys_9. These T-deprived animals failed to develop observable T-cell responses to α,Dnp-Lys_9 or PPD but were capable of responding to LPS, a known B-cell mitogen. However, these T-deprived strain 2 animals could be induced by α,Dnp-Lys_9 to form anti-Dnp IgG antibody of restricted clonality. Of great importance was the demonstration that these antibodies like those produced in non-responder animals and in strain 2 animals lacking T-cell responses, was incapable of distinguishing α,Dnp-Lys_9 from dinitrophenol. It must be emphasized that these animals possess the same B-cell repertoire as normal strain 2 guinea pigs, that is, clones capable of producing anti-α,Dnp-Lys_9 antibody of great specificity. Despite the presence of these clones they were neither selected for nor triggered in T-deprived animals. Thus, one could conclude that in the absence of sepcific T-cells, comparably specific B-cell responses were not generated, and perhaps more importantly, that specific T-cells facilitate the amplification of unique B-cell clones. The nature of this T-B interaction is not fully understood, but is consistent with the earlier studies demonstrating that T-cells could select B-cells of higher affinity (20-21).

Considerable data has been generated indicating that both B and T-cells bear similar antigenic recognition structures as defined by anti-idiotypic antibody and by isolation of V gene products (22-26). Similarly, studies in Dnp-oligolysine also indicate a comparable repertoire of specificities in both T and B-cells, i.e. both similar specificity in genetic responder animals and lack of specificity in non-responder animals (27). These studies also support the view that the repertoire of receptors for antigens in both T and B-cell populations are similar, if not identical. Given the diversity of antigen recognition by B and T-cells and the important role of T-cells in the amplification of precursor B-cells to restricted antigens in animals bearing the Ir gene, one cannot help but consider the possibility that uniquely specific T-cells can preferentially interact and trigger a clone of B-cells bearing similar if not identical receptors. The precise mechanism by which T-cells might regulate the selection of B-cell precursors of antibody-forming cells is not understood, but might occur as a consequence of release of specific antigen triggered T-cell factors specific for B-cells (28-30) or via an idiotype-anti-idiotype interaction such as that suggested by the network hypothesis (31). The role of macrophages and MHC gene products in triggering these specific T-cell responses and facilitating the interaction with B-cells is even less well understood at the present time (31).

BIBLIOGRAPHY

1. Levine, B.B., Ojeda, A., and Benacerraf, B. (1963) J. Exp. Med. 118, 953.

2. Schlossman, S.F., Yaron, A., Ben-Efraim, S., and Sober, H.A. (1965) Biochemistry 4, 1638.

3. Yaron, A. and Schlossman, S.F. (1968) Biochemistry 7, 2673.

4. Schlossman, S.F., Levine, H., and Yaron, A. (1968) Biochemistry 7, 1.

5. Schlossman, S.F. and Yaron, A. (1970) Ann. N.Y. Acad. Sci. 169, 108.

6. Levin, H.A., Levine, H., and Schlossman, S.F. (1971) J. Exp. Med. 133, 1199.

7. Civin, C.I., Levine, H.B., Williamson, A.R., and Schlossman, S.F. (1976) J. Immunol. 116, 1400.

8. Schlossman, S.F., Herman, J., and Yaron, A. (1969) J. Exp. Med. 130, 1031.

9. David, J.R. and Schlossman, S.F. (1968) J. Exp. Med. 128, 1451.

10. Schlossman, S.F. (1972) Transplant. Rev. 10, 97.

11. Kalir, R., Fridkin, M. and Patchornik, A. (1974) Eur. J. Biochem. 42, 151.

12. Schlossman, S.F., Ben-Efraim, S., Yaron, A., and Sober, H.A. (1966) J. Exp. Med. 123, 1083.

13. Von Boehmer, H. and Shortman, K. (1973) J. Imm. Methods 2, 293.

14. Civin, C.I., Levine, H.B., Williamson, A.R., and Schlossman, S.F. (1976) J. Immunol. 116, 1400.

15. Robbins, J.B., Haimovich, J., and Sela, M. (1967) Immunochemistry 4, 11.

16. Velick, S.F., Parker, S.W., and Eisen, H.N. (1960) Proc. Nat. Acad. Sci. U.S.A. 46, 1470.

17. Eisen, H. (1964) Methods Med. Res. 10, 115.

18. Stadecker, M.J., Bishop, G. and Wortis, H.H. (1973) J. Immunol. 111, 1834.

19. Stashenko, P.P. and Schlossman, S.F. (1977) J. Immunol. 118, 544.

20. Gershon, R.K. and Paul W.E. (1971) J. Immunol. 106, 872.

21. Mitchell, G.F. (1974) In Progress in Immunol. II Vol. 3, p. 89. (L. Brent and J. Holborow, eds., North-Holland Pub. Co., Amsterdam-Oxford).

22. Eichmann, K. and Rajewsky, K. (1975) Eur. J. Immunol. 5, 661.

23. Hämmerling, G.J., Black, S.J., Berek, C., Eichmann, K., and Rajewsky, K. (1976) J. Exp. Med. 143, 861.

24. Binz, H., Kimura, A. and Wigzell, H. (1975) Scand. J. Immunol. 4, 413.

25. Krawinkel, U., Cramer, M., Mage, R.G., Kelus, A.S., and Rajewsky, K. (1977). J. Exp. Med. 146, 792.

26. Geczy, A.F., Geczy, C.L., and deWeck, A.L. (1976) J. Exp. Med. 144, 226.

27. Jones, G. and Schlossman, S.F. (1974) In: Mechanisms of Cell-Mediated Immunity, p. 97. (R.J. McCluskey and S. Cohen, eds., John Wiley & Sons, Inc., New York).

28. Feldman, M. (1974). In: The Immune System: Genes, Receptors, Signals, p. 497. (E.E. Sercarz, A.R. Williamson, and C. Fox, eds., Academic Press, New York).

29. Mozes, E. (1976) In: The Role of Products of the Histocompatibility Gene Complex in Immune Responses, p. 485 (D.H. Katz and B. Benacerraf, eds., Academic Press, New York).

30. Taussig, M.J., Munro, A.J., and Luzzati, A.L. (1976) In: The Role of Products of the Histocompatibility Gene Complex in Immune Responses, p. 553. (D.H. Katz and B. Benacerraf, eds., Academic Press, New York).

31. Jerne, N.K. (1976) In: The Immune System, p. 259. (F. Melchers and K. Rajewsky, eds., 27 Colloquium-Mosbach. Springer-Verlag, Berlin, Heidelberg, New York).

32. Paul, W. and Benacerraf, B. (1977) Science 195, 1293.

This work was supported in part by National Institutes of Health grants AI-12069 and CA-06516 and by CAPES-Brazil.

We wish to thank Dr. Arieh Yaron for supplying us with the synthetic Dnp-peptides, and are also grateful to Ms Dorothy Whitkin for both excellent editorial and secretarial help.

L-GLUTAMIC ACID^{60}-L-ALANINE^{30}-L-TYROSINE^{10} (GAT): A PROBE FOR REGULATORY MECHANISMS IN ANTIBODY RESPONSES

Carl W. Pierce and Judith A. Kapp

Department of Pathology and Laboratory Medicine
The Jewish Hospital of St. Louis
and
Department of Pathology and
Department of Microbiology and Immunology
Washington University School of Medicine
St. Louis, Missouri 63110

INTRODUCTION

The interaction of foreign macromolecular antigen with immunocompetent, antigen-specific precursor lymphocytes initiates two distinct responses, cellular and humoral immunity. Cellular immune responses (delayed hypersensitivity and the various rejection phenomena) are mediated by T cells which recognize antigen by specific membrane receptors whose precise nature is yet to be defined. T cells respond primarily to protein or glycoprotein antigens rather than polysaccharides, and after stimulation, may release biologically active mediators which are responsible for the inflammatory response and tissue damage characteristic of delayed hypersensitivity reactions. Stimulation of T cells with membrane glycoprotein alloantigens on foreign cells leads to proliferative responses {the mixed lymphocyte reaction (MLR)} and the ability to specifically lyse target cells bearing the sensitizing antigen (the cytotoxic lymphocyte response). Humoral immune responses are mediated by lymphocytes which are functional homologs of bursa of Fabricius cells in birds. These precursors of antibody producing cells (B cells) recognize a wide variety of antigenic determinants by specific membrane Ig receptors and respond by synthesizing and secreting antibody specific for the stimulating antigenic determinant (Katz, 1977; Cantor and Weissman, 1975; Warner, 1974).

In the mouse, different subclasses of T cells have critical roles in the regulation of development and expression of both cellular and humoral immune responses. Antibody responses by B cells to complex multideterminant antigens (T cell-dependent antigens) require the active participation of concomitantly stimulated specific helper T cells (Katz, 1977). Development of cytotoxic lymphocyte responses also requires participation of a subclass of amplifier T cells which also participate in the MLR (Cantor and Weissman, 1975). Moreover, both cellular and humoral immune responses may be actively inhibited by specific or nonspecific suppressor T cells (Gershon, 1974; Pierce and Kapp, 1976). T cell subclasses mediating these various regulatory and effector cell functions have been characterized on the basis of membrane alloantigens of the Ly 1, 2,3 system. Ly 1^+ T cells have helper and amplifier regulatory functions and appear to be effector cells in delayed hypersensitivity reactions. Ly $2,3^+$ T cells mediate suppressor cell regulatory functions and are effector cells in cytotoxic lymphocyte responses. The function(s) of Ly $1,2,3^+$ T cells is yet to be defined, but these cells may be antigen-specific precursors of the Ly 1^+ or Ly $2,3^+$ T cells (Cantor and Boyse, 1977a,b). In addition to these antigen-specific lymphocytes, macrophages (Mø) have critical non-antigen specific functions in the initiation of immune responses which involve the uptake, catabolism and presentation of antigen in a configuration highly immunogenic for the responding T and B cells (Unanue, 1972; Pierce and Kapp, 1976b).

The importance of products of the major histocompatibility gene complex of the species (the H-2 complex in mice) in the initiation and regulation of immune responses has been demonstrated in several systems. The H-2 complex is a segment of genome in the IX linkage group on chromosome 17 which can be divided into 4 regions for this discussion. At the two ends are the K and D regions which encode the serologically defined (SD) specificities, or the major histocompatibility or transplantation antigens. These antigens are recognized predominantly by Ly $2,3^+$ precursor and effector cytotoxic lymphocytes and are involved to a lesser extent in stimulating MLR and graft-vs.-host responses (Shreffler and David, 1975; Klein, 1975). Inside the D region is the S region which encodes proteins of the complement sequence. Between the K and S regions (and probably between the S and D regions) is the I region which encodes the lymphocyte activating determinants (LAD) recognized by Ly 1^+ amplifier T cells in MLR and graft-vs.-host responses; these determinants may be identical to the Ia antigens also encoded by this region. The involvement of I region gene products in: 1) controlling immune responses to certain antigens (Ir genes); and, 2) mediating and regulating interactions among Mø, T cells and B cells in immune responses has made the study of the relationships of these I region products an active area of investigation.

Ir genes, which control responses to synthetic and natural protein and polypeptide antigens, have been mapped throughout the I region (Katz, 1977; Shreffler and David, 1975; Benacerraf, 1976). However, the nature of the Ir gene product and its specific function(s) are yet to be defined. Products of the I-A subregion (I region in guinea pigs) have been shown to restrict or control: 1) physiological interactions among T and B cells in the development of IgG antibody responses; 2) interactions between Mφ and T cells in the generation and functional expression of helper T cells *in vitro*, DNA synthetic responses to antigen in mice and guinea pigs, and secondary IgG antibody responses; and, 3) successful transfer of delayed hypersensitivity (Katz, 1977; Paul and Benacerraf, 1977).

IMMUNOBIOLOGY OF ANTIBODY RESPONSES TO AN ANTIGEN (GAT) CONTROLLED BY H-2 LINKED IR GENES

Antibody responses to a variety of synthetic and natural antigens are controlled by autosomal dominant, H-2 linked Ir gene(s) (Benacerraf, 1976). During the past few years in collaboration with Professor Baruj Benacerraf, the mechanisms by which these Ir genes regulate antibody responses have been probed using the random terpolymer of L-glutamic acid^{60}-L-alanine^{30}-L-tyrosine^{10} (GAT). *In vivo*, mice of the H-2^{a,b,d,f,j,k,r,u,v} haplotypes are "responders"; mice of the H-2^{p,q,s} haplotypes are "nonresponders". Both responder and nonresponder mice develop antibody responses to GAT when immunized with GAT complexed to the immunogenic carrier methylated bovine serum albumin (MBSA) or pigeon erythrocytes (PRBC). The gene(s) controlling these responses have been mapped to the I-A-I-B subregions.

The Mishell-Dutton culture system was used to study plaque-forming cell (PFC) responses to GAT and GAT-MBSA by spleen cells from responder and nonresponder mice. GAT stimulated primary and secondary IgG GAT-specific PFC responses by spleen cells from responder strains, but failed to stimulate responses by spleen cells from nonresponder strains. Spleen cells from F_1 hybrids of responders x nonresponders responded to GAT. GAT-MBSA and GAT-PRBC stimulated PFC responses by both responder and nonresponder spleen cells. Although IgM GAT-specific PFC were not detected under these culture conditions, anti μ antibody suppressed PFC responses to GAT indicating that μ^+ B cells were stimulated in these responses (Kapp et al, 1973a). These results correlated precisely with *in vivo* serological and PFC response data and this system was used to study cellular events regulated by Ir genes.

Mφ and helper T cells are required for development of IgG GAT-specific PFC responses to GAT and GAT-MBSA by responder B cells and for responses to GAT-MBSA by nonresponder B cells. Mφ from nonresponder mice supported development of PFC responses to GAT by responder lymphoid cells (T cells and B cells) indicating that the defect in nonresponder mice was not a Mϕ defect. Responder Mϕ supported PFC responses by nonresponder lymphoid cells to SRBC and GAT-MBSA, but not to GAT, indicating that Ir gene regulation of responses to GAT is expressed in lymphoid cells. Since nonresponder B cells synthesized antibody specific for GAT after stimulation with GAT-MBSA, and since the response to GAT was dependent on T cells, it appeared that nonresponder mice lacked appropriate GAT-specific helper T cell function (Kapp et al., 1973b).

Nonresponder spleen cells, after exposure to GAT *in vivo* or addition of GAT to culture, failed to respond to the normally immunogenic GAT-MBSA. Thus, interaction of nonresponder spleen cells with doses of GAT normally immunogenic for responder spleen cells (1-10 μg) induced a state of GAT-specific tolerance. Cell mixture experiments using X-irradiated, GAT-MBSA primed (C57BL/6 x B10.S)F_1 helper T cells and responder C57BL/6 or nonresponder B10.S B cells clearly demonstrated that GAT induced tolerance in nonresponder B cells (Kapp et al, 1974).

In an extension of these studies, the conditions for development of PFC responses to GAT in cultures containing responder C57BL/6 or nonresponder B10.S B cells and GAT primed, X-irradiated F_1 helper T cells were determined. The issue was whether primed F_1 T cells, which cooperate with parental B cells in responses to antigens not controlled by Ir genes, could cooperate with nonresponder B cells in responses to GAT. In other experimental systems (Katz, 1977), B cells lacking the Ir gene for an antigen failed to respond in the presence of functional primed F_1 T cells. PFC responses to GAT developed in cultures with primed F_1 T cells and responder B cells, but not with nonresponder B cells. By contrast, when GAT was presented on F_1 Mϕ or as GAT-MBSA, PFC responses by both responder and nonresponder B cells developed. Thus, B cells lacking the Ir gene for GAT responded in the presence of GAT-primed F_1 T cells when GAT was presented in an insoluble form (GAT-Mϕ or GAT-MBSA) to avoid B cell tolerance (Benacerraf et al, 1974).

Thus, GAT failed to elicit a GAT-specific PFC response in cultures of nonresponder spleen cells and induced tolerance in nonresponder B cells. However, nonresponder B cells, rendered unresponsive by exposure to GAT *in vivo*, responded to GAT-MBSA *in vitro* if carrier (MBSA) primed T cells were present. This unresponsiveness resulted from impaired carrier-specific helper T cell function in the GAT-primed nonresponder mice. Moreover, spleen cells from nonresponder mice primed with 1 to 100 μg GAT suppressed GAT-specific PFC responses to GAT-MBSA by normal syngeneic spleen cells from 3 days to 4 weeks after priming. This suppression was abrogated by treatment of GAT-primed spleen cells with anti-Thy 1 serum + C or X-irradiation. The B cells from these GAT-primed mice developed PFC responses to GAT-MBSA when cultured with appropriate helper T cells. Thus, the failure of genetic nonresponders to develop antibody responses to GAT appears to be due to a reversible B cell tolerance and more importantly to the preferential stimulation of GAT-specific suppressor T cells (rather than helper T cells) which actively inhibit development of PFC responses to immunogenic GAT-MBSA (Kapp et al, 1974b; Pierce and Kapp, 1976b).

To probe the mechanisms of action of these suppressor T cells, a soluble factor released into culture fluids by spleen cells from GAT-primed mice was sought; none was found. However, suppressor factors can be extracted from spleen, thymus, lymph node and purified T cells of GAT-primed nonresponder mice. This T cell product was a protein with a molecular weight of approximately 45,000 which specifically inhibited, in a dose-dependent manner, GAT-specific responses to GAT-MBSA and GAT-PRBC *in vivo* and *in vitro*. Interestingly, this factor inhibited responses to GAT-MBSA by spleen cells from histoincompatible strains of mice that are nonresponders to GAT, but not strains that are responders to GAT. The suppressive moiety contained a fragment of GAT and had binding sites for GAT and cross reactive copolymers GA and GT. Although the avidity of this factor for GAT was similar to that of anti-GAT antibody, it lacks detectable Ig determinants but has determinants encoded by the I region of the H-2 complex (Kapp et al, 1976; 1977).

Since nonresponder T cells recognize and respond to GAT by preferential development of suppressor T cells, a variety of manipulations were employed to determine what conditions, if any, led to generation of helper T cells in nonresponder mice. X-irradiated spleen cells from nonresponder mice primed with soluble GAT failed to provide helper T cell activity for PFC responses by syngeneic nonresponder and (responder x nonresponder)F_1 B cells. T cells from mice primed with GAT-MBSA had radioresistant helper T cell activity for nonresponder B cell responses to GAT-MBSA as expected, but also had helper cell activity for F_1 B cell responses to GAT and GAT-Mφ. T cells from mice primed with GAT-Mφ had GAT-specific helper cell activity for nonresponder B cell responses to GAT-MBSA and for F_1 B cell responses to GAT-MBSA and GAT-Mφ. Thus, GAT-specific helper T cells can be generated in nonresponder mice and presentation of GAT by Mφ is critical (Kapp et al., 1975).

GAT AS A PROBE TO STUDY THE ROLE OF Mφ IN ANTIBODY RESPONSES *IN VITRO*

Mφ are required for development of PFC responses in all Ig classes to all T cell-dependent antigens and to the T cell-independent antigen, TNP-Ficoll, but not TNP-LPS. Mϕ have at least two distinct functions; 1) to promote the survival of lymphoid cells in culture; and 2) to present antigen to responding T and B cells in an appropriate immunogenic configuration. The viability promoting function of Mϕ can be replaced by 2-mercaptoethanol and appears to promote the survival of virgin T cells in culture (Pierce and Kapp, 1976a).

The functions of peritoneal exudate Mϕ in antigen uptake, catabolism and presentation have been analyzed using ^{125}I-GAT. Optimal conditions for pulsing Mϕ with GAT have been determined; approximately 1-2 ng GAT was bound per 10^5 Mϕ after exposure of 2 x 10^6 Mϕ to 100 μg GAT (Pierce et al, 1974; Pierce et al, 1976, 1977a). After incubation for 24 hrs at 37°C, 90% of the GAT is lost from the Mϕ and is recovered in the culture fluid as acid soluble material. Incubation for an additional 6 days resulted in a loss of another 5% of the GAT from Mϕ (Pierce and Kapp, 1977a). 10^5 Mϕ bearing 1-2 ng of GAT and 5 to 10 μg soluble GAT stimulated comparable PFC responses by lymphoid cells, demonstrating the efficiency of antigen presentation by Mϕ. When GAT-Mϕ were reduced to 10^4 Mϕ/culture, minimal responses were stimulated; these responses were restored to normal by 5 x 10^{-5} M 2-mercaptoethanol or 9 x 10^4 non GAT-bearing Mϕ. Thus, 10^4 GAT-Mϕ had sufficient antigen to stimulate PFC responses, but were insufficient for the viability promoting function which was supplied by the normal Mϕ or 2-mercaptoethanol (Pierce and Kapp, 1977a).

Genetic restrictions regulate interactions among Mϕ and lymphocytes in other experimental models. However, syngeneic and allogeneic Mϕ supported development of comparable primary PFC responses to SRBC, soluble GAT and GAT-MBSA (Kapp et al, 1974b; Pierce and Kapp, 1976a; Pierce et al, 1976). Syngeneic and allogeneic GAT-Mϕ (1-2 ng GAT/10^5 Mϕ) also stimulated comparable PFC responses immediately after pulsing and after incubation for 24 hrs or 7 days during which >90% of the GAT initially associated with the Mϕ was released into the culture medium as acid soluble material. These latter observations suggested that transfer of GAT from allogeneic Mϕ to syngeneic Mϕ contaminating the lymphoid cells and that the PFC responses were actually stimulated by this GAT was unlikely. Allogeneic Mϕ did not stimulate a detectable mixed lymphocyte response by the lymphoid cells and stimulatory factors released as a result of an allogeneic interaction have not been detected. Thus, genetic restrictions do not appear to govern Mϕ-lymphoid cell interactions in the development of primary PFC responses *in vitro* (Pierce et al, 1976, 1977).

By contrast, immune spleen or lymphoid cells developed secondary PFC responses *in vitro* preferentially when stimulated with GAT-Mϕ syngeneic to the Mϕ used to present GAT during *in vivo* immunization. Thus, genetic restrictions govern efficient Mϕ-lymphocyte interactions in secondary PFC responses. These genetic restrictions are: a) antigen-specific; b) demonstrable for only a limited period of time (2 weeks to 8 weeks) after an immunization with limiting quantities of GAT on Mϕ; c) controlled by the I-A subregion of the H-2 complex; d) operative at the level of Mϕ-immune T cell interactions; and, e) involve an active suppressive mechanism (Pierce et al, 1976; 1977; Pierce and Kapp, 1977a,b). Control experiments have ruled antigen transfer as a mechanism of these restrictions and in systems involving Mϕ allogeneic to the responding T cells mixed lymphocyte responses and allogeneic effect-like factors have not been detected. Further, restrictions at the level of the B cell which may have been induced during immunization have not been detected.

Thus, T cells from mice immunized with syngeneic or allogeneic GAT-Mϕ function as helper cells in secondary PFC responses only when stimulated with GAT-Mϕ syngeneic at the I-A subregion of the H-2 complex with the immunizing Mϕ. T cells from these spleens specifically suppressed primary responses by virgin spleen cells stimulated by GAT-Mϕ which were nonidentical at I-A with the immunizing Mϕ. These restrictions on helper T and suppressor T cell activities were not altered with aged Mϕ, ruling out antigen transfer, or with highly purified Mϕ, ruling out a negative allogeneic effect mediated by T cells contaminating the Mϕ (Pierce and Kapp, 1977c,d).

The ability of virgin and immune (responder x nonresponder)F_1 spleen cells to develop PFC responses *in vitro* after stimulation with responder and nonresponder parental GAT-Mϕ was investigated. Virgin F_1 spleen cells developed comparable primary responses to both parental GAT-Mϕ. By contast, spleen cells from F_1 mice immunized with responder or nonresponder parental GAT-Mϕ developed secondary responses only to the parental Mϕ used for priming. Further, spleen cells from F_1 mice immunized with soluble GAT developed secondary responses only to responder parental GAT-Mϕ and failed to respond to nonresponder parental or third party GAT-Mϕ. Interestingly, F_1 spleen cells from mice primed with F_1 GAT-Mϕ responded to both responder and nonresponder parental GAT-Mϕ but not to third party GAT-Mϕ (Pierce et al, 1977b).

The experiments summarized above using GAT as a probe for regulatory mechanisms in immune responses have been highly informative with regard to mechanisms of Ir gene control of antibody responses and genetic restrictions governing Mϕ-T cell interactions. These data form the basis for experiments currently in progress investigating the mechanism(s) of action of the GAT-specific suppressor factor extracted from GAT-primed nonresponder mice and the mechanisms by which virgin T cells become restricted and function as helper cells only with the Mø-antigen complex used for immunization.

ABSTRACT

The synthetic random terpolymer of L-glutamic acid^{60}-L-alanine^{30}-L-tyrosine^{10} (GAT) has been used as a probe to investigate regulatory mechanisms in antibody responses in tissue culture systems. In this brief review, the mechanisms of H-2 linked Ir gene control of antibody responses to GAT and genetic restrictions governing Mø-immune T cell interactions in antibody responses to GAT are summarized.

ACKNOWLEDGEMENTS

These investigations were supported by U.S. Public Health Service Research Grants AI-13915, AI-13987, and AI-09920 from the National Institute of Allergy and Infectious Diseases and Biomedical Research Support Grant RR05491 to the Jewish Hospital of St. Louis from the Division of Research Resources, NIH. We thank Eleanor Menkhus for her skilled secretarial assistance in the preparation of this manuscript.

REFERENCES

Benacerraf, B., Editor, (1975) Immunogenetics and Immunodeficiency. Med. Techn. Publ. Col. Ltd., London.

Benacerraf, B., Kapp, J.A., Pierce, C.W., and Katz, D.H. (1974) J. Exp. Med. 140, 185.

Cantor, H., and Boyse, E.A. (1977a) Cold Spring Harbor Symp. Quant. Biol. 41, 23.

Cantor, H., and Boyse, E.A. (1977b) Contemp. Topics Immunobiol. 7, 47.

Cantor, H., and Weissman, I. (1975) Prog. Allergy 16, 300.

Gershon, R.K. (1974) Contemp. Topics Immunobiol. 3, 1.

Kapp, J.A., Pierce, C.W., and Benacerraf, B. (1973a) J. Exp. Med. 138, 1107.

Kapp, J.A., Pierce, C.W., and Benacerraf, B. (1973b) J. Exp. Med. 138, 1121.

Kapp, J.A., Pierce, C.W., and Benacerraf, B. (1974a) J. Exp. Med. 140, 172.

Kapp, J.A., Pierce, C.W., Schlossman, S., and Benacerraf, B. (1974b) J. Exp. Med. 140, 648.

Kapp, J.A., Pierce, C.W., and Benacerraf, B. (1975) J. Exp. Med. 142, 50.

Kapp, J.A., Pierce, C.W., de la Croix, F., and Benacerraf, B. (1976) J. Immunol. 116, 305.

Kapp, J.A., Pierce, C.W., and Benacerraf, B. (1977) J. Exp. Med. 145, 821.

Katz, D.H. (1977) Lymphocyte Differentiation, Recognition and Regulation, Academic Press, Inc., New York.

Klein, J. (1975) Biology of the Mouse Histocompatibility - 2 Complex, Springer-Verlag, New York.

Paul, W.E., and Benacerraf, B. (1977) Science 195, 1293.

Pierce, C.W., and Kapp, J.A. (1976a) In: Immunobiology of the Macrophage, Nelson, D.S., Editor, Academic Press, New York p.1.

Pierce, C.W., and Kapp, J.A. (1976b) Contemp. Topics Immunobiol. 5, 91.

Pierce, C.W., and Kapp, J.A. (1977a) Manuscript in Preparation.

Pierce, C.W., and Kapp, J.A. (1977b) In: Ir Genes and Ia Antigens McDevitt, H.O., Editor, Academic Press, Inc., New York (In Press).

Pierce, C.W., and Kapp, J.A. (1977c) Fed. Proc. (In Press).

Pierce, C.W., and Kapp, J.A. (1977d) Manuscript in Preparation.

Pierce, C.W., Kapp, J.A., Wood, D.D., and Benacerraf, B. (1974) J. Immunol. 112, 1181.

Pierce, C.W., Kapp, J.A., and Benacerraf, B. (1976) J. Exp. Med. 144, 371.

Pierce, C.W., Kapp, J.A., and Benacerraf, b. (1977a) Cold Spring Harbor Symp. Quant. Biol. 41, 563.

Pierce, C.W., Germain, R.N., Kapp, J.A., and Benacerraf, B. (1977b) J. Exp. Med. (In Press).

Shreffler, D.C., and David, C.S. (1975) Adv. Immunol. 20, 215.

Unanue, E.R. (1977) Adv. Immunol. 152, 95.

Warner, N.L. (1974) Adv. Immunol. 19, 67.

THE NATURE AND FUNCTIONS OF SPECIFIC IMMUNE RESPONSE GENES AND THEIR PRODUCTS

Edna Mozes

Department of Chemical Immunology, The Weizmann Institute of Science, Rehovot, Israel

ABSTRACT

Antibodies produced by inbred mouse strains immunized with the random synthetic polypeptide poly(Tyr,Glu)-poly(*DL*Ala)--polyLys denoted (T,G)-A--L were found to be specific mainly to the ordered peptide Tyr-Tyr-Glu-Glu.

Low responder $H\text{-}2^k$ mice, upon immunization with either the random (T,G)-A--L or the ordered (T-T-G-G)-A--L coupled to methylated bovine serum albumin (MBSA), produce antibodies with comparable titers to those observed in high responder $H\text{-}2^b$ mice following immunization with the antigens alone or with their complexes with MBSA. A comparison of the above antibodies have led to the conclusion that low responder mice, upon immunization with the synthetic antigens complexed with MBSA, produce antibodies of the same specificity and quality as those of high responders (as shown by the isoelectric focusing technique) and they also have the same affinity and heterogeneity as antibodies of $H\text{-}2^b$ mice (measured by equilibrium dialysis and antigen binding capacity assay).

Anti-idiotypic sera to anti-(T,G)-A--L antibodies of C3H.SW ($H\text{-}2^b$, $Ig\text{-}1^a$) mice were raised in guinea pigs. C3H.SW anti-(T,G)-A--L antibodies from different pools cross reacted idiotypically. Anti-(T,G)-A--L antibodies of CWB ($H\text{-}2^b$, $Ig\text{-}1^b$) mice did not react with the anti-idiotypic serum suggesting linkage between the genes coding for idiotypes and allotypes. C3H/DiSn ($H\text{-}2^k$, $Ig\text{-}1^a$) anti-(T,G)-A--L antibodies elicited by immunization with (T,G)-A--L complexed to MBSA reacted with the anti-idiotypic serum to the same degree as C3H.SW anti-(T,G)-A--L antibodies, confirming the similarity between the high and low responder anti-(T,G)-A--L antibodies.

C3H.SW ($H-2^b$) mice as well as C3H/HeJ or C3H/DiSn ($H-2^k$) mice were found to be capable of producing an antigen specific factor from "educated" T cells which replaces the helper effect of T cells in the process of antibody production. On the other hand B cells of $H-2^k$ mice were not triggered by a factor of either high or low responder specific T cells.

The activity of a C3H.SW (T,G)-A--L specific T cell factor was removed after passage on a Sepharose column coupled to the anti-idiotypic serum prepared against C3H.SW anti-(T,G)-A--L antibodies, suggesting similarity between the antigen specific T cell factor and the B cell recognition system. A (T,G)-A--L specific factor produced by C3H/DiSn ($H-2^k$, $Ig-1^a$) "educated" T cells reacted with the anti-idiotypic serum as well. Thus, C3H.SW high and C3H/DiSn low responder (T,G)-A--L specific T cell factors cross react at the level of their binding site for antigen.

INTRODUCTION

Synthetic polypeptide antigens have been a useful tool in the studies of genetic regulation of immune responsiveness. One of the antigens most extensively studied from the point of view of the genetic control of the immune responses it provokes, is the multichain polymer of α-amino acids, poly(*L*Tyr,*L*Glu)-poly(*DL*Ala)--poly(*L*Lys), denoted (T,G)-A--L (Sela *et al.*, 1962; McDevitt and Sela, 1965). This immunogen has been tested in many inbred strains of mice for its capacity to elicit antibody production. The response was found to be regulated by an autosomal, dominant gene(s) linked to the major histocompatibility (H-2) complex of the mouse (McDevitt and Sela, 1965; McDevitt and Tyan, 1968). Cellular analysis of the antibody response to (T,G)-A--L have revealed the involvement of several cell types and a soluble factor which are antigen specific and genetically controlled (Mozes and Shearer, 1972; Lichtenberg *et al.*, 1974; Taussig *et al.*, 1974).

We have attempted to determine the cell type(s) expressing the genetic defect in low responder mice through the analysis of both the B cell products, i.e., the specific anti-(T,G)-A--L antibodies and the T-cell products, i.e., the antigen specific T cell factors.

Properties of (T,G)-A--L Specific Antibodies

The polymer (T,G)-A--L is derived from multichain poly-*DL*-alanine to which short sequences of glutamic acid and tyrosine are attached. These short peptides are obtained by random polymerization of N-carboxyamino acid anhydrides (Sela *et al.*, 1962), and therefore they possess different sequence combinations. This raised the possibility that high and low responses to this antigen might be due to differences in: a) the specificity of the antibodies formed; b) the affinity of the antibodies produced; or c) the amounts of antibodies of the same specificity and affinity. In order to elucidate this problem we have prepared by stepwise method of peptide synthesis (Ramachandran *et al.*, 1971) several tetrapeptides each containing two tyrosines and two glutamic acid residues. Out of a series of ordered synthetic polypeptides (Tyr-Tyr-Glu-Glu) - poly(*DL*Ala)--poly(Lys) denoted (T-T-G-G)-A--L was found to resemble the properties of the random (T,G)-A--L most closely in the pattern of antibodies it elicited and in the genetic regulation of the immune responses provoked by this polymer (Mozes *et al.*, 1974; Schwartz *et al.*, 1975).

The response of low responder mice to (T,G)-A--L was shown to be restored following immunization with a complex of antigen with methylated bovine serum albumin (MBSA - McDevitt, 1968). However, the mechanism of this effect remained unknown, since it could not be ruled out that the antibodies produced by MBSA-reconstituted low responder mice might be directed against any of the possible determinants which exist in the random immunogen. An increase in the antibody titers of low responder mice to the complex of the ordered (T-T-G-G)-A--L polymer with MBSA would suggest that the antibodies produced by high and low responders to (T,G)-A--L are directed to the same determinant. As shown in Table 1, the antibody responses of low responder mice (H-2^k) were enhanced following immunization with (T-T-G-G)-A--L complexed with MBSA. Furthermore, similar titers were obtained for low responder antibodies to (T,G)-A--L + MBSA when titered with either (T,G)-A--L or (T-T-G-G)-A--L (Cramer *et al.*, 1976). These results indicated that the antibodies produced by high and low responders following immunization with the complex of (T,G)-A--L and MBSA are to the same determinant.

The possibility still existed, however, that antibodies of low and high responders to (T-T-G-G)-A--L, elicited upon immunization with either the random (T,G)-A--L or the ordered polypeptide complexed with MBSA, differ in other properties than specificity. Looking for such properties, we employed the technique of analytical isoelectric focusing (IEF), which was followed by an antigen binding assay of the focused antibodies (Cramer *et al.*, 1976).

When anti-(T-T-G-G)-A--L immune sera raised in the H-2^k low responder strains and in the H-2^b high responder mice were analyzed by IEF, striking differences were observed as demonstrated in Figure 1. While no IgG antibodies could be detected in the low responder sera, C3H.SW, high responder mice produced an antibody population with clearly resolved banding patterns as observed in every immune serum tested (Fig. 1).

Table 1

Enhancement of antibody responses to (T-T-G-G)-A--L in low responder strains upon immunization with a complex of antigen with MBSA

Mouse strain	H-2 type	Immunization with: (T-T-G-G)-A--L	(T-T-G-G)-A--L + MBSA
C3H.SW	b	5.37 ± 0.24[a)]	7.23 ± 0.34
C3H/HeJ	k	1.40 ± 0.30	7.09 ± 0.34
CWB	b	6.58 ± 0.25	7.53 ± 0.54
CKB	k	1.47 ± 0.19	6.05 ± 0.48

a) Average $\log_2$ of hemagglutination titers ± standard deviations of tests of 10 - 30 individual antisera. SRBC were coated with (T-T-G-G)-A--L for the hemagglutination assay.

The crucial finding, however, is depicted in Figure 2, where low (CKB) and high (CWB) responder strains were immunized with (T-T-G-G)-A--L + MBSA. Under these experimental conditions, as far as the high responder is concerned, there is no difference in the quality of the IEF spectrotypes whether MBSA was (Fig. 2) or was not (Fig. 1) used together with the antigen. Upon reconstitution with MBSA, however, the low responder IEF spectra are also characterized by discrete bands. The results demonstrated in Figure 2 indicate that high and low responder immune sera raised against (T-T-G-G)-A--L + MBSA are of a similar degree of restriction (Cramer *et al.*, 1976).

The same patterns of IEF spectrotypes were obtained for high and low responder mouse strains immunized with either (T,G)-A--L or its complex with MBSA when either ^{131}I-(T-T-G-G)-A--L or ^{131}I-(T,G)-A--L were used to bind to the focused antibodies (Cramer *et al.*, 1976).

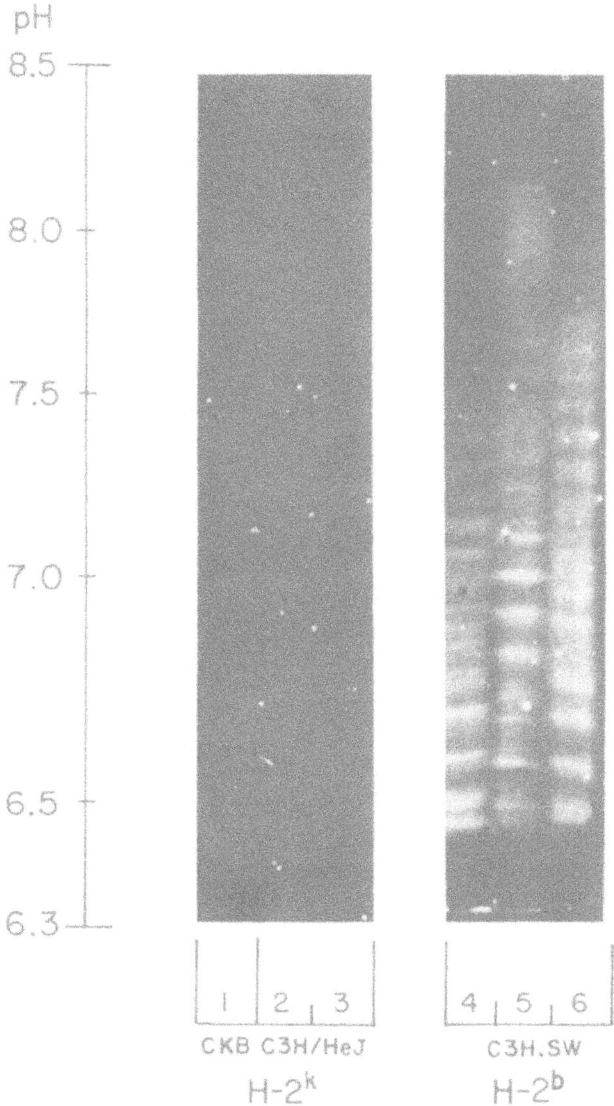

Fig. 1. IEF spectrotypes of representative immune sera of individual H-2^k CKB and C3H/HeJ low responder mice and H-2^b C3H.SW high responder mice to (T-T-G-G)-A--L. ^{131}I-(T-T-G-G)-A--L was used for development. Exposure time to the film: 24 h.

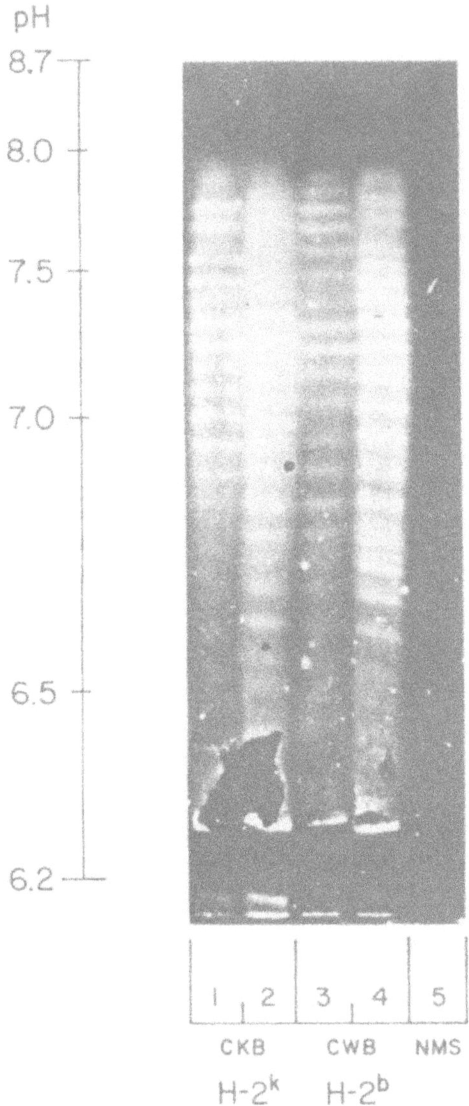

Fig. 2. IEF patterns of immune sera against (T-T-G-G)-A--L + MBSA produced by CKB ($H\text{-}2^k$) and CWB ($H\text{-}2^b$) mice. Normal mouse serum was added as control for specificity of binding. Sera were developed with ^{131}I-(T-T-G-G)-A--L, exposure time: 18 h.

The affinity of antibodies produced by high and low responder mouse strains to the ordered (T-T-G-G)-A--L and to the random (T,G)-A--L was measured following immunizations with the antigens alone or with the complexes of immunogens-MBSA. Determination of affinity values could not be performed by equilibrium dialysis as long as only the random polypeptide was available due to the lack of low molecular weight, dialyzable peptides, representing the antigenic determinants of the random (T,G)-A--L. The availability of the ordered polypeptide (T-T-G-G)-A--L, and the observation that the responses to the random (T,G)-A--L and to the complexes of the antigens with MBSA in high and low responders are directed to T-T-G-G (Mozes *et al.*, 1974; Schwartz *et al.*, 1975; Cramer *et al.*, 1976), enabled such measurements.

The results of equilibrium dialysis experiments performed with the tetrapeptide T-T-G-G to which *DL*-alanine-^{14}C was attached at the C-terminus indicated that the association constants of antibodies elicited by low responder C3H/HeJ mice to the complex of (T-T-G-G)-A--L with MBSA are of the same order of magnitude as of those produced by high responder C3H.SW mice either to the complex or to the antigen itself. The average values obtained for the three groups of antibodies were Ko = $4.5 \pm 1 \times 10^4$ M^{-1} and a = 1.0 ± 0.1.

The association constants of (T-T-G-G)-A--L specific antibodies were also measured by a binding capacity assay in which constant concentrations of antisera were mixed with different concentrations of ^{125}I-(T-T-G-G)-A--L. This assay was shown to be a reliable technique for comparison between different affinities of antibodies to common antigens (Steward and Petty, 1972). Using this technique, antibodies produced by high responder C3H.SW mice elicited against (T-T-G-G)-A--L and against (T-T-G-G)-A--L + MBSA and by low responder C3H/HeJ mice against the last complex were calculated to give a practically identical value of apparent Ko = 7×10^6 M^{-1}, with a = 1.0. The binding capacity of antibodies elicited against (T,G)-A--L and its MBSA complex were measured as well. Titrations were performed with ^{125}I-(T-T-G-G)-A--L and therefore the values obtained represented affinity of anti-(T,G)-A--L antibodies specific to the major determinant namely T-T-G-G. The apparent Ko values obtained for antisera of high responder immunized with either (T,G)-A--L alone or its MBSA complex and of low responder immunized with the complex of (T,G)-A--L MBSA were all similar with an average of - 1.2×10^6 M^{-1} and with an heterogeneity index of 0.9.

The Ko values as determined by the binding capacity assay using the whole polypeptide are of two orders of magnitude higher than those determined by equilibrium dialysis with the tetrapeptide. Such differences can be explained by taking into consideration that the determinant T-T-G-G is represented about 100 times in the ordered (T-T-G-G)-A--L. However the two assay systems led to the same conclusions, namely that the affinity values of the antibodies of low responders immunized with the antigen's complex with MBSA are comparable to those of high responders immunized with the antigen or with its MBSA complex (M. Schwartz, D. Lancet, E. Mozes and M. Sela).

Cross reactive idiotypic determinants on murine antibodies to (T,G)-A--L

Anti-idiotypic antibodies provided a powerful tool for identification of similarity of structures within the variable parts of the antibody molecules (Nisonoff *et al.*, 1975). In the mouse, idiotypes that are shared by different individuals of the same strain have been described for several antibody systems (Eichmann, 1972; Kuettner *et al.*, 1972; Cosenza and Kohler, 1972; Fathman and Sachs, 1976). It was, therefore, of interest to compare the idiotypic determinants of high and low responder antibodies specific to (T,G)-A--L. In order to do so, it was necessary to produce anti-idiotypic antibodies that will react with anti-(T,G)-A--L antibodies of different individuals of the same high responder mouse strain. Antisera were raised against purified anti-(T,G)-A--L antibodies (idiotypes) of C3H.SW high responder mice (McDevitt and Chinitz, 1969) in guinea pigs which were previously shown to respond well in the production of anti-idiotypes (Eichmann, 1972; Eichmann and Kindt, 1971). The guinea pigs (random bred DH albino) were first tolerized to C3H/HeJ IgG (which possess identical allotypes to that of C3H.SW) before immunization with the idiotypes. However, prior to assaying for anti-idiotypic activity, the guinea pig antisera were passed through a column of Sepharose to which C3H.SW IgG was attached to adsorb any residual anti Ig activity in the sera. Binding of ^{125}I-idiotype by specific anti-idiotypic serum of one of the guinea pigs at several dilutions is given in Figure 3. The anti-idiotypic sera bound 20 - 30% of the ^{125}I-idiotype. The low percentage of specific binding was expected as anti-(T,G)-A--L antibodies are not homogeneous (Fig. 1) and not all antibody species within the total population might express immunogenic idiotypic determinants.

Inhibition experiments were performed with the guinea pig anti-idiotypic serum presented in Figure 3, at a 1:300 dilution. Results of inhibition experiments presented in Figure 4 show that the unlabeled idiotype as well as C3H.SW anti-(T,G)-A--L antibodies isolated from a pool of sera other than that used for preparation of idiotype, reduced significantly the binding of ^{125}I-idiotype to the anti-idiotypic antibodies. Normal C3H.SW IgG at high concentration (500 μg/tube) did not inhibit the binding. C3H.SW anti-Nip-ovalbumin antibodies also did not affect the binding to a

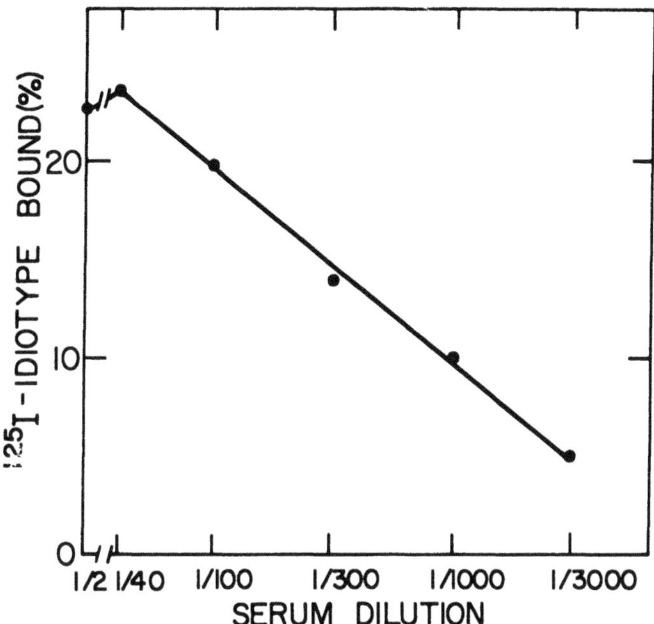

Fig. 3. Binding of ^{125}I-C3H.SW anti-(T,G)-A--L antibodies (5 ng) by a guinea pig anti-idiotypic serum. The average % binding of ^{125}I-idiotype by control normal guinea pig serum (6.7%) is substracted from each experimental value.

significant extent. It can, thus, be concluded that idiotypic determinants on C3H.SW antibodies used for immunization are found also in antibodies of the same specificity from other individuals of the same strain (J. Haimovich and E. Mozes).

The anti-idiotypic sera were used as inhibitors of the binding of anti-(T,G)-A--L antibodies to ^{125}I-(T,G)-A--L. In this case idiotypic specificities associated with the antibody combining sites were determined. Results presented in Table 2 show that the anti-idiotypic serum inhibited binding of ^{125}I-(T,G)-A--L to C3H.SW anti-(T,G)-A--L antibodies. On the other hand, the anti-idiotypic serum did not inhibit binding of (T,G)-A--L to anti-(T,G)-A--L antibodies from C57BL/6 mice. It also did not affect binding of ^{125}I-(T,G)-A--L to anti-(T,G)-A--L antibodies of CWB mice which are congenic with C3H.SW mice and differ only by allotypes. In contrast, the anti-idiotypic serum inhibited binding of antigen to

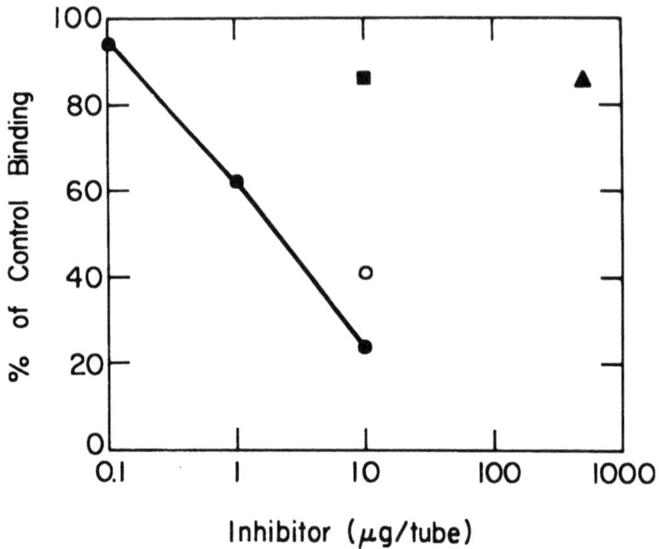

Fig. 4. Inhibition of binding of ^{125}I-C3H.SW anti-(T,G)-A--L antibodies to guinea pig anti-idiotypic serum by: ● - non iodinated idiotypic immunogen; o - C3H.SW antibodies to (T,G)-A--L isolated from a pool of sera other than that used for the preparation of the immunogen; ■ - C3H.SW antibodies to Nip-ovalbumin; ▲ - C3H.SW normal IgG.

anti-(T,G)-A--L antibodies of BALB.B10 which are of a different background than C3H.SW but possess the same Ig-1^{a} allotypes. These observations strongly suggest a possible linkage between the genes coding for idiotypes and allotypes. However, genetic analysis are now performed to establish whether linkage exists between anti-(T,G)-A--L idiotypic expression and heavy chain constant part allotypic markers.

The guinea pig anti-idiotypic serum was used as an inhibitor of the binding of ^{125}I-(T,G)-A--L to C3H.SW and C3H/DiSn antibodies raised with the complex of (T,G)-A--L-MBSA. As seen in Table 3 the binding of ^{125}I-(T,G)-A--L to C3H.SW anti (T,G)-A--L-MBSA antibodies was inhibited by the anti-idiotypic serum as well as the binding of C3H/DiSn anti-(T,G)-A--L-MBSA. Thus, C3H/DiSn low and C3H.SW high responder anti-(T,G)-A--L antibodies possess cross reacting idiotypic determinants.

Table 2

Inhibition of binding of anti-(T,G)-A--L sera to ^{125}I-(T,G)-A--L by anti-idiotypic serum[a]

Strain	H-2 type	Ig-1 allele	Immunogen	% inhibition
C3H.SW	b	a	(T,G)-A--L	31
CWB	b	b	(T,G)-A--L	0
C57BL/6	b	b	(T,G)-A--L	5
BALB.B10	b	a	(T,G)-A--L	40

a) The amount of antibodies and dilution of sera used were chosen to be in the range where binding of antigen was affected by further dilution (20-30% of antigen bound).

Table 3

Inhibition of binding of anti-(T,G)-A--L antibodies to ^{125}I-(T,G)-A--L by anti-idiotypic serum[a]

Strain	H-2 type	Ig-1 allele	Immunogen	% inhibition
C3H.SW	b	a	(T,G)-A--L	40
C3H.SW	b	a	(T,G)-A--L+MBSA	26
C3H/DiSn	k	a	(T,G)-A--L+MBSA	33.4

a) The binding was performed with antibodies purified on Sepharose-(T,G)-A--L. The amount of antibodies used was chosen to be in the range where binding of antigen was affected by further dilution (20-30% of antigen bound). Anti-idiotypic serum dilution of 1:5 was used for experiments described in Tables 2 and 3.

The reaction of the anti-idiotypic serum with C3H/DiSn H-2^k antibodies indicate the lack of linkage between the H-2 type of the animal and the idiotypic determinants expressed on the anti-(T,G)-A--L antibodies it produces. On the other hand, the fact that C3H/DiSn mice possess the Ig-1^a allele of C3H.SW strengthens the suggestion of linkage between genes coding for idiotypes and allotypes (R. Liphshitz, M. Schwartz, J. Haimovich and E. Mozes).

The results described up to now have shown that low responder H-2^k B cells have the potential to produce antibodies against the random (T,G)-A--L and the ordered (T-T-G-G)-A--L upon receiving the proper triggering signal. These antibodies are of the same specificity, affinity and heterogeneity as those of high responders and they share also idiotypic determinants with antibodies of high responder animals. Therefore, T cells of H-2^k low responder mice and their products were tested for their ability to react with (T,G)-A--L.

Functions and properties of T cell factors specific to (T,G)-A--L

One of the central functions of thymus derived (T) cells in the immune system is their helper effect in the process of antibody production by bone-marrow derived (B) cells to a variety of antigens (Claman *et al.*, 1966; Mitchell and Miller, 1968; Mitchison, 1971). However, the precise mechanism of T cell interaction with antibody forming cell precursors is still undefined. In order to understand better helper T cell function we have studied the products of these cells, namely, antigen specific T cell soluble factors which can replace T cell helper effect (Taussig, 1974; Taussig *et al.*, 1974). These antigen specific T cell factors are produced by antigen-"educated" thymocytes which are subsequently cultured for a short period *in vitro* in the presence of the inducing immunogen. The ability of a (T,G)-A--L specific T-cell factor produced by C3H.SW "educated" T cells to trigger syngeneic B cells for antibody production is demonstrated in Table 4. Since these T cell factors were found to cooperate efficiently with B cells for antibody production, T cells of different strains were tested for their ability to produce cooperating factors specific to (T,G)-A--L as a measure for their capacity to recognize and respond to this antigen. When "educated" T cells of C3H.SW high and C3H/HeJ low responder strains were compared for their ability to produce factors capable of cooperating with B cells in the response to (T,G)-A--L no interstrains differences were found as can be seen in Table 5. On the other hand, when B cells of the two strains were compared for their antibody response to (T,G)-A--L in the presence of active specific T-cell factors of either strain, only high responder C3H.SW B cells responded (Table 5). On the basis of these results the conclusion was drawn that the cellular

Table 4

Replacement of thymocytes by a specific T cell factor in eliciting an immune response to (T,G)-A--L

Cells and factors transferred into irradiated recipients	Mean P.F.C./ spleen ± S.D.	Average Log_2 of hemagglutination titers
10^7 C3H.SW B.M.	659 ± 349	0.8
10^7 C3H.SW B.M. + 10^8 C3H.SW thymocytes	11666 ± 2211	4.7
10^7 C3H.SW B.M. + C3H.SW T-cell factor[a]	9451 ± 1906	4.2

a) Produced by 1 spleen equivalent of "educated" T-cells.

Table 5

Antibody responses in irradiated recipients injected with 10^7 bone marrow cells, (T,G)-A--L and 10^8 thymocytes or specific T cell factor(s)

Donors of				
Bone marrow cells	Thymocytes	T cell factor(s)[a]	Mean PFC/ spleen±S.D.	Average Log_2 of hemagglutination titers
C3H/HeJ	-	-	171 ± 83	0.3
C3H/HeJ	C3H/HeJ	-	427 ± 317	0.7
C3H/HeJ	-	C3H/HeJ	718 ± 232	0.8
C3H/HeJ	-	C3H.SW	566 ± 378	0.6
C3H.SW	-	C3H/HeJ	8390 ± 2553	4.0
C3H.SW	-	C3H.SW	9451 ± 1906	4.2

a) Produced by 1 spleen equivalent of "educated" T cells.

difference between $H\text{-}2^k$ and $H\text{-}2^b$ mouse strains lies in the responsiveness of their B cells to specific signals or stimuli received from T cells (Taussig *et al.*, 1974).

An important feature of these T cell factors is their antigen specificity. The specificity of a T cell factor produced to (T,G)-A--L was demonstrated by the removal of its activity on specific antigen-Sepharose columns (Taussig and Munro, 1974). The eluate of such columns possesses the activity of the (T,G)-A--L specific T cell factor (Mozes *et al.*, 1975; Mozes, 1976). Further studies on the fine specificity of (T,G)-A--L specific T cell factors led to the conclusion that the specificity of these factors, although not identical, is similar to that of (T,G)-A--L specific antibodies (Isac and Mozes, 1977).

In view of the specificity for antigen of the T cell factors it is possible that they represent the soluble form of the T cell recognition system, since it seems most unlikely that T cells would release an antigen-specific product that was different in terms of antigen recognition from the T cell receptor. If this is the case, the molecular identification and characterization of the T cell factors may solve one of the most controversial topics in immunology.

Studies on the nature of T cell factors specific to synthetic polypeptide antigens have demonstrated that they are products of I region genes which are mapped at the I-A subregion of the major histocompatibility (H-2) complex of the mouse (Taussig *et al.*, 1975; Isac *et al.*, 1977). It has been suggested that the antigen specific T cell factors, by analogy with immunoglobulins, possess a constant region which is an I-region gene(s) product as well as an unidentified variable part, forming the binding site of these molecules (Mozes, 1976). Reports on sharing of idiotypes between T and B cells (Binz and Wigzell, 1975; Eichmann and Rajewsky, 1975), suggest that the V genes may in fact be those which code for the antibody binding site. It was, therefore, of interest to find out whether the T cell factors will cross-react with anti-idiotypic antibodies.

To approach this problem we have utilized our anti-idiotypic serum (described earlier in this report), which was produced against anti-(T,G)-A--L idiotypes. A factor prepared from (T,G)-A--L "educated" T cells of C3H.SW high responder mice was passed through a column of anti-idiotypic serum coupled to Sepharose (IgG of 1 ml serum per 1 gr of Sepharose). As demonstrated in Table 6, the activity of the specific factor was removed after passage through the anti-idiotypic IgG immunoadsorbent (Mozes, 1977). The activity of the same factor was not removed by a control column of guinea pig anti-mouse immunoglobulin.

Table 6

Removal of the activity of a (T,G)-A--L specific T-cell factor by anti-idiotypic serum

Cells and factors transferred into irradiated recipients	No. of mice	Average Log_2 of hemagglutination titers
2 x 10^7 C3H.SW B.M. + 10 μg (T,G)-A--L	11	1.2
2 x 10^7 C3H.SW B.M. + 10^8 C3H.SW thymocytes + 10 μg (T,G)-A--L	8	4.12
2 x 10^7 C3H.SW B.M. + C3H.SW factor[a] + 10 μg (T,G)-A--L	11	4.09
2 x 10^7 C3H.SW B.M. + C3H.SW factor-effluent from an anti-idiotypic IgG immuno-adsorbent + 10 μg (T,G)-A--L	10	1.2
2 x 10^7 C3H.SW B.M. + C3H.SW factor-effluent from a guinea-pig anti mouse Ig immunoadsorbent + 10 μg (T,G)-A--L	5	3.7
2 x 10^7 C3H.SW B.M. + C3H/DiSn factor + 10 μg (T,G)-A--L	11	3.8
2 x 10^7 C3H.SW B.M. + C3H/DiSn factor-effluent from an anti-idiotypic IgG immunoadsorbent + 10 μg (T,G)-A--L	11	0.64
2 x 10^7 C3H.SW B.M. + C3H/DiSn factor-effluent from a guinea-pig anti-mouse Ig immunoadsorbent + 10 μg (T,G)-A--L	12	3.75
2 x 10^7 C3H.SW B.M. + CWB factor + 10 μg (T,G)-A--L	6	4.0
2 x 10^7 C3H.SW B.M. + CWB factor-effluent from an anti-idiotypic IgG immunoadsorbent + 10 μg (T,G)-A--L	5	4.0

a) Produced by 1 spleen equivalent of "educated" T cells.

These results suggest that the (T,G)-A--L specific T cell factor share idiotypes or possess cross-reacting idiotypes with anti-(T,G)-A--L antibodies.

Since H-2^k C3H/DiSn low responder mice were found to produce an active (T,G)-A--L specific T cell factor (Taussig *et al.*, 1974), a factor produced by these mice was also passed through an anti-idiotypic serum immunoadsorbent. The results presented in Table 6 indicate that the ability of a C3H/DiSn (T,G)-A--L specific factor to trigger C3H.SW high responder B cells in the presence of antigen for antibody production, was removed following the reaction with the anti-idiotypic serum. It should be borne in mind that C3H/DiSn (T,G)-A--L specific antibodies elicited by immunization of these mice with the complex of (T,G)-A--L with MBSA reacted also with the same anti-idiotypic antiserum (Table 3). In contrast, a factor produced by CWB (H-2^b) high responder mice to (T,G)-A--L did not loose its biological activity when passed through the anti-idiotypic serum immunoadsorbent (Table 6, E. Mozes and J. Haimovich). CWB (H-2^b) mice are congenic with C3H.SW (H-2^b) mice and differ only by allotypes, however CWB (T,G)-A--L specific antibodies fail also to react with the anti-idiotypic serum produced against anti-(T,G)-A--L antibodies of the C3H.SW mice (Table 2).

It thus appears that B and T cell products possess cross-reacting V regions for antigen recognition. Since the antigen specific T cell helper factors have been shown to be products of I-region genes as well (Taussig *et al.*, 1975; Isac *et al.*, 1977), a mechanism would have to exist for binding Ig-V-genes to I-region C-genes.

CONCLUDING REMARKS

In order to understand better the mechanism by which specific immune responses are genetically regulated we have approached two of the cell types which their successful interaction is a prerequisite for mounting an efficient immune response. Comparison of the B cell products, namely, the antibodies of high and low responder mice to (T,G)-A--L have led to the conclusion that upon receiving the right triggering signal (achieved by immunization with a complex of (T,G)-A--L with MBSA), low responder B cells are capable of producing (T,G)-A--L specific antibodies which are similar in their affinity and specificity to those of high responder mice. Furthermore, H-2^k low responder mice which possess the same Ig-1 allele as the H-2^b high responder animals produce (T,G)-A--L specific antibodies with idiotypic determinants which cross react with those of high responder antibodies confirming the similarity of the two antibody populations.

On the other hand, low responder T cells are capable of

producing (T,G)-A--L specific T cell factors which trigger high responder but not low responder B cells for efficient antibody production. The similarity between low and high responder specific T cell factors has been further confirmed by showing that they possess the same idiotypic determinants which are cross reactive with those found on anti-(T,G)-A--L specific antibodies. Therefore, the genetic defect in response of H-2^k mice to (T,G)-A--L must be at the level of triggering of low responder B cell by a T cell signal, stimulated by antigen alone. Only sensitization with the MBSA complexed antigen provides a signal that bypasses the defect and stimulates these B cells to proliferation and production of antibodies. The exact nature of this defect is not yet known. However, further information on the T and B cell receptors which is expected to be achieved by studies utilizing the anti-idiotypic reagent as well as studies on the involvement of macrophages in the immune response to (T,G)-A--L will hopefully provide a clue for the yet unsolved problem of the cellular basis of the genetic regulation of specific immune responses.

ACKNOWLEDGEMENTS

The studies reported here were supported in part by grants 1RO1 AI 11405 and 1 RO1 AI CA 13200 from the National Institutes of Health, U.S. Public Health Service.

REFERENCES

Binz, H., and Wigzell, H. (1975) J. Exp. Med. 142, 197.
Claman, H.N., Chaperon, E.A., and Triplett, R.F. (1966) J. Immunol. 97, 828.
Cosenza, H., and Kohler, H. (1972) Proc. Natl. Acad. Sci. USA 69, 2701.
Cramer, M., Schwartz, M., Mozes, E., and Sela, M. (1976) Eur. J. Immunol. 6, 618.
Eichmann, K. (1972) Eur. J. Immunol. 2, 301.
Eichmann, K., and Kindt, T.J. (1971) J. Exp. Med. 134, 532.
Eichmann, K., and Rajewsky, K. (1975) Eur. J. Immunol. 5, 661.
Fathman, G.G., and Sachs, D.H. (1976) J. Immunol. 116, 959.
Isac, R., and Mozes, E. (1977) J. Immunol. 118, 584.
Isac, R., Dorf, M.E., and Mozes, E. (1977) Immunogenetics, in press.
Kuettner, M.G., Wang, A.L. and Nisonoff, A. (1972) J. Exp. Med. 135, 579.
Lichtenberg, L., Mozes, E., Shearer, G.M., and Sela, M. (1974) Eur. J. Immunol. 4, 430.
McDevitt, H.O. (1968) J. Immunol. 100, 485.
McDevitt, H.O., and Chinitz, A. (1969) Science 163, 1207.
McDevitt, H.O., and Sela, M. (1965) J. Exp. Med. 122, 517.

McDevitt, H.O., and Tyan, M.L. (1968) J. Exp. Med. 128, 1.
Mitchell, G.F., and Miller, J.F.A.P. (1968) J. Exp. Med. 128, 821.
Mitchison, N.A. (1971) Eur. J. Immunol. 1, 10.
Mozes, E. (1976) in "The Role of the Products of the Histocompatibility Gene Complex in Immune Responses" (D.H. Katz and B. Benacerraf, Eds.) p. 485. Academic Press, New York.
Mozes, E. (1977) in Proceedings of the 3rd Ir gene workshop. (H.O. McDevitt, Ed.) Academic Press, New York, in press.
Mozes, E., and Shearer, G.M. (1972). Curr. Top. Microbiol. Immunol. 59, 167.
Mozes, E., Schwartz, M., and Sela, M. (1974) J. Exp. Med. 140, 349.
Mozes, E., Isac, R., Givol, D., Zakut, R., and Beitsch, D. (1975) in "Immune Reactivity of Lymphocytes" (M. Feldman and A. Globerson, Eds.) Adv. Exp. Med. Biol. 66, 397. Plenum Press, New York.
Nisonoff, A., Hopper, J.E., and Spring, S.B. (1975) The antibody molecule. Academic Press, New York.
Ramachandran, J., Berger, A., and Katchalski, E. (1971) Biopolymers 10, 1829.
Schwartz, M., Mozes, E., and Sela, M. (1975) Eur. J. Immunol. 5, 866.
Sela, M., Fuchs, S., and Arnon, R. (1962) Biochem. J. 85, 223.
Steward, M.N., and Petty, R.E. (1972) Immunology 23, 881.
Taussig, M.J. (1974) Nature 248, 234.
Taussig, M.J., and Munro, A.J. (1974) Nature 251, 63.
Taussig, M.J., Mozes, E., and Isac, R. (1974) J. Exp. Med. 140, 301.
Taussig, M.J., Munro, A.J., Campbell, R., David, C.S., and Staines, N.A. (1975) J. Exp. Med. 142, 694.

GENETIC CONTROL OF THE IMMUNE RESPONSE TO INSULIN: ITS DEPENDENCE UPON A MACROPHAGE MEDIATED SELECTION OF DISTINCT ANTIGENIC SITES

Alan S. Rosenthal, Lanny J. Rosenwasser, Bonita L. Baskin, Joyce Schroer, James W. Thomas, and J. Thomas Blake

National Institute of Allergy and Infectious Diseases
National Institutes of Health
Bethesda, Maryland 20014

Current interest in the genetic control of the immune response to chemically well defined natural and synthetic polypeptides gives clear indication of the necessity for us to understand the contribution of structure to the antigenicity of proteins (1). Previously biochemist and immunologist alike had concerned themselves with the relationship of protein structure to the diversity and specificity of the antibody elicited following immunization. In view of our present appreciation of the complex cellular interactions which occur between macrophages, T lymphocytes (both helper and suppressor) and B lymphocytes, it is necessary to precisely define the influence of antigen structure on the initial step in the antigen recognition process, namely at the level of macrophage-T cell interaction.

Studies in our laboratory have used the insulin molecule as a model antigen. Data obtained in guinea pig, mouse, and man give clear indication of the profound influence of restricted molecular regions on the overall capacity of the animal to mount a thymus-dependent immune response to the whole molecule. The recognition of these regions is genetically determined and disparate between animals differing at genes linked to the major histocompatibility complex. More importantly, while T help or suppression of the antibody response is initiated by the recognition of the same determinants, no parallel restriction is seen at the B cell level with regards to either the amount of antibody or its specificity. Finally, the data will show that immune response (Ir) genes which play a regulatory role in the antigen recognition process operate at the level of the macrophage not at the level of the T lymphocyte.

I. IMMUNOLOGICALLY SPECIFIC INDUCTION OF T LYMPHOCYTE PROLIFERATION

Complex natural antigenic proteins such as tuberculin (PPD) as well as synthetic polymers such as the random copolymers of L-glutamic acid, L-lysine (GL) have neither defined secondary nor tertiary structure and thus it is difficult to define the precise intramolecular areas responsible for immunogenicity. By contrast, polypeptides of known structure such as insulin (2) offer a unique opportunity to characterize those regions of the molecule recognized by either the T cell receptor or antibody. The insulin monomer consists of two chains connected by interchain disulfides (Figure 1). The A chain has two helical portions separated by a loop region (α loop) formed by an intrachain disulfide between cysteine 7 and 11, while the B chain consists of pleated sheet segments at the amino and carboxy termini, joined by a central helical region. The following are a summary of our findings in both mouse and guinea pig delineating the immunodominant regions responsible for antigen specific activation of T cell function and generation of specific T help and suppression.

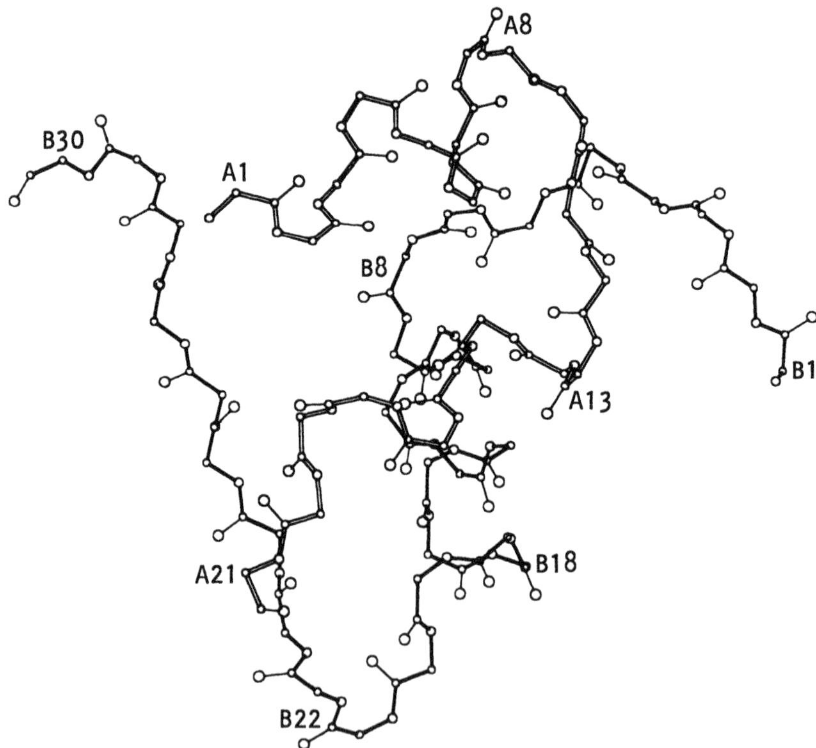

Figure 1. Structure of Beef Insulin (after Blundell).

T cells from both strain 2 and 13 guinea pigs immunized with pork insulin in complete Freund's adjuvant proliferate in vitro in response to insulin (3). The determinant recognized by the strain 13 guinea pig resides in the B chain region of the insulin molecule as evidenced by the capacity of insulin immune strain 13 but not strain 2 guinea pigs to respond to isolated oxidized B chain. When strain 2, 13 and F_1 (2 X 13) guinea pigs are immunized with oxidized B chain, strain 13 and F_1 but not strain 2 respond to either isolated B chain or native insulin. Genetic analysis of backcrossed and phenotypically characterized outbreds immunized to B chain showed that the relevant immune response gene defining response to the B chain determinant is linked to the strain 13 guinea pig histocompatibility complex. By contrast the strain 2 inbred guinea pig T cell recognizes insulin through a determinant present in insulin A chain. More specifically, they recognize the A chain loop and their T cell response is sensitive to amino acid changes in positions A8, A9 and A10. Insulins with total identity in this area completely cross-react in T cell proliferation and T helper cell activity. Insulins with partial or no identity in these amino acids residues show partial or no cross-reactivity respectively. In strain 13 animals, different species variants of insulin show cross-reactivity at a T cell level independent of their A chain loop constitution. As anticipated, F_1 T cells from insulin immune guinea pigs are able to recognize either determinant.

Keck, assessing in vivo antibody responses to dinitrophenylated pork and beef insulin, has also observed Ir gene control of the immune response to insulin in the mouse (4,5). In brief, $H2^b$ mice will respond when immunized with beef insulin but not when immunized with pork insulin. $H2^d$ mice will respond to both beef and pork insulin while $H2^k$ and $H2^a$ mice respond to neither. From these data one must conclude that the determinant on beef insulin recognized by $H2^b$ mice resides in the α loop of the A chain. In addition, Keck noted that the Ir gene controlling the response of $H2^b$ mice to beef insulin mapped to the left of IB, most probably in the IA subregion of the H-2 complex. We are currently extending such studies to a mouse in vitro model system (Thomas, J.W. and Rosenthal, A.S., unpublished observation).

The proliferative capacity of primed mouse peritoneal exudate T cells to respond to insulin was also assessed (6). We find that $H2^b$ mice will mount a T cell proliferative response to beef insulin if the mice have been primed with beef insulin in CFA (Table 1). Utilizing insulin "mutants" to test for cross reactions similar to that described in the guinea pig, we have found that neither pork nor sheep insulin will significantly cross react with beef insulin immune T cells. This established that the major determinant seen by the proliferating T cell in the $H2^b$ mouse resides in the amino acid sequence A8-A9-A10 of the A chain α loop since beef, sheep and pork insulin have identical amino acid sequences outside of this region.

TABLE 1
DNA Synthetic Response of Beef Insulin Immune $H2^b$ Mice to Beef and Other Species Variant Insulins

Antigen (10 μg/ml)	(Δcpm) X 10^{-3}
Beef Insulin	30.87
Pork Insulin	2.25
Sheep Insulin	2.62
PPD	89.10

The proliferative assay uses nylon wool column purified T cells obtained from sterile oil induced peritoneal exudates of primed mice. T cells, at 1 X 10^6/ml (200 μl/well) were cultured in microtiter trays for four days in the presence or absence of antigen. The DNA synthetic response was assessed after addition of 1 μCi of tritiated thymidine for the last 16-24 hours of culture.

An attempt to identify the determinant seen by $H2^d$ mice is shown in Table 2. Pork insulin immune $H2^d$ T cells were stimulated with pork insulin and several other species variants. As can be seen, beef, sheep and rabbit insulin all were able to cross react with pork immune T cells. However desoctapeptide pork insulin (pork insulin with the final 8 amino acids of its B chain cleaved off) did not cross react. Hence, this pattern of reactivity would suggest that either the major determinant seen by $H2^d$ mice resides in the last 8 amino acids of the B chain (most likely with an immunodominant lysine residue at position B29) or that recognition is critically dependent upon its presence.

Utilizing T cells from various recombinant strains of mice the DNA synthetic response to beef insulin maps to the left of IB, most likely in the IA subregion (Table 3). This table also demonstrates that the $H2^k$ and $H2^a$ haplotypes are nonresponders to beef insulin.

Thus, the immune T cell proliferative response to insulin in the responder strains, $H2^b$ and $H2^d$, is most likely governed by 2 distinct determinants ($H2^b$ = A chain determinant, $H2^d$ = B chain determinant); and the recognition of these is likely under Ir gene control. The pattern of recognition of determinants in $H2^b$ and $H2^d$ mice is remarkably similar to the determinant specificity exhibited by strain 2 and strain 13 guinea pigs respectively, suggesting a striking evolutionary conservation of Ir gene function between these two species.

TABLE 2
DNA Synthetic Response of Pork Insulin Immunized H2^d Mice to Pork Insulin and Other Species Variant Insulins

Antigen (10 μg/ml)	(Δcpm) X 10^{-3}
Beef Insulin	12.84
Pork Insulin	22.11
Sheep Insulin	14.38
Pork Desoctapeptide Insulin	1.68
Rabbit Insulin	15.62
PPD	138.30

TABLE 3
Mapping of the Location of Ir Gene Control of the Response to Beef Insulin (10 μg/ml) in Various Congenic Resistant Mouse Strains

Strain	Haplotype	(Δcpm) X 10^{-3}
B10.BR	k	>0<
B10.A	a	0.14
B10.A(2R)	h2	0.58
B10.A(4R)	h4	>0<
B10.A(5R)	i5	17.31
B10	b	22.97

II. HELPER T CELLS AND PROLIFERATING T CELLS RECOGNIZE THE SAME ANTIGENIC SPECIFICITIES

Since a fine T-cell specificity, with sensitivity for one amino acid difference is seen in strain 2 guinea pigs, this strain was used to compare the recognition specificity of helper T cells with that of the proliferating cell. A hapten-carrier system was employed to measure T-cell helper function. Strain 2 guinea pigs were primed i.p. with DNP-OVA and subsequently immunized with different insulins in CFA. The amount of anti-DNP antibodies was measured immediately before (day 0) and on days 7 and 21 after the boosting with DNP insulin. Two insulins that cross-react (rabbit and rat) with pork insulin at the level of T-cell proliferation and two which did not (sheep and fish) were assessed for their ability to prime T cells to function as helpers to DNP-OVA-primed B cells. Only those insulins that share A-chain α-loop identity with pork insulin are able to elicit a T-helper function similar to that elicited by pork insulin. Insulins different from pork insulin in the A-chain α-loop gave no significant response. Evidence that differences in this specific area of the molecule are enough to impair the ability of an insulin to help, is provided by the non-response observed with sheep insulin, which differs from pork insulin exclusively in amino acids A8, A9, and A10. Although these experiments do not discriminate whether or not T-helper and proliferating activities are the function of a single cell clone or distinct subpopulations of antigen-recognizing T cells, they do establish that such lymphocytes bear receptors with the same fine specificity.

III. SUPPRESSION OF ANTIBODY RESPONSE IS DETERMINANT SPECIFIC

Prior immunization of guinea pigs with antigens in incomplete Freund's adjuvant (IFA) suppresses delayed hypersensitivity skin reactions upon subsequent immunization of the guinea pig with the same antigen in complete Freund's adjuvant without alteration of the response to a second irrelevant antigen included in the immunizing mixture (7,8). When such an experimental manipulation is employed in F_1 guinea pigs pretreated with various species variants of insulin or B chain fragments in IFA, a striking determinant specific suppression of in vitro lymphocyte proliferation can be seen upon immunization with DNP-pork insulin (Baskin and Rosenthal, unpublished observations) (Table 4). If antibody responses are assessed in animals previously immunized with DNP on a heterologous carrier i.p. and in the footpads with IFA pork insulin, a suppression of anti-hapten DNP but not anti-carrier response is noted subsequent to immunization with DNP-pork insulin in CFA. Finding suppression of the proliferating T cell help for anti-hapten but not help for anti-carrier antibody raises the possibility either that distinctive T helper cells exist or that different "quantities" of helper cell activity may be required for anti-carrier as contrasted with anti-hapten responses.

TABLE 4
DETERMINANT SELECTIVE SUPPRESSION OF T LYMPHOCYTE PROLIFERATION IN INBRED GUINEA PIGS

Pretreatment with Antigen in IFA	Immunization with Antigen in CFA	Pork Insulin Initiated T Lymphocyte DNA Synthesis	
		Strain 2	Strain 13
		^{3}H-TdR Incorporation Δcpm X 10^{-3}	
None	Pork insulin	42.47	64.89
KLH	Pork insulin	41.26	66.30
Pork insulin	Pork insulin	<u>10.13</u>	<u>18.68</u>
Sheep insulin	Pork insulin	35.95	<u>20.38</u>
Oxidized B chain	Pork insulin	46.26	<u>19.71</u>

Pretreatment of guinea pigs 10-14 days prior to immunization with pork insulin in CFA. T lymphocyte synthesis was assessed as described in Table 5. Underlined values indicate suppressed ^{3}H-thymidine incorporation.

IV. STRAIN 2 AND STRAIN 13 ANTI-PORK INSULIN ANTIBODIES SHARE SPECIFICITIES

Having defined the specificity for T-cell proliferation in both inbred strains of guinea pig, as two dinstinct sites on the pork insulin molecule, operationally under the control of relevant Ir genes, and having shown that at least in one strain the same specificities initiate T-cell helper function, we examined the fine specificity of anti-insulin antibodies generated in strain 2 and 13 guinea pigs. Both antibody populations present similar isoelectric-focusing patterns, revealing restricted heterogeneity (Schroer and Rosenthal, unpublished observation). Inhibition assays of the binding of ^{125}I-labeled pork insulin to strain 2 and 13 anti-pork insulin antibodies by different insulin variants were performed. All the variants tested were able to inhibit the above mentioned reactions, irrespective of their α loop amino acid sequence. These data differ considerably from those of Arquilla and Finn (9), who by means of an hemolytic assay showed differences in the ability of strain 2 and strain 13 anti-beef insulin to combine to insulin coupled to sheep red blood cells to which rabbit anti-insulin antibodies had already bound. These authors concluded that configurational differences existed between the antibodies produced by the two inbred strains of guinea pig. The apparent disagreement with our results could be due to the fact that those authors used as their indicator the binding of antibodies to the insulin hexamer, while in our radioimmune assay, the insulin is present in monomeric form.

V. MACROPHAGES AS THE CELL EXPRESSING THE IR GENE PRODUCT

If Ir gene function operates exclusively at the level of the responding lymphocyte, both determinants should be simultaneously recognized by F_1 T cells independently of which parental macrophage (Mϕ) is "presenting" the antigen. Conversely, if the definition of which determinant is actually recognized depends on the genetic profile of the antigen presenting Mϕ, then Ir gene function must also be operating at this cell level. The data favor the latter assumption (10). Mϕ from both inbred strains of guinea pig are able to "present" pork insulin to pork insulin immune F_1 (2 X 13) lymphocytes. As with PPD, a strong proliferative response is observed when pork insulin pulsed Mϕ from either strain of guinea pig are added to F_1 PELs. However, when different species variants of intact insulin are presented to the same pork immune insulin F_1 PELs by either strain 2 or 13 Mϕ, two different patterns of response are seen. An A chain loop pattern of cross-reactivity is observed when the antigens are presented on strain 2 Mϕ. This pattern of cross-reactivity is characterized by partial cross-reactivity between pork and beef insulin (partial identity in the loop) and little cross-reactivity between pork and sheep insulin (no identities in the loop). In order to corroborate the above finding and to show that a specific B chain determinant is being selected when the whole insulin molecule is presented by strain 13 Mϕ, we studied the response of oxidized insulin B chain immune F_1 (2 X 13) PELs to parental Mϕ pulsed with native insulin or isolated B chain. As can be seen in Table 5, only strain 13 Mϕ can present native insulin to B chain immune F_1 (2 X 13) PELs. Despite the capacity of strain 2 Mϕ to present the same insulin to insulin immune F_1 T cells, they cannot initiate DNA synthesis in B chain immune F_1 T cells.

The possibility exists that in F_1 (2 X 13) animals immunized to insulin, two distinct sets of clones of T cells are generated: one that recognizes the α loop antigenic determinant "Processed" by or "presented" by the strain 2 specific cell structures in the F_1 Mϕ, and one that recognizes the B chain determinant generated by the 13 counterpart of the system. This hypothesis has been examined by bromodeoxyurindine (BUdR) and light elimination experiments in F_1 guinea pigs.

As shown in Table 6, initial culture of insulin bearing parental macrophages with insulin immune F_1 T cells in the presence of BUdR and light selectively decreases responsiveness, on subsequent exposure to insulin bearing macrophages identical to those originally

TABLE 5
DNA Synthetic Response of T Cells from Oxidized B Chain Immunized F_1 (2 X 13) Guinea Pigs to Parental Macrophage Pulsed with Native Insulin and Isolated B Chain

Macrophages Pulsed with:	Macrophage Genetic Background Strain 2	Strain 13
	^{3}H-TdR incorporation Δcpm X 10^{-3}	
PPD	145,810	98,010
Pork Insulin	100	13,160

Mean ± S.E. of 5 experiments.
F_1 (2 X 13) guinea pigs were immunized with 10 μg of B chain in CFA, 2-3 weeks prior to use. Oil induced, macrophage-rich peritoneal exudate cells were pulsed with 100 μg/ml of antigen and 40 μg/ml of mitomycin-C at 37°C for 60 minutes. After four washes 1.2 X 10^5 of these cells were added to 2.4 X 10^5 responding peritoneal exudate lymphocytes depleted of adherent cells (PELs) in 200 μl of 5% heat inactivated male guinea pig serum in RPMI-1640 plus 2.5 X 10^{-5}M of 2-Mercaptoethanol in round bottom microtiter plates. After 48 hours of culture 1 μc of ^{3}H-methyl-thymidine (New England Nuclear, sp. act. 6.7 c/mM) was added to each well for an additional 24 hours of culture. At this time cells were harvested on glass fiber filters with a simi-automated microharvester (Adaps Corporation, Boston, MA) and ^{3}H-thymidine incorporation determined by liquid scintillation spectrometry.

used to elicit cell activation. Thus, preculture of F_1 T cells with strain 2 macrophages bearing insulin significantly depresses (96%) their response to antigen on strain 2 macrophages on subsequent cultures without comparably effecting responsiveness to insulin presented by strain 13 macrophages. Conversely, exposure of F_1 T cells to strain 13 macrophages bearing pork insulin eliminates 97% of responsiveness on repeated culture to pork insulin on strain 13 macrophages but does not effect the response of F_1 T cells to strain 2 macrophages bearing pork insulin. Such data shown that at least two distinct clones of insulin reactive T cells exist in F_1 animals.

These data and others (11-20) support the concept that macrophages play a fundamental role in selecting, in a complex antigen, the moiety(ies) to be recognized by immune T cells. The T cell bearing either a single or dual receptor would thus have availably to it only a restricted region of the native molecule. The T cell

TABLE 6
BUdR and Light Elimination of Antigen Specific F_1 T Cell Proliferation: Intramolecular Determinant Selection by Pork Insulin-Bearing Parental Macrophages

Macrophages Used in 1st Culture	% Elimination of F_1 T Cell DNA Synthetic Response on 2nd Culture	
	Macrophage used:	
	Strain 2	Strain 13
Strain 2	96	12
Strain 13	0	97

Immune PELs at a concentration of 1 X 10^6/ml were cultured 1st with 3 X 10^5 mitomycin C treated insulin pulsed Mϕ for 48 hours in 12 X 75 mm capped plastic tubes. At the end of this time 2 μg/ml of freshly prepared 5-bromodeoxyuridine (BUdR) was added to the cultures. Twenty-four hours later, the cell pellets were exposed to light by placing the culture tubes directly on an array of three fluorescent light bulbs (Cool-Ray GE) for 90 minutes. After four washes of the cell pellet with Hanks BSS, the BUdR and light treated cells were cultured a second time in microtiter plates (as described in Table 5) in the presence of added pork insulin-pulsed Mϕ. Data are expressed as % inhibition of DNA synthesis remaining after BUdR and light treatment. BUdR is a thymidine analog which if present during the S phase of the cell cycle is incorporated into newly synthesized DNA and cross-links DNA strands upon light activation. Treatment of activated lymphocytes with BUdR and light leads to an irreversible block in cell replication (21).

might possess a dual receptor of either of two types: one for antigen and a second independent receptor for H-linked surface molecules or alternatively a "compound antigen determinant" consisting of antigen in unique association with an Ia antigen not antigen alone, is recognized by a single T cell receptor. Our studies of the immune response to insulin further indicate that a selected amino acid sequence and/or conformation within the antigen itself is seen by the T cell receptor and that generation or display of such antigenic determinants is a function of immune response genes operating at the level of the antigen presenting cell. Two general mechanisms by which macrophages may function can be suggested One possibility is that immune response genes define a class of receptors or broad specificity which recognize molecular shape and thus have the unique ability to focus or orient distinct regions of the antigen for presentation to the T cell. A second possibility is that immune response gene products are or regulate the activity of families of enzymes which modify or metabolize polypeptide antigens. In this latter situation, the repertoire of Ir genes associated with a given haplotype would define restricted areas of the molecule as available for display to the T cell receptor. There are unique advantages to a determinant selection model in that while not excluding dual receptor models, it nonetheless is the only current hypothesis which does not require them. More importantly, even if more than a single T cell receptor exists, determinant selection provides a precise description of the function of the immune response gene product.

VI. SUMMARY

The immune response to insulin, in both mouse and guinea pig, is under control of H-linked immune response genes. When immunized with either pork or beef insulin in CFA, both strain 2 and 13 guinea pigs respond by antigen-specific lymphocyte proliferation and synthesis of specific antibody. The specificity of the elicited antibodies are indistinguishable between these inbred strains. By contrast, strain 2 T cells recognize a distinct region of the A chain α loop consisting of amino acids residues 8, 9 and 10, while strain 13 T cells see an as yet undefined region of the B chain. $H2^b$ (A chain α loop responder) and $H2^d$ (B chain responder) mice similarly discriminate which area of the molecule are recognized by their T lymphocytes. The function of the Ir gene, in both the guinea pig and mouse appears to be an intramolecular selection of discrete regions within the antigen for recognition by the T cell. The data presented suggest that this function operates at the level of the macrophage.

VII. REFERENCES

1. Shreffler, D.C., and David, C.S., Adv. Immunol. 20, 125 (1975).

2. Blundell, T., Dodson, G., Hodgkins, D., and Mercola, D., Adv. Protein Chem. 26, 279 (1972).

3. Barcinski, M.A., and Rosenthal, A.S., J. Exp. Med. 145, 726, (1977).

4. Keck, K., Eur. J. Immunol. 5, 801 (1975).

5. Kolb, H., Keck, K., Momayezi, M., Schicker, C., and Trissl, D., J. Immunol. 118, 427 (1977).

6. Rosenwasser, L.J., Schwartz, R.H., and Rosenthal, A.S., (manuscript in preparation).

7. Bullock, W., Katz, D.H., and Benacerraf, B., J. Exp. Med. 142, 261 (1975).

8. Neta, R., and Salvin, S.B., J. Immunol. 117, 2014 (1976).

9. Arquilla, E., and Finn, J., J. Exp. Med. 122, 771 (1965).

10. Rosenthal, A.S., Barcinski, M.A., and Blake, J.T., Nature 267, 156 (1977).

11. Rosenthal, A.S., and Shevach, E.M., J. Exp. Med. 138, 1194 (1973).

12. Erb, P., Meier, B., and Feldmann, M., Nature 263, 601 (1976).

13. Katz, D.H., and Benacerraf, B., Transplant Rev. 22, 175 (1976).

14. Shevach, E.M., and Rosenthal, A.S., J. Exp. Med. 138, 1213 (1973).

15. Shevach, E.M., J. Immunol. 116, 1582 (1976).

16. Schwartz, R.H., David, C.S., Sachs, D.H., and Paul, W.E., J. Immunol. 117, 531 (1976).

17. Greineder, D.K., Shevach, E.M., and Rosenthal, A.S., J. Immunol. 117, 1261 (1976).

18. Pierce, C.W., Kapp, J.A., and Benacerraf, B., J. Exp. Med. 144, 371 (1976).

19. Miller, J.F.A.P., Vadas, M.A., Whitelaw, A., and Gamble, J., Proc. Nat. Acad. Sci. (USA) 73, 2486 (1976).

20. Thomas, D.W., and Shevach, E.M., J. Exp. Med. 144, 1263 (1976).

21. Zoschke, D.C., and Bach, F.H., Science 170, 1404 (1976).

IMMUNE RESPONSES OF INBRED GUINEA PIGS AND MICE TO HELICAL SEQUENTIAL POLYMERS OF AMINO ACIDS

Paul H. Maurer, Allen R. Zeiger, Carmen F. Merryman and Chang-Hai Lai

Thomas Jefferson University, Dept. of Biochemistry
Philadelphia, Pennsylvania 19107

ABSTRACT

The immune responses against the sequential polypeptides; $(T\text{-}G\text{-}A\text{-}Gly)_n$, $(T\text{-}A\text{-}G\text{-}Gly)_n$, $(Phe\text{-}G\text{-}A\text{-}Gly)_n$ and $(Phe\text{-}A\text{-}G\text{-}Gly)_n$ were studied in inbred guinea pigs and mice. Strain 13 guinea pigs responded to $(Phe\text{-}G\text{-}A\text{-}Gly)_n$ and $(T\text{-}G\text{-}A\text{-}Gly)_n$ whereas strain 2 guinea pigs responded to $(T\text{-}A\text{-}G\text{-}Gly)_n$ and $(Phe\text{-}A\text{-}G\text{-}Gly)_n$. These responses which are linked to MHC, are only against the helical form of the polymers which have conformational determinants. Significant cross reactions at the humoral and T cell levels (PELS) are exhibited with the following reciprocal combinations: $(Phe\text{-}G\text{-}A\text{-}Gly)_n$ and $(T\text{-}G\text{-}A\text{-}Gly)_n$; $(T\text{-}A\text{-}G\text{-}Gly)_n$ and $(Phe\text{-}A\text{-}G\text{-}Gly)_n$.

With mice, the polymers were shown to be T dependent with the following response patterns: mice of $H\text{-}2^b$ haplotype respond against $(T\text{-}G\text{-}A\text{-}Gly)_n$; those of $H\text{-}2^{b,f}$ and r haplotypes respond against $(T\text{-}A\text{-}G\text{-}Gly)_n$. There are no responders against $(Phe\text{-}G\text{-}A\text{-}Gly)_n$ and only mice of $H\text{-}2^f$ respond against $(Phe\text{-}A\text{-}G\text{-}Gly)_n$. "Nonresponders" respond against the MBSA aggregates of all of these polymers. The Ir gene(s) controlling these T cell dependent H-linked responses mapped to the IA subregion. Antibody responses against (T-G-A-Gly) and (T-A-G-Gly) were quite variable, and were most marked in, F1 mice of (responder and nonresponder) and in backcross populations of (F1 x R) and (F1 x NR). However, the T cell proliferative responses performed with nylon wool purified T cells gave clear cut and predictable distinctions between "responders" and nonresponders and linkage with responding haplotype.

Hypotheses advanced to explain these findings relate to the poor immunogenicity (antibody) of these polymers, which have a restricted number of repeating determinants, the B cell mitogenic properties of these polymers and the possible involvement of suppressor cells.

The specificities of the humoral responses, i.e. cross reactions, were similar to those found in guinea pigs. However, in contrast to the guinea pig studies cross stimulation with structurally related polymers occurred only in those situations where the immunizing and "cross reacting" polymers were both immunogenic in mice of the same haplotype, i.e., $(T\text{-}A\text{-}G\text{-}Gly)_n$ and $(Phe\text{-}A\text{-}G\text{-}Gly)_n$ in mice of $H\text{-}2^f$ haplotypes.

Introduction: Major contributions to our understanding of the genetic control of the immune response have been made employing random synthetic and multichain polymers of amino acids. (Benacerraf and McDevitt, 1972; Benacerraf and Katz, 1975) However, significant differences in results have been noted from laboratory to laboratory and within the same laboratory with a number of polymer preparations having similar amino acid compositions (Maurer, et al., 1977, Koch and Simonsen, 1977). Associated with these discordant results might be that the nature of the determinants involved in either T cell activation of the specificity of the humoral responses might indeed be altered or different in various preparations. Synthetic polymers can exhibit intrachain heterogeity and amino acid composition variability from chain to chain associated with differing polymerization rates of the amino acid anhydrides. (Liberti and Vickerman, 1977) Therefore, for a number of years our laboratory has been involved with synthesizing polymers whose amino acid sequence and composition are known (Zeiger, et al., 1975). It was hoped that by dealing with more homogeneous polymers we might indeed be able to better define the nature of the determinants involved in phases of the immune responses.

The use of biophysical techniques allows characterization of the properties of these high molecular weight, sequential polymers. (Zeiger and Maurer, 1977) The limited primary and secondary structures may also result in restricted antigenic determinants which may be defined by specificity studies at both the humoral and cellular levels. Although we have studied a number of the polymers containing three of four amino acids in repeating sequences, this presentation will only deal with four of the sequential polymers of amino acids that have been used to study Ir gene function in guinea pigs and mice as it relates to the recognition phenomenon at the T cell level as well as the specificity of the antibody produced.

Materials and Methods: The sequential polymers employed are shown in Table 1. All of these polymers were of high molecular weight and exhibited considerable α helicity in their polymeric form. The oligopeptides of $(T\text{-}G\text{-}A\text{-}Gly)_n$ and some of the random polymers of amino acids used are also listed.

TABLE 1: Polymers of α-L-Amino Acids Employed in Present Study.

Known Sequence Polymers	Abbreviations	Molecular Weight (Approx.)	Helicity
Poly(Tyrosine-Glutamic Acid-Alanine-Glycine)	$(T\text{-}G\text{-}A\text{-}Gly)_n$	53,000	++++
Fractions of $(T\text{-}G\text{-}A\text{-}Gly)_n$	Fraction I	22,600	++++
	Fraction II	9,700	+++
	Fraction III	1,300	-
	Fraction IV	900	-
Poly(Tyrosine-Alanine-Glutamic Acid-Glycine)	$(T\text{-}A\text{-}G\text{-}Gly)_n$	33,000	++++
Poly(Phenylalanine-Glutamic Acid-Alanine-Glycine)	$(Phe\text{-}G\text{-}A\text{-}Gly)_n$	90,000	++++
Poly(Phenylalanine-Alanine-Glutamic Acid-Glycine)	$(Phe\text{-}A\text{-}G\text{-}Gly)_n$	24,000	++++
<u>Random Copolymers</u>			
Poly(Glutamic Acid^{60}, Alanine^{40})	GA	35,000	+
Poly(Glutamic Acid^{50}, Tyrosine^{50})	GT	22,600	-
Poly(Glutamic Acid^{60}, Alanine^{30}, Tyrosine^{10})	GAT^{10}	55,000	++

<u>Guinea Pigs</u>: Inbred strain 2 and 13 guinea pigs were immunized with 2.5-500 μg of the polymers in complete Freund's adjuvant. Two weeks later they were bled, skin tested for immediate and delayed reaction, and boosted intraperitoneally with the same dose of polymer. In addition to immunization with the polymers per se, aggregates of the appropriate polymers were made with methylated bovine serum albumin (MBSA) and injected into "nonresponder" animals.

<u>Antibody Assays</u>: Sera was assayed for antibody against $(T\text{-}G\text{-}A\text{-}Gly)_n$, $(T\text{-}A\text{-}G\text{-}Gly)_n$, (Phe-G-A-Gly)n and $(Phe\text{-}A\text{-}G\text{-}Gly)_n$ as well as the other random polymers employing an antigen binding assay with the ^{125}I labelled polymers. For the measurements of the $(Phe\text{-}G\text{-}A\text{-}Gly)_n$ and

(Phe-A-G-Gly) responses tyrosine analogs were employed along with a polyvalent sheep anti-guinea pig globulin antisera as described (Maurer et al. 1973). The percent of added antigen bound was used as an index of responsiveness. Binding values greater than 15% were considered positive. Passive cutaneous reaction in guinea pigs were also used to detect antibody against the polymers as well as the cross reactions.

In Vitro Antigen Stimulation: Guinea pig peritoneal exudate lymphocytes (PELS) were produced and harvested for the *in vitro* antigen stimulation studies according to Rosenstreich et al. 1971. The purified PELS were cultured with or without the appropriate antigens at 37° for 72 hours in 5% CO_2 and 95% air. Four hours before harvesting, tritiated thymidine was added. The cells were collected on filter discs and washed in cold saline containing thymidine. Radioactivity was counted in a liquid scintillation counter. Stimulation indices as presented were calculated as follows:

$$\text{Stimulation index} = (\text{S.I.}) = \frac{\text{CPM experiment - background}}{\text{CPM control - background}}$$

Results: Tables 2 and 3 present summaries of the responses of the inbred guinea pigs to the sequential polymers. Responders are defined not only by the percent binding of the I^{125} labeled antigen but also by the positive skin reactions (not shown) and the stimulation indices. Strain 13 guinea pigs responded to the $(\text{Tyr-Glu-Ala-Gly})_n$ (Maurer, et al. 1973) and $(\text{Phe-Glu-Ala-Gly})_n$

TABLE 2: Humoral Responses of Inbred Guinea Pigs to Sequential Polymers*

Strain	Immunogen	% Antigen Bound ± S.E	Immunogen	% Antigen Bound ± S.E.
2	$(\text{T-G-A-Gly})_n$	0	$(\text{Phe-G-A-Gly})_n$	1± 1
	$(\text{T-A-G-Gly})_n$	64.5±18.5	$(\text{Phe-A-G-Gly})_n$	33±12
	$(\text{T-G-A-Gly})_n$· MBSA	48 ± 2		
13	$(\text{T-G-A-Gly})_n$**	75.5±5.0	$(\text{Phe-G-A-Gly})_n$	57±14
	$(\text{T-A-G-Gly})_n$	0	$(\text{Phe-A-G-Gly})_n$	0
	$(\text{T-A-G-Gly})_n$· MBSA	33±20		

** Strain 13 guinea pigs also responded to 2.5 μg of $(\text{T-G-A-Gly})_n$ and Fractions I and II of oligopeptides.

* Percent 0.001 μg N labeled polymer bound by 1:5 dilution of serum.

TABLE 3

In Vitro Antigen Stimulation of Guinea Pig Peritoneal Exudate Lymphocyte Cultures as Measured by 3H Thymidine Incorporation

Strain	Immunogen	Stimulation Index $(T\text{-}G\text{-}A\text{-}Gly)_n$	Stimulation Index $(Phe\text{-}G\text{-}A\text{-}Gly)_n$	Immunogen	Stimulation Index $(T\text{-}A\text{-}G\text{-}Gly)_n$	Stimulation Index $(Phe\text{-}A\text{-}G\text{-}Gly)_n$
2	$(T\text{-}G\text{-}A\text{-}Gly)_n$	0.8	-	$(T\text{-}A\text{-}G\text{-}Gly)_n$	5.4	-
	$(Phe\text{-}G\text{-}A\text{-}Gly)_n$	1.3	0.4	$(Phe\text{-}A\text{-}G\text{-}Gly)_n$	3.5	3.8
13	$(T\text{-}G\text{-}A\text{-}Gly)_n$	40	25	$(T\text{-}A\text{-}G\text{-}Gly)_n$	0.8	-
	$(Phe\text{-}G\text{-}A\text{-}Gly)_n$	3	4	$(Phe\text{-}A\text{-}G\text{-}Gly)_n$	0.9	1.3

* The oligomers of $(T\text{-}G\text{-}A\text{-}Gly)_n$ Fractions I and II were stimulatory, Fractions III and IV were not.

TABLE 4

Inhibition of Guinea Pig Anti-$(T\text{-}G\text{-}A\text{-}Gly)_n$ by Homologous Polymer, Oligomers and Random Polymers

Inhibitor	Inhibitor Concentration* 10 (% Inhibition)	Inhibitor Concentration* 500 (% Inhibition)	Inhibitor	Inhibitor Concentration 500 (5 Inhibition)	Inhibitor Concentration 2000 (5 Inhibition)
$(T\text{-}G\text{-}A\text{-}Gly)_n$	69	100	$(Phe\text{-}G\text{-}A\text{-}Gly)_n$	27	40
Fraction I	47	90	GA	0	0
II	22	87	GT	0	0
$(T\text{-}A\text{-}G\text{-}Gly)_n$	0	10	GAT10	0	0

* Concentrations of inhibitors are expressed as the "fold". 0.001 μg $(T\text{-}G\text{-}A\text{-}Gly)_n$ equals one fold. Fractions III and IV do not inhibit.

the interchange of glutamic acid and alanine in the tetrapeptide caused a tremendous change in the immune response patterns of the guinea pigs which were linked to the MHC. However, there was little difference in the immune response pattern (recognition) by interchange of tyrosine and phenylalanine, i.e., strain 13 guinea pigs responded to $(T\text{-}G\text{-}A\text{-}Gly)_n$ and $(Phe\text{-}G\text{-}A\text{-}Gly)_n$ and strain 2 guinea pigs responded to $(T\text{-}A\text{-}G\text{-}Gly)_n$ and $(Phe\text{-}A\text{-}G\text{-}Gly)_n$. The tyrosine delayed skin reactions or *in vitro* antigen stimulation of PELS with the appropriate polymers could be elicited. From studies with outbred Hartley as well as the inbred guinea pigs, the ability to respond to $(T\text{-}G\text{-}A\text{-}Gly)_n$ and $(Phe\text{-}G\text{-}A\text{-}Gly)_n$ was shown to be linked to the Strain 13 histocompatibility (H) locus (Lai et al., 1977) and the ability to respond to $(T\text{-}A\text{-}G\text{-}Gly)_n$ and $(Phe\text{-}A\text{-}G\text{-}Gly)_n$ was linked to the strain 2 MHC. The Ir gene controlling the responses was dominantly expressed.

Oligomers of $(T\text{-}G\text{-}A\text{-}Gly)_n$ were studied for immunogenicity in strain 13 guinea pigs. The guinea pigs did not respond to low molecular weight fractions of 1300 daltons or less which also were non-helical. This appears to indicate the importance of the helical structure of the oligomers or the polymers for the immunogenicity of the polymers (Lai and Maurer, 1977).

The inhibition of binding of the $^{125}I(T\text{-}G\text{-}A\text{-}Gly)_n$ by oligomers of (T-G-A-Gly) as well as a number of other polymers is shown in Table 4. A unique specificity against these polymers is shown in that the $(T\text{-}G\text{-}A\text{-}Gly)_n$ antibody is not inhibited by $(T\text{-}A\text{-}G\text{-}Gly)_n$, $(Phe\text{-}A\text{-}G\text{-}Gly)_n$ or the random copolymers GA, GT, GAT^{10}. However, there is significant but weak inhibition with the $(Phe\text{-}G\text{-}A\text{-}Gly)_n$ polymer. The unique specificity of anti-$(T\text{-}A\text{-}G\text{-}Gly)_n$ was also evident in that it was not inhibited by $(T\text{-}G\text{-}A\text{-}Gly)_n$ or the polymers GA, GT, GAT^{10} but could be inhibited to a limited extent by $(Phe\text{-}A\text{-}G\text{-}Gly)_n$. That differences do exist beteen the structures of $(T\text{-}A\text{-}G\text{-}Gly)_n$ and $(Phe\text{-}A\text{-}G\text{-}Gly)_n$ was shown by the fact that although the anti-$(T\text{-}A\text{-}G\text{-}Gly)_n$ bound 65% $(T\text{-}A\text{-}G\text{-}Gly)_n$ at the same concentration, only 15% of $(Phe\text{-}A\text{-}G\text{-}Gly)_n$ was bound. The anti-$(Phe\text{-}A\text{-}G\text{-}Gly)_n$ bound the $(T\text{-}A\text{-}G\text{-}Gly)_n$ as well as the homologous polymer.

In addition to measuring the antibody specificities, the ability of the various sequential polymers to cause *in vitro* stimulation of PELS was studied. (Table 3) Here too, a unique kind of specificity was shown. PELS from responder animals immunized with (T-G-A-Gly) could be stimulated by (T-G-A-Gly) and $(Phe\text{-}G\text{-}A\text{-}Gly)_n$ but not by $(T\text{-}A\text{-}G\text{-}Gly)_n$ or $(Phe\text{-}A\text{-}G\text{-}Gly)_n$.Similarly, the PELS from strain 2 guinea pigs immunized with $(Phe\text{-}A\text{-}G\text{-}Gly)_n$ could be cross stimulated by $(T\text{-}A\text{-}G\text{-}Gly)_n$.

The important points presented are as follows: Although all four sequential polymers presented here are helical in structure, but not to $(Tyr\text{-}Ala\text{-}Glu\text{-}Gly)_n$ or $(Phe\text{-}Ala\text{-}Glu\text{-}Gly)_n$; whereas Strain 2 guinea pigs responded to the latter but not to the former 2 polymers. (Zeiger and Maurer, 1976) When the Strain 13 guinea pigs that could not respond to $(T\text{-}A\text{-}G\text{-}Gly)_n$ were immunized with the MBSA aggregate, they responded. Similarly, Strain 2 guinea pigs which were nonresponders to $(T\text{-}G\text{-}A\text{-}Gly)_n$ responded (antibody) to the MBSA aggregate. However, in these "MBSA situations", no analogues were more immunogenic then the phenylalanine polymers, and $(T\text{-}G\text{-}A\text{-}Gly)_n$ was more immunogenic than $(T\text{-}A\text{-}G\text{-}Gly)_n$. The specificities of the antibodies were directed predominantly against the conformational (helical) determinants in the polymer. The interchange of glutamic acid and alanine caused significant changes in the specificity of the antibody produced. Of considerable significance was that cross *in vitro* stimulation of PELS could be elicited by the phenylalanine or tyrosine analogs of the specific polymers, i.e. PELS from guinea pigs immunized with $(T\text{-}G\text{-}A\text{-}Gly)_n$ or $(Phe\text{-}G\text{-}A\text{-}Gly)_n$ could be cross stimulated. The structural relationships shown between $(Phe\text{-}G\text{-}A\text{-}Gly)_n$ and $(T\text{-}G\text{-}A\text{-}Gly)_n$ at the humoral level could also be demonstrated in the *in vitro* proliferative responses. It would appear therefore that in the guinea pig systems the specificities of recognition with these polymers at the B cell level and at the T cell or macrophage level are similar.

However, as will be shown below with the mouse studies, one cannot extrapolate these findings to other species, and that an important factor in addition to having close structural relationships among immunogens as measured by cross reactions at the B cell level (antibody), the specific polymers must be immunogenic in a specific strain in order to elicit cross T cell proliferative responses.

Whether the polymers that cross react at the B cell level in the guinea pig systems are indeed reacting with the same "T cell receptor" or Ir gene product is yet to be determined. It would be of interest to determine whether separate genes are indeed controlling the responses to the closely related polymers $(T\text{-}G\text{-}A\text{-}Gly)_n$ and $(Phe\text{-}G\text{-}A\text{-}Gly)_n$ in strain 13 guinea pigs and $(T\text{-}A\text{-}G\text{-}Gly)_n$ and $(Phe\text{-}A\text{-}G\text{-}Gly)_n$ in strain 2 guinea pigs.

Mouse Studies: In the mouse unigenic and multigenic immune response (Ir) dominant gene control for a number of synthetic polymers (Merryman, et al. 1975) as well as some protein antigens have been mapped to the I region of the MHC (Klein, 1975).

Materials and Methods: In our mouse studies groups of mice were immunized with 100 μg of the polymers in complete Freund's adjuvant. Three weeks later the mice were boosted with the same amount of antigen given in aqueous solution. Usually the animals were bled three weeks after the initial adjuvant injection and ten days after the booster injection.

Antibody Assays: The responses were measured using a modified ^{125}I antigen binding assay and polyvalent goat anti-mouse gamma globulin serum. Generally the values presented indicate the percent of 0.0003 μg N of I-125 labelled polymer bound by 25 μl of a 1:2 dilution of antiserum. Less than 10% binding was regarded as not significant (Merryman, et al. 1975).

Inhibition of ^{125}I Antigen Binding: The antiserum dilution which bound 50% of the added antigen was used in inhibition studies. To 25 μl of the appropriately diluted antiserum different amounts of inhibitors were added. After incubation the radiolabelled homologous polymer was added and the above procedure for measuring the antigen binding was followed.

In Vitro Antigen Stimulation (T Cell Proliferative Responses) Varying times after immunization, mice were killed and peritoneal exudate cells were harvested for culturing. The peritoneal exudate cells were produced by injecting the mice with 10% Brewer's thioglycolate four days before killing. Four days later the cells were harvested by flushing the peritoneal cavity with RPMI 1640 containing heparin, the cells washed and passed through an appropiately prepared rayon-wool column. The 30 ml plastic syringe was washed with 50 ml of Dulbecoo's phosphate buffered saline followed by 50 ml RPMI-1640. The column containing the cells and medium was incubated at 37° C, and the nonadherent cells which were eluted with warm medium were passed over nylon wool columns according to Schwartz et al., 1975. The resulting PETLES (1×10^5) were then cultured in 200 μl of modified EHAA medium supplemented with 50 μmoles of 2ME and 10% heat inactivated FCS in sterile U-bottom polystyrene microculture plates. Antigens or mitogens were added and cultures were maintained at 37° in a humidified atmosphere of 2% CO_2 and 98% air for four days. Four to 16 hours before harvesting, 1 μCi of tritiated thymidine was added. Cultures were harvested with a MASH-2 automated harvester, washed, and the dried filter discs counted in a scintillation counter. Stimulation indices were calculated as in the guinea pig studies.

Results: Table 5 presents a summary of the secondary antibody responses to the sequential polymers. Only mice of H-2^b and ^{bc} haplotypes responded to (T-G-A-Gly)$_n$. There were no responders to (Phe-G-A-Gly)$_n$; mice of H-2 b, f and ^{r} haplotypes responded to (T-A-G-Gly)$_n$; and only mice of H-2^f haplotype responded to (Phe-G-A-Gly)$_n$. In all situations where nonresponsiveness to the polymer per se was shown, the mice did respond to the MBSA aggregates of the specific polymers (Data not shown).

TABLE 5: Responses of Inbred, Congenic, and F1 Mice to Sequential Polymers*

Strain	H-2 Haplotype	$(T\text{-}G\text{-}A\text{-}Gly)_n$	$(T\text{-}A\text{-}G\text{-}Gly)_n$	$(Phe\text{-}A\text{-}G\text{-}Gly)_n$
		Percent Antigen Bound		
A.By/Sn	b	43 ± 10	40 ± 13	10 ± 3
C57BL/10Sn	b	51 ± 15	61 ± 8	7 ± 3
129	bc	59 ± 8		
B10.M/Sn	f		47 ± 14	31 ± 2
A.CA/Sn	f	3 ± 4	49 ± 14	36 ± 1
B10.RIII	r	5 ± 1	63 ± 16	5 ± 4
F1 Hybrids				
(C57B1/6 X BALB/c)	(b x d)	41 ± 14		
(C57B1/6 X DBA/1)	(b x q)	42 ± 6	44 ± 7	13 ± 3
(C57B1/6 X A.CA	(b x f)	28 ± 16	54 ± 5	
(B10.M-$H\text{-}2^{fb}$ X CBA F_1)	(fb x k)			20 ± 4
		Non-Responder Haplotypes		
		a,d,f,k j,ja;p,q s	a,d,k q,s	a,b,d,k p,q,r,s

* None of the mice responded to $(Phe\text{-}G\text{-}A\text{-}Gly)_n$.

Representative data (Table 5) with F1 mice of (R X NR) indicated that the genes controlling responsiveness were dominant. However, as will be presented separately, the levels of antibody in many F1 mice were lower than anticipated, an area which we are presently investigating.

The responses of recombinant inbred strains of mice of the sequential polymers are shown in (Table 6). The data indicate that the Ir gene(s) controlling the responses mapped to the left of IB; i.e. in IA and/or K regions. More extensive studies were undertaken with $(T\text{-}G\text{-}A\text{-}Gly)_n$ and $(T\text{-}A\text{-}G\text{-}Gly)_n$.

$(T\text{-}G\text{-}A\text{-}Gly)_n$: Individual sera from the $H\text{-}2^b$ mice studied at the 1:2 dilution exhibited a wide variability in antigen bound (10-84%). Insignificant binding was present even when the strong sera were diluted 1:50 to 1:100. Attempts to reduce the variability in antibody levels by reimmunization were unsuccessful (Merryman, et al. (mss in prep).

TABLE 6

Mapping of Responses of Recombinant Inbred Mice to Sequential Polymers

Strain	H-2 Type	PERCENT ANTIGEN BOUND			
		$(T\text{-}G\text{-}A\text{-}Gly)_n$	$(Phe\text{-}G\text{-}A\text{-}Gly)_n$	$(T\text{-}A\text{-}G\text{-}Gly)_n$	$(Phe\text{-}A\text{-}G\text{-}Gly)_n$
ATFR.3	ap3			47 ± 3	33 ± 2
D2.GD	g2	2 ± 2	6 ± 2	2 ± 2	
B10.A(4R)	h4	7 ± 1	8 ± 5	4 ± 3	18 ± 1
B10.A(3R)	i3	47 ± 29			
B10.A(5R)	i5	34 ± 14	7 ± 2	54 ± 9	7 ± 3
21R		52 ± 21			

TABLE 7

Responses of (C57B1/6 X BALB/c) F1 Mice to 100 μg $(T\text{-}G\text{-}A\text{-}Gly)_n$*

Responder Classification	No. of Mice	Days After Immunization: 21	34	44	Stimulation Index (Day 44)
		Per Cent Antigen Bound ± S.E.			
High	8	22.4 ± 9.6	40.7 ± 13.6	44.4 ± 16.7	23.5
Medium	8	12.4 ± 4	10.6 ± 4.9	17.2 ± 8.1	25.9
Low	7	7.0 ± 2.3	5.4 ± 2.8	9.0 ± 4.6	11.6

*Only one injection of polymer was given.

In view of the consistently positive T cell responses in responder mice discussed below, a "kinetic" study of the antibody response was undertaken. Mice were immunized with 100μg of $(T\text{-}G\text{-}A\text{-}Gly)_n$ and bled for 8 consecutive weeks. Our findings indicated that a number of mice did not respond (antibody) until week four and in general the maximum antibody response was not reached until week 5 or 6. Similar findings were noted in studies with (C57Bl/6 X BALB/C) F1 mice. Twenty three F1 mice were bled 21, 34 and 44 days after immunization and based upon the values obtained on day 44 divided into high, medium or intermediate responders. As summarized (Table 7) the level of antigen bound in the high responders increased from 22.4% to 44.4%; with the medium responders the values were 12% on day 21 and 17% day 44 and with the low responders 7% antigen was bound on day 21 and 9% on day 44. Also shown in the Table are the T cell stimulation indexes.

As with the guinea pig studies, mice responded to the $(T\text{-}G\text{-}A\text{-}Gly)_n$ oligomers Fraction 1 (38 ± 16) and Fraction 2 (42 ± 16) but not to the nonhelical fractions 3 and 4. T cell dependency of the responses was shown by the following: 1) nonresponder A/J and BALB/C mice produced levels of antibody of 50 ± 7% and 53 ± 9% antigen bound respectively when immunized with the $(T\text{-}G\text{-}A\text{-}Gly)_n$-MBSA complex. 2) When C57Bl/6 nu/nu and Nu/nu littermates were immunized, only the Nu/nu heterozygote mice responded (39% ± 4%).

The homologous $(T\text{-}G\text{-}A\text{-}Gly)_n$, Fractions 1 and 2 and $(Phe\text{-}G\text{-}A\text{-}Gly)_n$ inhibited the anti-$(T\text{-}G\text{-}A\text{-}Gly)_n$ antibody. However, there was little inhibition with Fraction 3 or 4, $(T\text{-}A\text{-}G\text{-}Gly)_n$ or the random polymers GA, GT, GAT[10], and a number of multichain polymers of amino acids. The important observation was that anti-$(T\text{-}G\text{-}A\text{-}Gly)_n$ could react with $(Phe\text{-}G\text{-}A\text{-}Gly)_n$. However, 500 X more of $(Phe\text{-}G\text{-}A\text{-}Gly)_n$ was needed to inhibit the homologous reaction 50% compared with $(T\text{-}G\text{-}A\text{-}Gly)_n$. This would indicate, as was determined before, the close structural and conformational relationships between $(T\text{-}G\text{-}A\text{-}Gly)_n$ and $(Phe\text{-}G\text{-}A\text{-}Gly)_n$ although they are both different.

The T cell proliferative responses of the C57Bl/6 mice were positive. The PETLES from $(T\text{-}G\text{-}A\text{-}Gly)_n$ responder mice ($H\text{-}2^b$) could be stimulated only by the homologous $(T\text{-}G\text{-}A\text{-}Gly)_n$ and not by: $(Phe\text{-}G\text{-}A\text{-}Gly)_n$ which was shown above to cross react at the humoral level; or $(T\text{-}A\text{-}G\text{-}Gly)_n$ or any of the other random polymers of amino acids (Table 8).

<u>(T-A-G-Gly)</u>: Mice of $H\text{-}2^{b,f,r}$ halotypes responded to this polymer (Table 5). We have reported that the responses might be controlled by at least two genes - one linked to the H-2 haplotype which controls the ability to respond (T cell), and non H-2 gene(s) which controls the antibody level. The response to this polymer was also shown to be under dominant Ir gene control, and no evidence of complementation of genes governing the response was

noted (Merryman, et al. 1977).

Antibody studies with the offspring obtained from the backcross between the F1 hybrid X the low responder parental strain, (C57Bl/6 X DBA/1) X DBA/1, did not show the expected segregation for a dominant trait between heterozygous responder animals (bq) and homozygous nonresponder mice (qq). Only 1/10 mice, a heterozygote (b,q) produced detectable antibody (47% antigen bound). The responses of the backcross offspring derived by crossing the F1 and the parental responder (C57Bl/6) were also unusual in that only 5/10 rather than 10/10 mice produced antibody. These findings were obtained before we had employed the T cell proliferative responses as indicators of responsiveness. As mentioned in the studies with $(T\text{-}G\text{-}A\text{-}Gly)_n$, positive T cell proliferative responses have been consistently obtained even in the presence of low levels of antibody. C57Bl/6, A·BY, B10-M and A·CA mice that are responders to $(T\text{-}A\text{-}G\text{-}Gly)_n$ exhibit good T cell proliferative responses (Table 8). The T cells from 2 responder haplotypes ($H\text{-}2^{b,f}$) were studied for in vitro responses with "homologous" and "related" polymers. Although cells from the above mice were stimulated by $(T\text{-}A\text{-}G\text{-}Gly)_n$ only cells from $H\text{-}2^f$ mice could be cross stimulated by $(Phe\text{-}A\text{-}G\text{-}Gly)_n$. In contrast to this, as shown below, antibody against $(T\text{-}A\text{-}G\text{-}Gly)_n$ could react with the $(Phe\text{-}A\text{-}G\text{-}Gly)_n$ polymer.

The specificity of the $(T\text{-}A\text{-}G\text{-}Gly)_n$ antibody was studied by measuring cross reactions (or inhibition) with the following polymers: $(T\text{-}G\text{-}A\text{-}Gly)_n$, $(Phe\text{-}A\text{-}G\text{-}Gly)_n$, GA, GT, and GAT^{10}. The antisera bound the homologous polymer and $(Phe\text{-}A\text{-}G\text{-}Gly)_n$ showing that the specificities were directed against the immunizing $(T\text{-}A\text{-}G\text{-}Gly)_n$ polymer and the closely related polymer $(Phe\text{-}A\text{-}G\text{-}Gly)_n$.

$(Phe\text{-}A\text{-}G\text{-}Gly)_n$: Only mice of $H\text{-}2^f$ haplotype responded (Table 5). It was possible to cross stimulate the T cells of responder mice with the structurally related $(T\text{-}A\text{-}G\text{-}Gly)_n$, against which mice with this haplotype could respond.

General Discussion: It is apparent that with the sequential helical polymers with which we are dealing, restricted response patterns are obtained, i.e.: the number of responding haplotypes and the specificity of the antibody. The genes controlling the recognition of these T cell dependent polymers mapped to the K or IA subregion. The unexpected variability in the magnitude of the antibody responses found may be a general property of "weak immunogens". In fact, it required a minimum of 100 μg of polymer to elicit responses in mice in contrast to our studies with other polymers where 1-10 μg were sufficient. The variability was more striking in F1 (responder x nonresponder), backcross and F_2 mice immunized with $(T\text{-}G\text{-}A\text{-}Gly)_n$ and $(T\text{-}A\text{-}G\text{-}Gly)_n$. In contrast to this, consistently positive T cell proliferative responses were

TABLE 8

Homologous and Heterologous Proliferative Responses of PETLES with Sequential Polymers*

Strain	H-2	IMMUNOGEN $(T\text{-}G\text{-}A\text{-}Gly)_n$			$(T\text{-}A\text{-}G\text{-}Gly)_n$		$(Phe\text{-}A\text{-}Gly)_n$	
		$(T\text{-}G\text{-}A\text{-}Gly)_n$**	$(Phe\text{-}G\text{-}A\text{-}Gly)_n$	$(T\text{-}A\text{-}G\text{-}Gly)_n$	$(T\text{-}A\text{-}G\text{-}Gly)_n$**	$(Phe\text{-}A\text{-}G\text{-}Gly)_n$	$(Phe\text{-}A\text{-}G\text{-}Gly)_n$**	$(T\text{-}A\text{-}G\text{-}Gly)_n$
C57B1/6	b	26	1.0	1.3	7.5			
A.BY	b	8.2	0.1	1.2	8.8	1.7		
B10.M	f				3.4	7.3	7.4	6.3
A.CA	f				7.3	8.5	9.8	5.7

* Stimulation index

** Homologous polymer

obtained in all mice posessing a responder haplotype in their genome. That low levels of antibody were produced was confirmed by the fact that at 1:50 dilution of serum even the strongest sera no longer bound antigen. In addition, the maximum antibody response generally appeared at 5-6 weeks rather than at the third week as noted with many other immunogens.

Although we do not yet have an adequate explanation for these findings with these immunogens which consist of a restricted number of determinants, some possible explanations are in order. 1) We may be dealing with an important non H-2 gene dosage effect controlling the level of antibody which is reduced in the F1 mice. 2) These sequential helical polymers have been shown to be B cell (non polyclonal) mitogens in all mice, i.e.: responders and nonresponders. That B cell mitogens might signal T cells for suppression has been suggested (Calkins, et al. 1976). 3) Whether activation of suppressor T cells or the presence of a restricted repertoire of specific B cell clones recognizing the polymers might be accounting for the poor immunogenicity of the polymer is presently under investigation.

The guinea pig and mouse studies indicate that there are specific requirements for a polymer to induce a heterologous T cell proliferative response in vitro. Structural relationships as measured by the ability of the specific polymer to cross react with antibody appears to be a necessary but not sufficient criterion. The other important requisite is that the "cross reacting polymer" also be immunogenic in the specific strain whose T cells are being studied. The sequential polymers, $(T\text{-}G\text{-}A\text{-}Gly)_n$ and $(Phe\text{-}G\text{-}A\text{-}Gly)_n$ both of which are immunogenic in strain 13 guinea pigs, induce cross T cell proliferative responses. Similarly, with $(T\text{-}A\text{-}G\text{-}Gly)_n$ and $(Phe\text{-}A\text{-}G\text{-}Gly)_n$ which are immunogenic in strain 2 guinea pigs cross stimulation responses can be elicited. In these situations the ability to cross react at the humoral level is also manifested at the T cell level.

In the mice studies, the requirement for a cross-reacting polymer to also be immunogenic in order to elicit cross T cell proliferative responses is evident. T cells from $H\text{-}2^b$ mice immunized with $(T\text{-}G\text{-}A\text{-}Gly)_n$ cannot be stimulated with $(Phe\text{-}G\text{-}A\text{-}Gly)_n$ which is nonimmunogenic, although the latter polymer can cross react with anti-$(T\text{-}G\text{-}A\text{-}Gly)_n$. The most informative data came from the responses of $H\text{-}2^f$ mice to both $(T\text{-}A\text{-}G\text{-}Gly)_n$ and $(Phe\text{-}A\text{-}G\text{-}Gly)_n$. $H\text{-}2^f$ mice respond to both polymers and associated with this is the ability to also exhibit cross proliferative T cell responses. However, mice of $H\text{-}2^b$ haplotype, when immunized with $(T\text{-}A\text{-}G\text{-}Gly)_n$ do not exhibit cross T cell responses with $(Phe\text{-}A\text{-}G\text{-}Gly)_n$ which is nonimmunogenic for $H\text{-}2^b$ mice.

Similar kinds of observations were also noted with the random polymers of amino acids. That is, in addition to the important requirement for a cross reacting polymer to have structural similarities with the immunizing antigen, the cross reacting polymer must also be immunogenic in the specific responding strain in which the studies are being conducted. 1)T cells from mice immunized with GAT[10] can be stimulated *in vitro* with GA, which is immunogenic in the same inbred strains of mice, but not with the nonimmunogenic GT. 2)BALB/c mice (H-2^d) respond against the random polymers GLPhe[5] and GLT[5]. Appropriate T cells show cross stimulation with either immunogenic polymer but not with GL; which is nonimmunogenic; although most of the antibody specificity is directed against this polymer. 3)Mice of H-2^p haplotype respond to GLPhe[9] but not to GLT[5]. T cells from mice immunized with GLPhe[9] could not be stimulated with the highly cross reactive (antibody) but nonimmunogenic GLT[5].

Several important questions we would like to answer are: 1) whether in those situations where closely related polymers either sequential or random, induce cross stimulation at the T cell level, we are dealing with a single receptor recognizing both polymers, or separate T cell receptors; 2) the basis for the difference between T cell and B cell specificities; and 3) whether the restricted responses to the sequential polymers are associated with activation of suppressor T cells. Studies underway with these unique compounds may answer these questions.

ACKNOWLEDGEMENTS

This research was supported by Research Grant A107825 from the National Institute of Allergy and Infectious Diseases and by Research Grant IM5D from the American Cancer Society and Grant I-492 from the National Foundation.

REFERENCES

Benacerraf, B., and McDevitt, H.O., (1972) Science 175 273.

Benacerraf, B., and Katz, D.H. (1975) In: Immunogenetics and Immunodeficiency, Ed. by B. Benacerraf, p. 117, University Park Press, Baltimore, Md.

Calkins, C.E., Orbach-Arbouys, S., Stutman, O., and Gershon, R.K. (1976), J. Exp. Med. 143 1421.

Klein, J. (1975) In: The Biology of the Mouse Histocompatibility - 2 Complex Springer-Verlag, N,Y.

Koch, C., and Simonsen, M. (1977) Immunogenetics 5, 161.

Lai, C.H., and Maurer, P.H., (1977) J. Immunol., 119, 842

Lai, C.H., Maurer, P.H., and Shevach, E.M. (1977) J. Immunol., 119 906

Liberti, P.A., and Vickerman, C. (1977) Immunochem., 14 543.

Maurer, P.H., Merryman, C.F., Ganfield, D., and Lai, C.H. (1977) Third Ir Gene Workshop, Asilomar, Ca.

Maurer, P.H., Odstrchel, G., and Merryman, C.F. (1973) J. Immunol. 111, 1018

Merryman, C.F., Maurer, P.H., and Stimpfling, J.H. (1975) Immunogenetics 2, 441.
Merryman, C.F., Maurer, P.H., and Zeiger, A.R. (1977) Immunogenetics 4, 373.
Merryman, C.F., Maurer, P.H., Lai, C.H., and Zeiger, A.R., In preparation.
Rosenstreich, D.L., Blake, J.T., and Rosenthal, A.S.(1971) J. Exp. Med. 134 1170.
Schwartz, R.H., Jackson, L., and Paul, W.E. (1975) J. Immunol. 115 1330.
Zeiger, A.R., Lange, A., and Maurer, P.H. (1973) Biopolymers 12, 2135.
Zeiger, A.R., Lai, C.H., and Maurer, P.H. (1975) Biopolymers, 14, 2281.
Zeiger, A.R., and Maurer, P.H. (1976) J. Immunol. 117 708
Zeiger, A.R., and Maurer, P.H. (1977) Biochem. 16, 3514.

Lymphocyte Membrane Structure

INTRODUCTION

Leon Wofsy

Department of Bacteriology and Immunology
University of California
Berkeley, California 94720

I won't try to take you back as far as Dr. Krause did last night, all the way to Amphioxus. Instead, I want to look only fleetingly back to the 1967 Cold Spring Harbor meeting, where Neils Jerne described a world divided between cis- and trans-immunologists (1). Actually, another division was hidden there: Gaul was really divided into three parts, because the trans-immunologists were also divided Way back then, there were those who approached things from the point of view of antigenic structure and those who looked at problems from the point of view of antibody, or immunoglobulin, structure.

Little did we know at that time that we would all fall into the hands of the geneticists. Those of us who worked on antibody structure got there first with the genetics of antibody diversity, but eventually the genetics of the immune response and of lymphocyte diversity engulfed us all. Now, we've all come together essentially at the level of the cell surface. While the geneticists, as we see again at this symposium, seem to glory in working their way through the tangles of cellular immunology, we antigen and antibody protein chemists sometimes feel just a little bewildered and in need of a hand to hold. So, I thought I might try, in this brief introduction to the papers on lymphocyte membrane receptors, to build some self-confidence by reminding us of one major contribution from the chemists, the immunochemists in particular, to cell biology and immunology: namely, the ability to look at a cell surface and see something there. Immunospecific labeling of cellular antigens with markers suitable for fluorescence (2), electron microscopy (3), or radioautography (4) has become important for distinguishing lymphocyte subsets, as well as for identifying and isolating cell surface receptors. It has become important, and promises to become more so, in the difficult task of specific purification of diverse lymphocyte subpopulations (5).

Since this is the last session of our symposium, and no one has yet shown any slides picturing cells, I think it may be appropriate for a chemist to do so. I would like to illustrate briefly a method that our laboratory has developed for visualizing membrane antigens, namely, hapten-sandwich labeling (6). This method seems valuable especially in circumstances where amplification is required for observing alloantigens, or where simultaneous labeling of two or more antigens is desired, as well as in a number of other suggested applications (7-9). One use of the hapten-sandwich labeling technique, to identify T cells, has already been mentioned at this meeting in Dr. Joel Goodman's talk. We use the amidination reaction to link covalently about twenty hapten groups to any anti-cell surface antibody (Ig fraction) with virtually no loss of antibody activity (6). The hapten is first azocoupled to a bifunctional phenolimidoester reagent, which is then reacted with the antibody preparation to amidinate amino groups exclusively (Figure 1). The hapten-antibody conjugate is

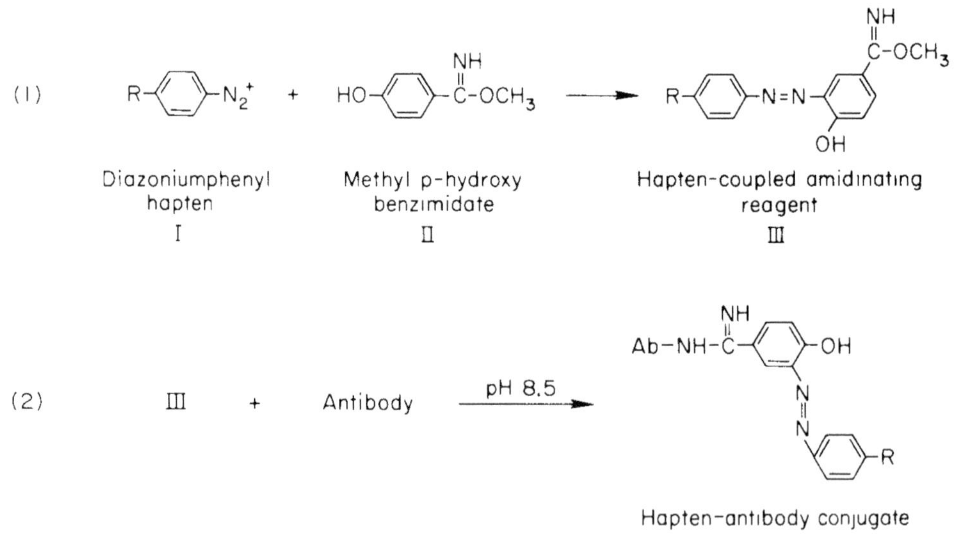

(1) $R-C_6H_4-N_2^+$ + $HO-C_6H_4-C(=NH)-OCH_3$ ⟶ $R-C_6H_4-N{=}N-C_6H_3(OH)-C(=NH)-OCH_3$

Diazoniumphenyl hapten I — Methyl p-hydroxy benzimidate II — Hapten-coupled amidinating reagent III

(2) III + Antibody $\xrightarrow{pH\ 8.5}$ $Ab-NH-C(=NH)-C_6H_3(OH)-N{=}N-C_6H_4-R$

Hapten-antibody conjugate

Fig. 1. Use of bifunctional phenolimidoester reagent (II) to prepare active hapten-antibody conjugates (6).

then available as a first-layer reagent to label cell surface antigens, which may then be detected with a high degree of amplification using purified anti-hapten antibodies that bear fluorescent, electron dense, radioisotopic or other markers.

A few photographs will demonstrate the effectiveness of the technique. In Figure 2, we see sharp discrimination between B and T lymphocytes in a mouse lymph node cell suspension: B cells are labeled with azophenyl β-lactoside (lac) hapten-coupled anti-μ chain, amplified with rhodamine-anti-lac antibody (center); T cells are labeled with azobenzene arsonate (ars) hapten-coupled anti-mouse brain, followed by fluorescein-anti-ars antibody (right).

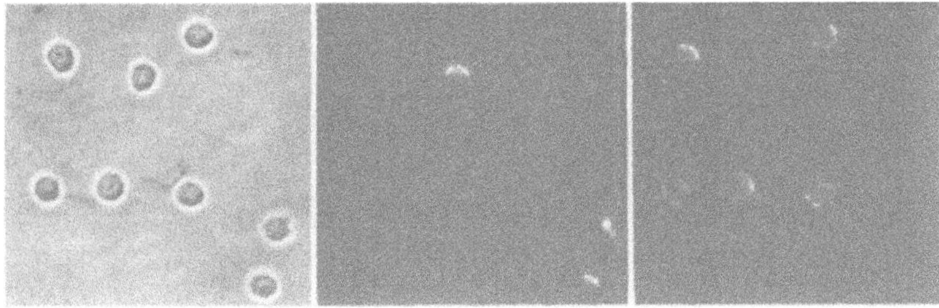

Fig. 2. Selective fluorescent labeling of mouse B and T lymphocytes with hapten-sandwich reagents. Lymph node cells were treated with lac-anti-μ and ars-anti-mouse brain, followed by Rh-anti-lac and Fl-anti-ars antibodies. Left, phase; center, rhodamine; right, fluorescein.

Ia alloantigens can readily be visualized with ars-coupled mouse Fab-anti-Ia, amplified with rabbit $(Fab')_2$ anti-ars antibody to which fluorescein (Figure 3) or keyhole limpet hemocyanin (KLH) (Figures 4a and 4b) markers are attached. This is especially useful for studies in which it is necessary to avoid ambiguities that may result from binding to Fc receptors (10). With this reagent system, we have been able to demonstrate Ia antigens on the membranes of macrophages (Figure 4b) (C. Henry, E. Chan, J. Kimura, and J. Goodman, to be published) and of some thymocytes and T cells (B. Mayhew Doe, C. Henry, J. Kimura, and J. North, to be published).

I hope you will forgive me for being less well-behaved than those who chaired the earlier sessions, most of whom did not use their prerogative to slip in slides on their own work. At least I can follow their example by leaving the major topics for the session to be presented by our speakers.

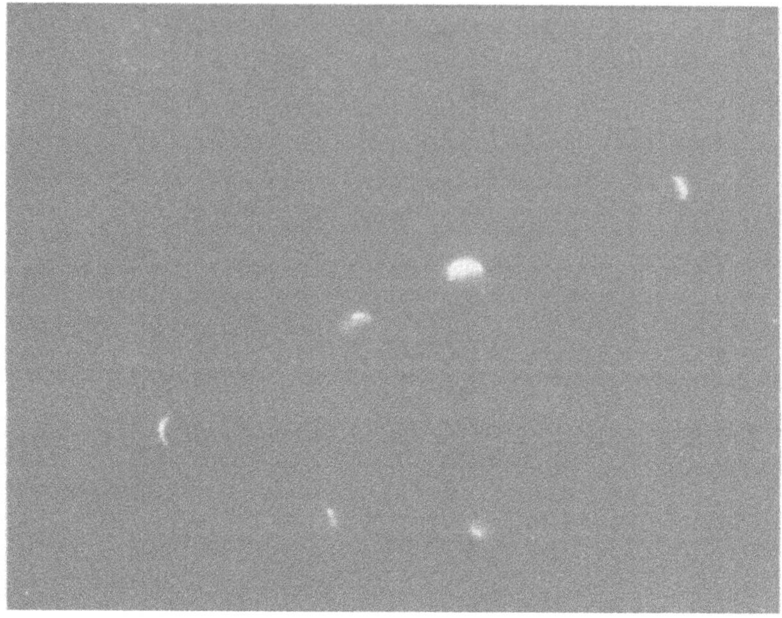

Fig. 3. C_3H/DiSn mouse spleen cells labeled with ars-Fab-anti-Ia^k followed by Fl-$(Fab')_2$-anti-ars antibodies (capping conditions).

Dr. Warner and Dr. Sachs have an interesting task today. They are going to be presenting matters that have actually been assumed through much of the discussion at the symposium: differentiation antigens, membrane receptors and their significance in learning about lymphocyte diversity. So our speakers at this closing session will not really be introducing a new subject. Rather, they will be putting into some perspective the study of the lymphocyte surface as the common meeting ground for many of us who are recent graduates from the schools of cis- and trans-immunology.

Fig. 4. C_3H/DiSn mouse spleen cells labeled with ars-Fab-anti-Ia^k and $(Fab')_2$-anti-ars coupled to KLH: a) a lymphocyte, b) a macrophage. Arrows identify KLH markers. Electron microscopy was performed by Dr. Joseph Goodman, Dept. of Pediatrics, University of California Medical Center and Veterans' Administration, San Francisco.

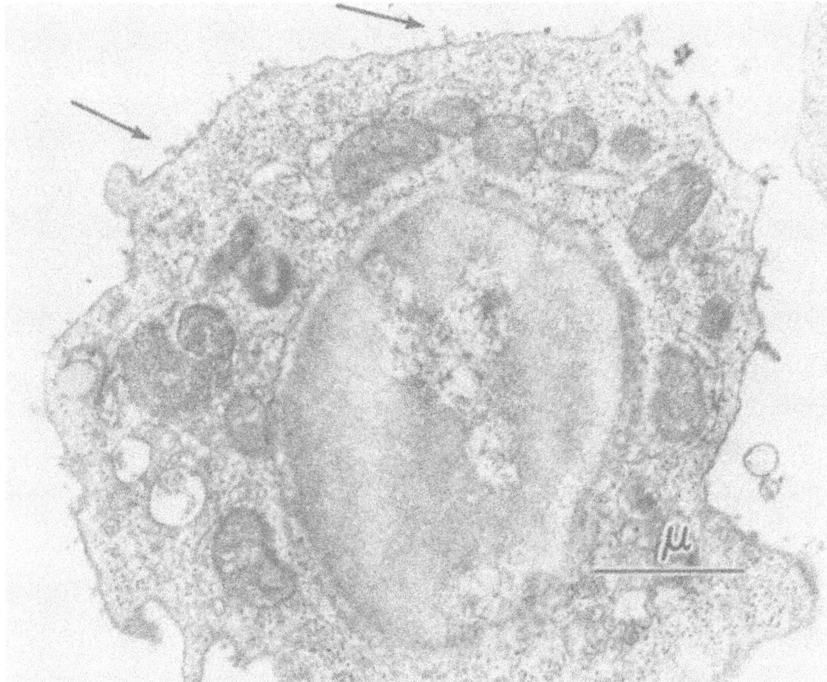

Fig. 4a

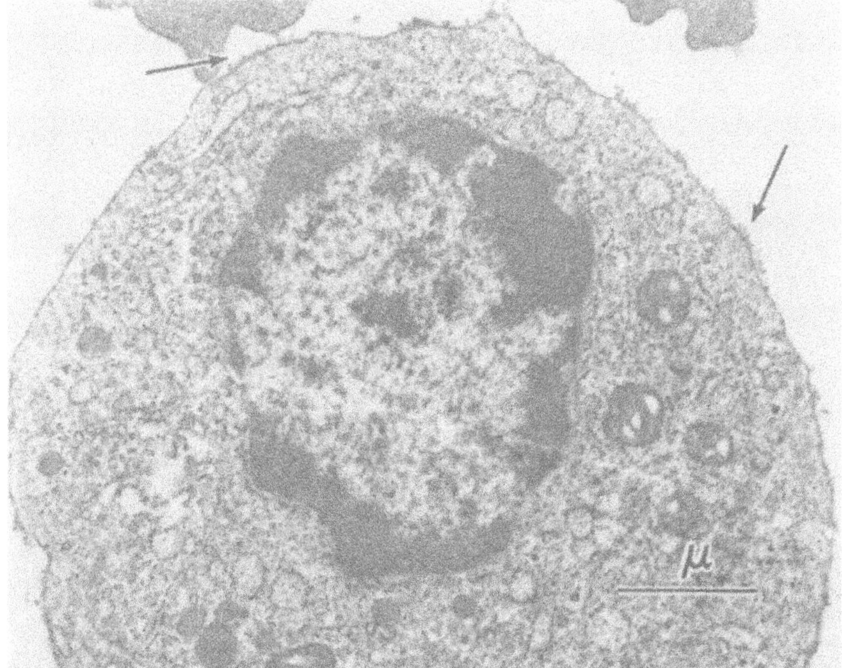

Fig. 4b

REFERENCES

1. Jerne, N. K. (1967) Cold Spring Harbor Symp. Quant. Biol. 32:591.

2. Coons, A.H., Creech, H.J. Jones, R.N. and Berliner, E. (1942) J. Immunol. 45:159.

3. Singer, S.J. and Schick, A.F. (1961) J. Biophys. Biochem. Cytol. 9:519.

4. McFarlane, A.S. (1958) Nature, Lond. 182:53.

5. Hulett, H.R., Bonner, W.A., Barrett, J. and Herzenberg, L.A. (1969) Science 166:747.

6. Cammisuli, S. and Wofsy, L. (1976) J. Immunol. 117:1695.

7. Lamm, M.E., Koo, G.C., Stackpole, C.W. and Hämmerling, U. (1972) Proc. Natl. Acad. Sci., USA 69:3732.

8. Wofsy, L., Baker, P.C., Thompson, K., Goodman, J., Kimura, J. and Henry, C. (1974) J. Exp. Med. 140:523.

9. Nemanic, M.K., Carter, D.P., Pitelka, D.R. and Wofsy, L. (1975) J. Cell. Biol. 64:311.

10. Wofsy, L., McDevitt, H.O. and Henry, C. (1977) J. Immunol. 119:61.

LYMPHOCYTE DIFFERENTIATION AS ANALYZED BY THE EXPRESSION OF DEFINED CELL SURFACE MARKERS

Noel L. Warner, Alan W. Harris, I.F.C. McKenzie,
D. De Luca and G. Gutman
Department of Pathology, University of New Mexico School of Medicine, Albuquerque, NM; The Walter and Eliza Hall Institute of Medical Research, Melbourne Australia; and Department of Medicine, Austin Hospital, Heidelberg, Australia

The general subject of this presentation concerns aspects of lymphocyte differentiation as analyzed through the use of murine lymphomas. It might first be questioned whether this general topic has particular relevance to the theme of the immunobiology of proteins and peptides. Throughout this symposium, considerable emphasis has been placed on the nature of the immunogenic stimulus as presented to different populations of T cells and B cells, and on the possible role of macrophages. Thus, the relevance of considering the stages and pathways of lymphocyte differentiation and the specific gene products that are expressed by cells at these different stages, is to provide the basis for determining the following points which are of specific relevance to this symposium:

(i) The nature of antigen receptors on these different cell types;
(ii) The cell surface components and factors that may be released by these cells and may be involved in cell interactions;
(iii) The nature of cell surface components that may play a direct role in antigen presentation, such as the possible role of H2 gene products which in association with specific antigens may form the appropriate immunogenic stimulus for the activation of cytotoxic T cells (Zinkernagel and Doherty, 1976).

In studying normal lymphocyte differentiation it has become evident over recent years that there are multiple pathways of both T and B cell differentiation, and that within each differentiation lineage, multiple stages of differentiation may be clearly defined.

Because of this extensive heterogeneity of lymphocyte subpopulations, analysis of any one cell lineage or any one stage in differentiation is relatively difficult with cell populations isolated from normal tissues, unless very specific markers can be used in an appropriate manner to isolate these subpopulations. An alternative approach that has begun to receive considerably greater attention in the last year or two, is the use of murine lymphoid tumors. Such tumors have been extensively used in experimental tumor research for many years principally in relation to virological aspects and to studies of tumor immunity. However it has recently become evident that many lymphoid tumors may each represent the monoclonal neoplastic proliferation of a cell that belongs to a specific T or B cell subpopulation, and is arrested in its differentiation at a particular stage. Thus analysis of a series of lymphoid tumors may provide representatives of these different stages of arrest within several differentiation lineages, and may provide suitable models for studying not only the cell surface markers that provide the approach to then analyzing the normal counterpart cells, but may in fact provide direct models for studying functional properties. Several specific examples of these possibilities with lymphoid or hematopoietic tumors will now be described to indicate some of the potential of this particular field of research.

MACROPHAGE TUMORS

One of the main aspects of the immunobiology of proteins and peptides concerns the initial role of macrophage subpopulations in the handling and presentation of antigens for initiation of immune responses. From a variety of experimental studies it is becoming evident that the term macrophage might be thought of in the same context as the term lymphocyte, namely a generic name for a family of related cells, related through their differentiation ancestry, but having differentiated into distinctly different functional subpopulations. One approach to this problem is to study a series of murine macrophage tumors to determine whether they have characteristics that may be shared between them, such as specific cell surface markers that may define their cell differentiation lineage, but may nevertheless have distinct differences in functional properties. Several reports in the literature (Koren and Hodes, 1977; Muschel, et. al., 1977) have indicated that certain macrophage tumors can mediate some of the normal functions ascribed to macrophage subpopulations.

We have recently commenced to study in detail several tumor lines that show some potential of belonging to a macrophage lineage. The results in Table 1 document in a summarized fashion our observations relating to the tumor PU-5-1R. This tumor which was derived from the Salk Institute collection and has in some instances been referred to as a B cell lymphoma, appears to have had an unusual

TABLE 1

Properties of Cultured PU-5-IR Cells

Assay	Observation
M.Ig (direct I.F., K, μ, γ, α)	Negative
M.Ig (indirect I.F.)	Negative (occ. weak pos.)
MTLA (indirect I.F.)	Negative
Thy-1.2 (indirect I.F.)	Weak positive
Fc Receptor (Rabbit Ig)	Strongly positive
Fc Receptor (Mouse Ig)	Strongly positive
Inhibition of FcR	Preferentially by IgG_{2a}
Phagocytosis (latex)	Positive
Phagocytosis (sensitized RBC)	Positive
Culture Growth Behavior	Adherent Cell
Steroid Inhibition (Hydrocortisone)	Resistant
Thymidine Inhibition	Intermediate
Unusual Growth Requirement	Asparagine
Macrophage Ag (indirect I.F.)	Strongly positive

I.F., immunofluorescence; M.Ig., membrane immunoglobulin; MTLA, mouse T lymphocyte antigen.

history, in that the original tumor induced by Asofsky showed many characteristics that would indeed appear indicative of a B lymphoma (Asofsky, personal communication). However at some stage along the line of its transplantation history, some changes appear to have occurred, and it is to be stressed that the properties described in this table directly relate to the tumor line that is now maintained, but it is still uncertain whether this present tumor line was directly derived from the original tumor, or whether at some stage a new tumor arose in a mouse during a transplantation of the original parent line.

When studied by direct or indirect immunofluorescence with a range of anti-immunoglobulin reagents, this line has consistently been totally negative by all direct immunofluorescence procedures, but has on occassion shown weak positive reactions with indirect immunofluorescence. In the latter case, when the reagents are first subjected to ultracentrifugation, consistently negative results are then obtained. The weak positive results may thus be due to Fc receptor binding of the reagents. In similar fashion with two different T cell specific reagents, a totally negative result was obtained with a heterologous MTLA serum, whereas with a conventional Thy-1.2 antiserum a weak positive reaction was occassionally observed, which again disappeared on ultracentrifugation of the reagent. These results are probably explained by the observations made on Fc receptor activity. In a standard Fc rosette assay using sheep erythrocytes sensitized with subagglutinating doses of rabbit anti sheep cell antibody, this tumor line shows one of the most avid expressions of Fc receptors that we have yet encountered. The results from a typical experiment shown in Table 2, indicate the percent of rosette forming cells observed with red cells sensitized with several different concentrations of antibody. The tumor lines indicated are all Fc receptor positive, but show marked differences in percent of rosettes with these very low concentrations of sensitizing antibody, which may be associated with the avidity of Fc receptors; this in turn may either be ascribable to a true affinity difference of Fc receptor:antibody binding, or perhaps more likely, to the number of Fc receptors found on the cell surface. Previous studies on the specificity of Fc receptors for different immunoglobulin classes has demonstrated distinct specificity differences for Fc receptors of different cell lineages (Warner, 1974; Dickler, 1976). In previous studies we have shown that mastocytoma cells primarily react to immunoglobulins of IgE or IgG1 types (Warner and Ovary, 1972), whereas the Fc receptors of either Fc receptor positive T lymphocyte subpopulations or of B cells, react preferentially with IgG1 and to a certain extent with both classes of IgG2 (Warner, et.al., 1975). In distinction the Fc receptors of macrophages predominately react with IgG_{2a} immunoglobulin (Cline, et.al., 1972). In similar studies on the inhibition of Fc receptor formation with the PU-5 tumor we have observed that this Fc receptor is preferentially inhibited by IgG_{2a} immunoglobulin, which would indicate on this basis that the Fc receptor behaved more in the fashion as that of macrophage type.

This latter conclusion was then further reinforced by studies of the phagocytic properties of this tumor line which was shown to be capable of phagocytosing both latex particles and antibody coated sheep erythrocytes (but not non-antibody coated erythrocytes). The cultured tumor grew as an adherent cell which again would be expected should the cell be of macrophage lineage, and in studies on corticosteroid sensitivity and sensitivity to thymidine, showed respectively resistant or intermediate properties. It was noted that this

TABLE 2

Fc Receptor Expression by Several Tumor Lines in Relation to Dose of Erythrocyte Sensitizing Antibody

Tumor Line	Type	Percent Rosettes at Indicated Sensitizing Concentrations*		
		51200	12800	800
PU-5-IR	Macrophage	68	77	96
S.49	T Lymphoma	5	24	94
P-815	Mastocytoma	<1	12	82
2PK-3	B Lymphoma	<1	<1	10

* Sheep erythrocytes (SRBC) were sensitized with the indicated reciprocal dilution of mouse anti-SRBC antiserum; were washed extensively and used for Fc receptor detection by a rosette assay.

particular tumor also showed an unusual growth requirement for the addition of the non essential amino acid asparagine. Using a specific rabbit antimacrophage antiserum obtained from Drs. K. Shortman and J. Fidler, which showed absolutely no reaction by indirect immunofluorescence with any of our established T or B cell tumors, strongly positive reactions were observed by indirect immunofluorescence with cells of the PU-5-IR line. This latter positive reaction persisted after ultracentrifugation of the serological reagents, and we thus conclude that this tumor expresses surface antigens specific for those of macrophage lineage, and the cell expresses the Fc receptors characteristic of macrophages.

Thus, this neoplastic cell expresses many properties of normal macrophages. The question that must then be asked is whether this cell line expresses any functional properties indicative of a macrophage lineage. Such studies on the role of antigen processing and presentation are currently in progress. Preliminary studies with Dr. Robert Burton have, however, indicated that this tumor line possesses inherent cytotoxic activity and is capable of lysing many other chromium labeled tumor cell lines, possibly in a fashion analogous to that described by many non specifically activated macrophage subpopulations.

TABLE 3

Growth Requirement for 2-Mercaptoethanol

Tumor Line	Type	Requirement for 2ME [a]
WEHI-267	Ig secreting B lymphoma	Yes
2PK-3	"	Yes
ABE-8	Pre B cell lymphoma	Yes
WEHI-231	B lymphoma	Yes
WEHI-279	"	Yes
S-49	T lymphoma	No
WEHI-7	"	No
WEHI-22	"	No
WEHI-265	Myeloid leukemia	No
WEHI-274	"	No

[a] Tumor lines were established in the presence of 2-mercaptoethanol and remained dependent on its presence for satisfactory in vitro growth (Yes); or were readily established in permanent culture without the need for 2-ME addition (No).

LYMPHOMA CELL LINES

Current research in this area is attempting to evaluate whether a series of lymphoid tumors all show distinctly different phenotypic properties that in turn will be representative of normal lymphocyte subpopulations. The following presents a series of examples from our current studies on lymphoid tumors with several markers, that indicate that marked heterogeneity exists between lymphoid tumors and that in all cases this is paralleled by similar differences in normal lymphocyte subpopulations.

In attempting to establish a series of lymphoid tumors into culture, it was noted that all B cell lines that were successfully established in culture required the addition of 2-mercaptoethanol to the tissue culture medium for the permanent establishment of these cell lines. The results summarized in Table 3 show that for both ABE-8 (which is classified as a pre-B cell lymphoma), WEHI-231 and -279 (B lymphomas), and WEHI-267 and 2PK3 , which are established Ig secreting B cell lymphomas, 2-mercaptoethanol was absolutely essential for their maintenance in culture. In contrast neither the myeloid leukemias nor thymic nor peripheral derived T cell lymphomas studied showed this requirement. Since several studies have indicated that macrophage factors can directly influence B cell proliferation, it is possible that this is paralleled in these observations indicating that neoplasias of the B cell system are similarly susceptible to macrophage type factors, which in turn can be substituted in some unknown manner by mercaptoethanol.

Studies on the expression of Fc receptors on a variety of murine tumor lines are summarized in Table 4. These results show marked analogy with that for normal lymphocyte populations, in that all B cell lymphomas studied have shown Fc receptor activity, whereas in T lymphoma populations only three of 28 T cell lymphomas expressed these receptors (Warner, et.al., 1975). At the terminal end of B cell differentiation, plasma cell tumors generally show only a marginal expression of Fc receptors(Harris, 1977) and it is not clear whether this indicates a repression of the gene coding for the Fc receptor, or whether other cell surface components may

TABLE 4

Fc Receptor Expression on Murine Tumor Lines

Tumor Type	No. Lines Tested	No. Lines with Fc Receptor Expression
B Lymphoma	5	5
Plasmacytoma	18	5
T Lymphoma	28	3
Non Lymphoid Hematopoietic*	6	6

* Includes mastocytoma, myeloid and macrophage tumors.

be expressed that mask the availability of Fc receptors. Further studies are in progress to determine whether the 5 of 18 plasmacytoma lines that demonstrate Fc receptor expression may show other parameters that would be indicative of a more immature stage of plasma cell differentiation, as contrasted to the non Fc receptor bearing plasma cell tumors. This receptor may thus be useful in defining stages within B cell differentiation, and distinguishing between certain T cell populations, although as noted in the last line of this table, other hemopoietic tumors of non lymphoid type may also express Fc receptors. These can frequently be distinguished however in terms of the immunoglobulin class specificity of the receptor, as noted above in relation to macrophage tumors.

Studies have been initiated on the expression of several cell surface alloantigens that may be indicative of B cell differentiation. The results summarized in Table 5 relate to the markers Ly4.1 and Ly7.2 which are both expressed on virtually all normal B cell populations (McKenzie, et.al., 1977), and in the case of Ly-7, an additional subpopulation of T cells also appear to express this marker. In studying tumor cell lines with these alloantisera, neither marker has been found to be present on a myeloid leukemia, a mastocytoma, nor T lymphomas with one notable exception, namely the tumor S.49 which expresses the Ly-7 marker. This tumor may therefore be representative of the normal T cell subpopulation that expresses the Ly-7 marker, and it is of note that the S.49 tumor arose in peripheral lymphoid tissue, in contrast to thymic origin which is the more frequent site of origin of T cell tumors. The alloantigen Ly4.1, which has been found only on normal B cell populations, similarly has been shown to be present on all 4 B cell lymphomas studied and not on any of other tumor types. Of particular interest however was the observation that the Ly-7 antigen was present on only 3 of the four B cell tumors, and the tumor lacking this marker is distinct from the other three in many ways, in representing a more immature stage of B cell differentiation. From these studies it might therefore be suggested that the Ly-4 gene product is expressed early in B cell differentiation and is followed by expression of the Ly-7 gene. The tumor ABE-8 is known to express only very marginal amounts of membrane immunoglobulin and to have no Ig secretory activity, whereas the tumors WEHI-231 and -279 have extremely high density membrane immunoglobulins of IgM types but no secretory activity:Tumor 2PK-3 in contrast, has cell surface IgG2 immunoglobulin and a modest amount of Ig secretory activity (Gutman, G., Warner, N.L., Harris, A.W., manuscript in preparation). A further distinction between these 4 tumors is shown in Table 6, with preliminary data on I region expression by these tumors. Tumor ABE-8 again shows only very marginal, if any, expression of I region antigens, whereas tumors WEHI-231 and -279 each show a proportion of cells expressing I region determinants. In the case of WEHI-231, only a very small subpopulation expresses this

TABLE 5

Expression of B Cell Alloantigenic Markers on Murine Tumors

Tumor Line	Type	Expression of Marker *	
		Ly 4.1	Ly 7.2
ABE-8	Pre B Lymphoma	+	-
WEHI-231	B Lymphoma	+	+
WEHI-279	"	+	+
2PK-3	"	nt	+
WEHI-22	T Lymphoma	-	-
WEHI-7	"	-	-
S.49	"	-	+
WEHI-265	Myeloid Leukemia	-	-
P815	Mastocytoma	-	-

* Evaluated by microcytotoxicity titration with rabbit complement, and/or by indirect immunofluorescence with fluorescein conjugated anti IgG_1/IgG_2 as second reagent. nt, not tested.

antigen. In contrast, tumor 2PK-3 shows virtually complete expression of I region antigens on all cells with a very high intensity, as judged by immunofluorescence and cytotoxicity studies with these antisera. At the present stage we have not determined which I subregion is expressed on these tumors. It is also to be noted that in general, plasma cell tumors have been found to only marginally express I region antigens both by immunofluorescence studies and in collaboration with Dr. J. Goding by cytotoxicity.

These studies thus suggest that through a combination of various Ly alloantigens, membrane immunoglobulin, and I region antigen expression, distinct stages in B cell differentiation may be clearly defined, and with the development of further series of Ly-B alloantigens, the versatility in defining specific stages in B cell differentiation will in all likelihood considerably increase.

TABLE 6

I Region Expression on B Cell Tumors

Tumor Line	Type	Ia Expression *
ABE-8	Pre B Lymphoma	Negative
WEHI-231	B Lymphoma	2-3% Cells +++
WEHI-279	"	50% Cells +++
WEHI-301	Ig Secreting B Lymphoma	>80% +++
2PK-3	"	>80% +++
HPC-108	Plasmacytoma	>80% +
HPC-6	"	Negative
C118	"	Negative

* Ia expression evaluated by indirect immunofluorescence with alloantiserum and fluorescein conjugated anti IgG. Approximate intensity of staining is indicated.

A final example in the possible use of lymphomas in studying lymphocyte subpopulations concerns antigen binding properties by such tumors. A series of B lymphoma and plasma cell tumors have been screened by immunofluorescence using fluorescein or rhodamine conjugated antigens. The results for the available information are summarized in Table 7, and several points might be noted. Firstly, an unexpected observation was that 5 of these tumors all demonstrated clear binding of horse spleen ferritin. The binding of ferritin was shown to be inhibitable by pretreatment of the cells with anti-immunoglobulin sera, which was shown in control studies to be specifically due to the anti-immunoglobulin activity in those sera. In several instances cocapping studies were performed, and membrane immunoglobulin gave at least partial cocapping with the fluorescent antigen. Thus in these cases it appears possible that the ferritin is binding to immunoglobulin on the surface of these cells. Whether this binding is however due to an interaction of antigen with a V region site is debatable in view of the observation that all of

TABLE 7

Tumor Line	Type	FITC - Antigen Binding			
		DNP-POL	HSF	KLH	NIP-POL
ABE-8.1	pre B Lymphoma	-	+	-	-
WEHI-231	B Lymphoma	-	+	-	-
WEHI-259	"	-	+	-	-
WEHI-279	"	-	+	+	-
WEHI-301	"	+	+	-	-
WEHI-267	"		-	-	
2PK-3	"		-	-	
HPC-108	Plasmacytoma		-	-	
MPC-11	"		-	-	
MOPC-315	"	+	-	-	-

Fluorescein conjugated antigens include Dinitrophenylated flagellin (DNP-POL), horse spleen ferritin (HSF), hemocyanin (KLH), and NIP haptenated flagellin (NIP-POL). Binding (+) or lack of binding (-) to the tumors is indicated.

these tumors with high density membrane immunoglobulin showed this binding. It may be that ferritin binds to another portion of the molecule, perhaps analogous to Staph A binding to the Fc region of immunoglobulin (Grov, et.al., 1970) and this is particularly best demonstrated in cells with high density membrane immunoglobulin of IgM type. Further studies on this aspect are under investigation.

In contrast to this observation however, are the several instances where a given tumor appears to be almost unique in binding a specific antigen, and in these instances binding to a V region site of the membrane immunoglobulin might be a more likely explanation. In the case of tumor MOPC-315 as would be anticipated from other studies (Eisen, et.al., 1968) binding of DNP-POL occurred. This was also found in the case of tumor WEHI-301, and preliminary studies on the IgM of this tumor have indicated that the IgM may be of a rheumatoid factor type, which in several other studies, has been shown to cross react with DNP (Hannestad, 1969). In another instance, binding of hemocyanin was observed, and in view of the lack of binding of other fluorescent antigens to this tumor (with the exception of ferritin, see above), and the lack of binding of fluorescein KLH to all of the other tumors, it might be suggested that the immunoglobulin of this tumor had binding activity to a component of hemocyanin. Further examination of these instances of specific binding are being pursued to determine whether antigen binding B cell lymphomas may, in fact, provide models for studies of the initial events following specific antigen union with a lymphoid cell.

From these limited examples shown in this paper, we feel that the concept of arrest of differentiation is applicable to this series of lymphoid tumors, and that most of these tumors represent an equivalent normal T, B, or macrophage cell subpopulation, which may be arrested at a particular stage of differentiation. Further studies of these tumors may thus serve several purposes, in both providing a rational basis for the characterization of lymphomas; in providing suitable experimental models for further investigating the nature of cell surface components; and in providing models for the specific interaction of antigen with distinct lymphoid subpopulations.

REFERENCES

Cline, M.J. Warner, N.L., and Metcalf, D. (1972) Blood, 39, 326.

Dickler, H.B. (1976) Adv. Immunol., 24, 167.

Eisen, H.N., Simms, E.S., and Potter, M. (1968) Biochemistry, 7, 4126.

Grov, A., Oeding, P., Myklestad, B., and Ausen, J. (1970) Acta. Path. Microbiol. Scand., 78B, 106.

Hannestad, K. (1969) Clin. Exp. Immunol., 4, 555.

Harris, A.W. (1977) Protides of the biological fluids. 25th Colloquim. H. Peeters, Ed., Pergamon Press. In press.

Koren, H.S. and Hodes, R.J. (1977) Eur. J. Immunol., 7, 394.

McKenzie, I.F.C., Gardiner, J., Cherry, M., and Snell, G.D. (1977) Transpl. Proc., 9, 667.

Muschel, R.J., Rosen, N., Rosen, O.M., and Bloom B.R. (1977) J. Immunol., 119, 1813.

Warner, N.L. (1974) Adv. Immunol., 19, 67.

Warner, N.L., and Ovary, Z. (1972) Scand. J. Immunol., 1, 41.

Warner, N.L., Harris, A.W., and Gutman, G. (1975) in Membrane Receptors of Lymphocytes. (Eds. M. Seligmann, J-L Preud'homme, and F.M. Kourilsky) North Holland. P. 203.

Zinkernagel, R.M., and Doherty, P.C. (1977) Contemp. Topics in Immunobiology. 7, 179.

CONTRIBUTORS

M. Z. ATASSI, Mayo Medical School, Rochester, Minnesota; University of Minnesota Medical School, Minneapolis, Minnesota

M. BALTZ, ICRF Tumor Immunology Unit, Department of Zoology, University College London, London, England

B. L. BASKIN, National Institute of Allergy and Infectious Diseases, National Institutes of Health, Bethesda, Maryland

D. C. BENJAMIN, Department of Microbiology, University of Virginia School of Medicine, Charlottesville, Virginia

E. BENJAMINI, Department of Medical Microbiology, University of California, Davis, School of Medicine, Davis, California

J. A. BERZOFSKY, Metabolism Branch, National Cancer Institute, National Institutes of Health, Bethesda, Maryland

J. T. BLAKE, National Institute of Allergy and Infectious Diseases, National Institutes of Health, Bethesda, Maryland

A. CAMPOS-NETO, Department of Medicine, Harvard Medical School, Boston, Massachusetts

J. M. DAVIE, Washington University School of Medicine, St. Louis, Missouri

D. De LUCA, Department of Pathology, University of New Mexico School of Medicine, Albuquerque, New Mexico

G. Der BALIAN, Department of Microbiology, University of California at San Francisco, San Francisco, California

J. ENG, State University of New York at Buffalo School of Medicine, Veterans Administration Hospital, Buffalo, New York

P. ERB, ICRF Tumour Immunology Unit, Department of Zoology, University College London, London, England

E. H. EYLAR, Playfair Neuroscience Unit and Department of Biochemistry, University of Toronto, Toronto, Ontario, Canada

M. FELDMANN, ICRF Tumour Immunology Unit, Department of Zoology, University College London, London, England

S. FONG, Department of Microbiology, University of California at San Francisco, San Francisco, California

G. T. GOOCH, Department of Microbiology, School of Medicine, Case Western Reserve University, Cleveland, Ohio

J. W. GOODMAN, Department of Microbiology, University of California at San Francisco, San Francisco, California

R. C. GRIFFITH, Washington University School of Medicine, St. Louis, Missouri

G. GUTMAN, The Walter and Eliza Hall Institute of Medical Research, Melbourne, Australia

A.F.S.A. HABEEB, Department of Biochemistry and Nutrition, Medical Sciences Campus, University of Puerto Rico, San Juan, Puerto Rico

W. W. HAROLD, Department of Microbiology, School of Medicine, Case Western Reserve University, Cleveland, Ohio

A. HARRIS, Department of Pathology, University of New Mexico School of Medicine, Albuquerque, New Mexico

A. HOWIE, ICRF Tumour Immunology Unit, Department of Zoology, University College London, London, England

R. JEMMERSON, Department of Biochemistry and Molecular Biology, Northwestern University, Evanston, Illinois

E. A. KABAT, Departments of Microbiology and Human Genetics and Development and Neurology, Columbia University, New York, New York, and National Cancer Institute, Bethesda, Maryland

R. KAMIN, Department of Microbiology, University of California at San Francisco, San Francisco, California

J. A. KAPP, Department of Pathology and of Microbiology and Immunology, Washington University School of Medicine, St. Louis, Missouri

D. H. KATZ, Department of Cellular and Developmental Immunology, Scripps Clinic and Research Foundation, La Jolla, California

A. L. KAZIM, Mayo Medical School, Rochester, Minnesota; University of Minnesota Medical School, Minneapolis, Minnesota

B. KELLY, Department of Microbiology, University of British Columbia, Vancouver, British Columbia, Canada

V. KLINGMANN, Department of Medical Microbiology, School of Medicine, University of California, Davis, California

S. KONTIAINEN, ICRF Tumour Immunology Unit, Department of Zoology, University College London, London, England

R. M. KRAUSE, National Institute of Allergy and Infectious Diseases, National Institutes of Health, Bethesda, Maryland

C.-H. LAI, Thomas Jefferson University, Department of Biochemistry, Philadelphia, Pennsylvania

S. LESKOWITZ, Department of Pathology, Tufts Medical School, Boston, Massachusetts

C. Y. LEUNG, Department of Medical Microbiology, School of Medicine, University of California, Davis, California

H. LEVINE, Department of Medicine, Harvard Medical School, Boston, Massachusetts

J. G. LEVY, Department of Microbiology, University of British Columbia, Vancouver, British Columbia, Canada

G. K. LEWIS, Department of Microbiology and Immunology, University of California, San Francisco, Medical Center, San Francisco, California

G. L. MANDERINO, Department of Microbiology, School of Medicine, Case Western Reserve University, Cleveland, Ohio

E. MARGOLIASH, Department of Biochemistry and Molecular Biology, Northwestern University, Evanston, Illinois

P. H. MAURER, Department of Biochemistry, Thomas Jefferson University, Philadelphia, Pennsylvania

I. F. C. McKENZIE, Department of Medicine, Austin Hospital, Heidelberg, Australia

C. F. MERRYMAN, Department of Biochemistry, Thomas Jefferson University, Philadelphia, Pennsylvania

A. MILLER, Department of Bacteriology, University of California, Los Angeles, California

E. MOZES, Department of Clinical Immunology, The Weizmann Institute of Science, Rehovot, Israel

D. E. NITECKI, Department of Microbiology, University of California at San Francisco, San Francisco, California

R. P. PELLEY, Division of Geographic Medicine, Department of Medicine, School of Medicine, Case Western Reserve University, Cleveland, Ohio

C. W. PIERCE, Department of Pathology and Laboratory Medicine, The Jewish Hospital of St. Louis, Washington University School of Medicine, St. Louis, Missouri

D. S. PISETSKY, National Institutes of Health, Bethesda, Maryland

R. RANKEN, Department of Microbiology and Immunology, University of California, San Francisco, Medical Center, San Francisco, California

M. REICHLIN, State University of New York at Buffalo School of Medicine, Buffalo, New York

D. M. RENNICK, Department of Medical Microbiology, University of California, Davis, School of Medicine, Davis, California

M. B. RITTENBERG, Department of Microbiology and Immunology, University of Oregon Health Sciences Center, Portland, Oregon

A. ROSENTHAL, National Institute of Allergy and Infectious Diseases, National Institutes of Health, Bethesda, Maryland

L. J. ROSENWASSER, National Institute of Allergy and Infectious Diseases, National Institutes of Health, Bethesda, Maryland

D. H. SACHS, National Cancer Institute, National Institutes of Health, Bethesda, Maryland

A. N. SCHECHTER, National Institute of Arthritis, Metabolism and Digestive Diseases, National Institutes of Health, Bethesda, Maryland

S. F. SCHLOSSMAN, Department of Medicine, Harvard Medical School, Boston, Massachusetts

J. SCHROER, National Institute of Allergy and Infectious Diseases, National Institutes of Health, Bethesda, Maryland

R. H. SCHWARTŽ, Laboratory of Immunology, National Institute of Allergy and Infectious Diseases, National Institutes of Health, Bethesda, Maryland

R. J. SCIBIENSKI, Department of Medical Microbiology, University of California, Davis, School of Medicine, Davis, California

A. M. SOLINGER, The Laboratory of Immunology, National Institute of Allergy and Infectious Diseases, National Institutes of Health, Bethesda, Maryland

A. B. STAVITSKY, Department of Microbiology, Case Western Reserve University, School of Medicine, Cleveland, Ohio

J. W. THOMAS, National Institute of Allergy and Infectious Diseases, National Institutes of Health, Bethesda, Maryland

K. THOMPSON, Department of Medical Microbiology, University of California, Davis, School of Medicine, Davis, California

T. V. TITTLE, Department of Microbiology and Immunology, University of Oregon Health Sciences Center, Portland, Oregon

A. TORANO, ICRF Tumour Immunology Unit, Department of Zoology, University College London, London, England

M. ULTEE, Laboratory of Immunology, National Institute of Allergy and Infectious Diseases, National Institutes of Health, Bethesda, Maryland

N. L. WARNER, Department of Pathology, University of New Mexico School of Medicine, Albuquerque, New Mexico

R. W. WARREN, Washington University, School of Medicine, St. Louis, Missouri

L. WOFSY, Department of Bacteriology and Immunology, University of California, Berkeley, California

A. ZEIGER, Department of Biochemistry, Thomas Jefferson University, Philadelphia, Pennsylvania

SUBJECT INDEX

GPSR Compliance
The European Union's (EU) General Product Safety Regulation (GPSR) is a set of rules that requires consumer products to be safe and our obligations to ensure this.

If you have any concerns about our products, you can contact us on

ProductSafety@springernature.com

In case Publisher is established outside the EU, the EU authorized representative is:

Springer Nature Customer Service Center GmbH
Europaplatz 3
69115 Heidelberg, Germany

www.ingramcontent.com/pod-product-compliance
Ingram Content Group UK Ltd.
Pitfield, Milton Keynes, MK11 3LW, UK
UKHW051127260726
13967UKWH00010B/2912

* 9 7 8 1 4 6 1 5 8 8 5 9 7 *